from
Silence
to Voice

A VOLUME IN THE SERIES

The Culture and Politics of Health Care Work

Edited by Suzanne Gordon and Sioban Nelson

Nobody's Home: Candid Reflections of a Nursing Home Aide
    by Thomas Edward Gass

Nursing against the Odds: How Health Care Cost Cutting, Media Stereotypes, and Medical Hubris Undermine Nurses and Patient Care
    by Suzanne Gordon

Nurses on the Move: Migration and the Global Health Care Economy
    by Mireille Kingma

Code Green: Money-Driven Hospitals and the Dismantling of Nursing
    by Dana Weinberg

from Silence to Voice

What Nurses Know and Must Communicate to the Public

Bernice Buresh

Suzanne Gordon

Foreword by
Patricia Benner, RN, PhD, FAAN

ILR Press
AN IMPRINT OF CORNELL UNIVERSITY PRESS
ITHACA AND LONDON

First printing, Cornell Paperbacks, 2006

Printed in the United States of America

Library of Congress Cataloging-in-Publication Data

Buresh, Bernice, 1941–
    From silence to voice : what nurses know and must communicate to the public / Bernice Buresh
and Suzanne Gordon ; foreword by Patricia Benner.—2nd ed.
        p. cm. — (The culture and politics of health care work)
    Includes bibliographical references and index.
    ISBN-13: 978-0-8014-7258-9 (pbk. : alk. paper)
    ISBN-10: 0-8014-7258-X (pbk. : alk. paper)
    1. Nursing.   2. Communication in nursing.   3. Mass media.   4. Public opinion.
5. Nursing—Social aspects.   I. Gordon, Suzanne, 1945–   II. Title.   III. Series.
    RT42.B83 2006
    610.73--dc22   2005032183

Cornell University Press strives to use environmentally
responsible suppliers and materials to the fullest extent
possible in the publishing of its books. Such materials include
vegetable-based, low-VOC inks and acid-free papers that are
recycled, totally chlorine-free, or partly composed of nonwood
fibers. For further information, visit our website at
www.cornellpress.cornell.edu.

Paperback printing   10 9 8 7 6 5 4 3 2

For Our Mothers

Contents

Foreword by Patricia Benner   ix

Acknowledgments to the Second Edition   xiii

Introduction   1

Part I Silent No More

1   Ending the Silence   11

2   Creating a Voice of Agency   25

3   Presenting Yourself as a Nurse   42

4   Tell the World What You Do   64

5   Creating Anecdotes and Arguments   82

Part II Communicating with the Media and the Public

6   How the News Media Work   109

7   Reaching Out to the News Media   137

8   Working with Public Relations Professionals   166

9   Constructing Campaigns That Work   179

10   In Your Own Voice: Letters to the Editor, Op-Eds, and Blogs   204

11   Appearing on Television and Radio   228

12 Promoting Nursing Research   249

13 Conclusion   272

References   279

Index   289

Foreword

In the second edition of *From Silence to Voice*, Bernice Buresh and Suzanne Gordon, two widely known feminist journalists, once again have given nurses:

1. a gift of clearly stated respect for the worth of nursing work;
2. a manifesto calling on nurses to apply their courage and develop their skills to speak out forcefully and effectively to the public and in the media; and
3. a practical step-by-step guide providing inspiring, confident approaches to increasing nurses' visibility and voice in media and policy arenas.

I came to this text with full appreciation for the power that nurses acquire when they articulate the skill and knowledge that is embedded in their practice. For many years, part of my work has been to help nurses construct clinical narratives that are self-informing both professionally and personally. Nurses can, of course, perform their work without standing back and analyzing its components. But we found that discerning and describing the knowledge, competence, and skill that goes into day-to-day nursing work allows nurses themselves to comprehend their work in a more empowering way. It increases nurses' mastery and appreciation of their own work and, by extension, nurses' ability to better care for patients. The articulation of nursing work can not only spur hospital management to value and reward nursing, it contributes to nurses valuing themselves and each other.

This book has had a wide impact in the international nursing community since it was first published in 2000. Thousands of nurses worldwide have used it as a guide to understand how public communication and the media actually work and have put its advice into practice to engage in public outreach. *From Silence to Voice* is assigned reading in many nursing schools. Nursing organizations consult it for guidance as they work to promote nurses' work to a broader public.

Some organizations—such as the Swiss Nurses Association—have mounted visibility campaigns that they explicitly attribute to the book's influence. Nursing organizations throughout the world have invited the authors to discuss how to move from silence to voice in their particular country and culture. The book's audience continues to grow. To date it has been translated into Japanese, Portuguese, and German.

This new edition reflects the authors' extensive interactions with real nurses who are dealing with today's challenges. It draws on the give-and-take that is a feature of their presentations and workshops and, as a result, offers concrete, reality-based advice on how nurses can tell their stories and avoid sentimental clichés that trivialize their important caregiving skills and oversimplify their complex practice. Since expertise is based on practice, the authors have added exercises that nurses can use to build their public communication skills and confidence in using them.

Today, the need for nurses to talk about their work is ever more urgent. Cost-cutters in many countries are threatening the integrity of nursing practice, nursing education, and even nursing research. If patients are to get the care they need, nurses must tell their stories in credible, effective ways.

Buresh and Gordon are powerful voices for nursing and teach us how nursing can be heard in the mass media. *From Silence to Voice* is a practical guide. From it nurses can learn how to get their stories, insights, research, and expert opinions into the media. The authors give away many insider secrets on how the media—print, the Internet, radio and television—work, how they are interrelated, and, most important, how to influence them.

Reading this book gave me an expanded vision and renewed enthusiasm for improving health care by making nursing practice visible to the public and the media. The authors convincingly explain why nurses must take the risk to be heard and to be visible. They show why it is essential for nurses to bridge the communication gap between the profession and the greater public. Nothing less than living in a safer and healthier society is at stake.

Without the authors' passionate vision for the worth of nursing work, this particular book could not have been written. They take nursing and nursing work seriously. They do not trivialize nursing by dressing it up in others' power suits. They oppose the sham of false advertising, selling nursing as the latest hot commodity in a fickle marketplace. Rather, they direct the reader to the real societal worth of nurses' knowledgeable care of the vulnerable, the sick, and the injured. They point to both the wisdom of the heart and mind in nursing practice. They are sure, as they put it, that: "Nurses can articulate their thoughts, find the right words to describe their work, do so in a confident way that doesn't sound boastful or self-aggrandizing, believe in their own knowledge and ability to acquire more, answer tough questions, and tolerate making the occasional mistake. In doing so, nurses will reveal what it really means to be 'just a nurse.'"

I commend this book to every nurse. It is a must-read for nurse educators, nurse executives, and all practicing nurses. It should be a required text for all levels of nursing students.

PATRICIA BENNER, RN, PhD, FAAN

Professor and Chair, Department of Social and Behavioral Sciences, University of California, San Francisco, School of Nursing

Acknowledgments
to the Second Edition

It was not until Suzanne Gordon and I were engaged in writing this book that I understood how central the theme, From Silence to Voice, has been to my life and work. To be sure, the struggle for voice is not limited to women. Anyone involved in the three areas that have occupied my professional life—journalism, education, and writing—grapples with external and internal restraints on free expression. Still, we must not overlook those cultural constraints that have stilled the authentic voices, and writing hands, of so many women.

Women artists and writers began to explore these constraints in earnest in the 1970s. I joined my first women's writers' group then and have since belonged to others. While these groups often focused on practical matters (how to approach an editor or agent with a particular project, for example), they were primarily vehicles for women to make the transition from silence to voice in their own art. I wish, now, to thank members of those groups who contributed so much to my understanding of these issues. I am particularly grateful to Janet H. Murray, Diana Korzenik, and Katherine Butler Jones for their interest in and thoughtful suggestions for this book.

The genesis of this book occurred in a setting dedicated to fostering democratic discourse and political participation—the Joan Shorenstein Center on the Press, Politics, and Public Policy at Harvard University's John F. Kennedy School of Government. I was a fellow there in 1989 and was exploring a question that I had found intriguing while covering political movements and in my previous teaching at Boston University. It was: Why are women so underrepresented as "newsmakers" and as expert sources in the media?

The canonical answer was that women would appear in the news when more of them achieved "newsworthy" positions. But that answer raised more questions. Why were certain positions worthy of coverage and others not? What of the professions where women already were in the majority, such as health care (as nurses as opposed to doctors), education (as teachers as opposed to professors) and social and caregiving work (as care providers as opposed to policy makers)? Why weren't the activities of these women also worthy of journalistic attention? These sorts of questions led to my professional association with Suzanne Gordon and to our exploration of who in our society gets to be seen and heard. I am grateful to Marvin Kalb of the Shorenstein Center for providing a launching site for this inquiry and to Nancy Palmer for her many kindnesses. I would especially like to thank Lawrence K. Grossman for extending his expertise and encouragement for all of these years.

A considerable amount of the writing, editing, and thinking that I have done in connection with this book took place in the Writers' Room of Boston, a place that provides the silence that writers need to hear their own voices. My heartfelt thanks go to all of the writers who have contributed to the special nature of the Writers' Room. In particular, I would like to thank Ivan Gold, Nancy Kassell, Nan Fornal, and Donald E. Cecich, with whom I have had the pleasure of working closely, for all they have done to make the Writers' Room possible. There are two other people I want to mention for contributing to "voice" in other ways: Barry Kesselman and Helen Soussou.

The first nurse I ever knew was my aunt Theresa H. Reineck whose work was a source of family pride. Now there are other nurses in the family, my niece, Cathy Buresh, and my cousin Beth Halusan. My mother, Erna H. Byrne, has followed the progress of this book every inch of the way. I am grateful to her and to my brother Theodore F. Buresh and my sister Gail Schank for their support. My greatest thanks go to Irwin Oppenheim, my husband, and to Josh Buresh-Oppenheim, my son, for being never-ending sources of love, strength, and sanctuary.

Finally, it may seem peculiar to acknowledge the coauthor of a coauthored book, but Suzanne Gordon has been a valued friend and colleague, and, by thinking up the title, *From Silence to Voice*, has crystallized for me, for other women, and for caregivers, the passage we must continue to make.

BERNICE BURESH

Cambridge, Massachusetts

For more than a decade and a half, Bernice Buresh and I have been holding a vibrant conversation that has informed this book. Our ability to not only agree, but to disagree—even fight over words, phrases, and concepts—has helped me to clarify my ideas about nurses' and women's issues. I am deeply grateful to nursing for bringing me together with this true colleague and dear friend.

I also want to thank my oldest friend, Isabel Marcus, for the intellectual companionship that has been so important to this and to other work.

Claire Fagin and Joan Lynaugh have been two of my tireless guides into the world of nursing. I also want to thank Patricia Benner for her extraordinary ability to describe what nurses know and do. There have been countless exchanges with Victoria Palmer Erbs, Charlene Harrington, Connie Barden, Trish Gibbons, Peggy O'Malley, Ellen Baer, Tom Keighley, and Tom Smith for which I am grateful. Kathleen Dracup not only taught me about nursing, she allowed me to be her "nurse" when she needed care. That experience enriched my understanding of how difficult it is to think like a nurse. And I want to thank Joyce Clifford for access to the Beth Israel Hospital, Nancy Rumplik, Jeannie Chaisson, and Ellen Kitchen for allowing me to observe their nursing practice.

I'd like to thank Laurie Gottlieb for the opportunity to teach nurses at the McGill School of Nursing, and Genevieve E. Chandler for numerous opportunities to share her ideas and meet with her students at the University of Massachusetts School of Nursing at Amherst.

I am deeply grateful to Sioban Nelson for helping me to understand the history of nursing silence.

SUZANNE GORDON

Arlington, Massachusetts

We wish to thank the Canadian Nurses Association for publishing the original version of this book. We are enormously grateful to Frances Benson, our editor, and to Cornell University Press for extending the reach of the first edition and for making it possible for us to bring the knowledge and experience we've gained from working with nurses internationally to this new edition. It has been a pleasure to work with Ange Romeo-Hall, Andrea Fleck Clardy, Nancy Ferguson, and other members of this highly skilled staff.

We wish to thank the following people for responding so generously to our many requests in the midst of their demanding schedules: Chuck Idelson at the California Nurses Association, David Schildmeier at the Massachusetts Nurses Association, Joan Meehan Hurwitz at the American Nurses Association, Art Moses at the British Columbia Nurses Union, Jamie Cohen at the Service Employees International Union, Andrew Williamson at Southern Health in Melbourne, Doris Grinspun and Sine MacKinnon at the Registered Nurses Association of Ontario, Karen McCarthy at the Canadian Nurses Association, Ramón Lavandero and Dana Woods at the American Association of Critical-Care Nurses, Robert Rosseter at the American Association of Colleges and Nursing, Joy McIntyre and Ross Koppel at the University of Pennsylvania School of Nursing, Maureen McInaney at the University of California San Francisco Medical Center, and Diana Mason at the *American Journal of Nursing.*

We are extremely grateful to our colleague and friend Masako Hayano for her superb Japanese translations of our work and for her guidance into Japanese culture. We wish to express our appreciation to the Japanese Nurses Association, Ariadne Editora, Lda., and Verlag Hans Huber for publishing translations in Japanese, Portuguese, and German.

Our thanks go to Shinya Sato, Yumiko Katsuhara, Inger Holter, Ro Licata, Susie Kim, Peggy Wong, Natalie Ashcroft, Sue Ramsey, Di Twigg, Sanchia Aranda, Meiner Krishnaswamehy, Lisa FitzPatrick, Kim Sykes, Sandra Dunn, Jennie Beutel, Pierre-André Wagner, Elsbeth Wandler, Ana Albuquerque Queirós, Shigeko Takayama, Andreas Büscher, Angelika Zegelin, and Franz Wagner for helping to give this new edition an international scope as nurses mount a global challenge to the myth that caregivers must be silent and invisible.

B.B. AND S.G.

May 2005

from
Silence
to Voice

Introduction

Our inquiry into nursing and public communication began in 1989 when we served as news media consultants to the Nurses of America (NOA) project, a national public relations campaign to rectify *that* nursing shortage by attracting high-quality candidates into the field. As journalists and writers all of our professional lives, we have written about social and political actions in the United States including the civil rights, women's, antiwar, gay rights, labor, and community organizing movements. We have also covered mainstream elective politics. We have seen how marginalized groups managed to bring their agendas to the forefront of public attention and win important legal and social victories. So when NOA asked us to help, we were delighted to accept.

The Nurses of America project was funded by almost a million dollars from the Pew Charitable Trusts and administered by a council of representatives from major nursing organizations. It sponsored activities designed to analyze public attitudes toward nurses and to project a positive image of contemporary nursing. The project undertook studies, monitored the media, distributed press materials, and "media-trained" nurses so that they would be more skilled in talking to reporters, appearing on television, and developing "media events" to stimulate coverage of nursing.

We were particularly interested in press coverage of nursing. We wanted to know whether and to what degree journalists used nurses and nursing organizations as sources of information on health and health care. We devised a study to examine the representation of nurses in the health coverage of three major newspapers. This is an important line of inquiry because a profession's public status and credibility are enhanced by having its expertise acknowledged in the journalistic media.

We were quite sure that nursing—the largest health care profession by far—would be shown to be vastly underrepresented in news coverage. But we didn't expect nursing to be virtually missing from health reportage. This is what the study, "Who Counts in News Coverage of Health Care?" documented.[1]

We found that practically everyone had more of a public voice on health and health care than nurses. When we analyzed the sources of 908 direct quotations by "occupation," we found that physicians were by far the most frequently quoted occupational group. They accounted for nearly one-third of the quotations. But nurses were not a close second, third, or even fourth. After physicians, eleven other groups were quoted more frequently than nurses. These included sources from government, business, nonprofit organizations, education, public relations, and medical organizations, as well as patients, family members, and an assortment of professional and nonprofessional health care workers. Nurses were at the bottom of the list, accounting for only ten, or 1.1 percent, of the quotations. No matter how we analyzed public visibility, nurses were either in or tied for last place.

This was an astounding discovery and one with far-reaching implications. If there was little trace of nursing in the serious coverage of health and health care, then how could anyone, including those in a position to supply nursing with needed resources, understand and recognize its value? When medicine is consistently depicted as the center of the health care universe, physicians get credit for every contribution to health care, even in those instances when it should go to nursing or another profession.

Concerned about what might be a systematic journalistic bias against nursing, we were determined to acquaint our fellow journalists, particularly those who specialize in health and medical reporting, with this serious omission in their reporting. Armed with the study, we and small groups of nurses met with journalists to discuss the fact that they seemed to be ignoring nurses as sources of health care information and nursing issues as news. We made sure our study was widely circulated. It was distributed to journalists at conferences and its findings appeared in the journalism trade press.

Many journalists acknowledged they knew nothing about nursing. To help them get a better grasp of the field, we prepared a media packet that contained information on nursing and on newsworthy nursing projects, and biographies of nurses. These materials linked nursing with contemporary health care issues, suggested potential stories, and gave reporters the names of expert nurses to talk to.

Later on, with the support of major nursing organizations, we created a nursing source directory for journalists so that they would have the names of nurses (instead of only physicians) whom they could call for information on health care.[2] This project was suggested and partially funded by the Ms. Foundation for Communication and Education, Inc.

In general, reporters and editors welcomed this material. Some readily acknowledged that they had not paid much attention to nursing. Many said they were interested in doing stories that included nurses. When groups of nurses provided them with materials on current health care issues, many in fact did stories that included nurses as primary spokespersons. In most cases, when nurses sought meetings with editorial boards to discuss health coverage, they received positive responses and discussed how coverage could be improved.

At this point, approaches to increasing the visibility of nursing seemed straightforward enough. The news media constituted the major conduit. Nurses had to work on educating journalists about nursing so that they would be more receptive to covering the profession. Nurses and nursing organizations had to be much more active in presenting journalists with newsworthy material. All this could be accomplished if more nurses developed public communication skills. Indeed we would write a public communication book for nurses that would help them develop these skills.

We anticipated that the Nurses of America project would provide the foundation for a cooperative communication program by nursing organizations, and there was some discussion of such a plan. We also expected nurses who had been media trained to take an active role in media outreach. We ourselves wrote articles about nursing and thought that more journalists would routinely cover nursing.

But these expectations did not come to fruition at the time. Rather, nursing was thrust onto the public stage in connection with the health care upheaval of the mid-1990s. Many nurses became alarmed when hospital restructuring experiments endangered their patients, and some courageous nurses did speak up. Still journalists covering this story had a difficult time finding nurses who would talk with them about these events or even about routine nursing practice so that they could understand the changes that were going on.

Journalists still complain that they are frustrated in their attempts to find nurses who will do even the basics of communication—return phone calls or answer simple questions about their work. These complaints are echoed by public relations specialists in nursing organizations, nursing schools, and hospitals and medical centers. They tell us they might interest a journalist in an idea for a story only to discover that they can't find nurses willing to talk to reporters, even about noncontroversial subjects.

These experiences made us realize that we had underestimated the significance of cultural issues in the relationship between nursing and the external public world. Whereas we once thought that nursing could become significantly more visible by using more or less generic public relations techniques, we now believe that communication considerations specific to nursing must be addressed. Our metaphors also changed over time. Initially we thought in terms of the "invisibility" and "visibility" of nursing. Now we strongly feel the operative terms are "silence" and "voice." That is why we call this book *From Silence to Voice* and why we focus, in this edition, on moving beyond a "virtue script" that idealizes nursing toward messages that accurately depict nursing and its importance in health care.

Therefore, throughout this book we focus on communication challenges that exist on three levels:

1. Not enough nurses are willing to talk about their work.
2. When nurses and nursing organizations do talk about their work, too often they unintentionally project an inaccurate picture of nursing by using a "virtue" instead of a "knowledge" script.[3]
3. When nursing groups give voice to nursing, they sometimes bypass, downplay, or even devalue the basic nursing work that occurs in direct care of the sick while elevating an image of "elite" nurses in advanced practice, administration, and academia. This contributes to social stereotypes that deride anyone who is "just a nurse."

How serious are these problems? If there aren't enough nurses willing to talk about their work, the results will be catastrophic for nursing. Nursing, like every other profession in today's world, must justify its existence and compete for resources. If nursing is misunderstood by the public and those with influence, it will continue to be disproportionately vulnerable to the budget ax, and new resources for nursing education and practice will not be forthcoming at sufficient levels.

If nursing's script continues to emphasize the virtues of the nurse as a person to the detriment of the knowledgeable work that nurses do, then nurses themselves offer a rationale for limiting resources for nursing. Focusing on who the nurse is rather than on what the nurse does could be an invitation to seek not the best and the brightest recruits, but the most virtuous, meekest, and self-sacrificing who will try to do more and more with less and less.

Finally, nursing's major strength is in its numbers and the influence it can bring to bear through those numbers. Communication efforts that seek gain for certain groups of nurses at the expense of other nurses potentially damage the profession itself. Such efforts highlight nursing's failure to work out standardized educational requirements for practice entry, recertification, and advanced degrees, and risk undermining the provision of resources for bedside nursing. Most important, they fail to harness the latent power of nursing's numbers. Approaches that incorporate the richness and diversity of nursing while explaining the importance of hands-on nursing are much more likely to generate greater support for the nursing profession as a whole.

These challenges are evident in the kind of coverage that nursing receives today. Even though nursing is still perceived to be largely invisible in the media,[4] we observe that nursing has a much larger presence in the news than it did when we first started monitoring the news. But how is nursing visible? It is in the news largely in connection with the nursing shortage, debate about staff ratios, and patient problems. The public must know about these things. But this "problem" narrative is not balanced in the media by a "practice" narrative that would help the public understand what it is that nurses do.[5]

Nursing practice stories occasionally get into the news through strong efforts by a nursing organization, medical center, or editor of a nursing journal. But reporters still tell us that nurses they encounter seem terrified of talking about their work and expressing their opinions. In general, nurses don't reach out to journalists and don't make journalists' work easier, or even possible, by providing necessary information and by returning telephone calls before deadlines. And this applies even to some of the nurses whose names are given to journalists as expert sources on various aspects of nursing and health care. This has also been our experience in trying to interview nurses for articles and books.

Public communication skills are important to nurses. That's why half of this book is devoted to them. But the willingness of nurses to use these skills is even more important. Over the last decade and a half, we have come to believe that a profound ambivalence exists in nursing about whether it is even advisable to be more visible, more vocal, and to assume a larger role on the public stage.

Therefore, the first chapter, "Ending the Silence," envisions the benefits to nurses and to health care if the public knew and understood the importance of nursing.

In Chapter 2 we take a serious look at the systematic, though often unacknowledged, conditioning that goes on within nursing to inhibit the kind of public communication that would make nursing known. We introduce our concept of a "voice of agency" that could make it possible for nurses to comfortably move from silence to voice.

Learning to be more public is an incremental process that begins in the workplace, in the home, and in the community. Even nurses who never have contact with the news media are public communicators by the way they present themselves. Therefore, Chapter 3 concentrates on self-presentation and first impressions.

In Chapter 4, "Tell the World What You Do," we define "the world" as being those whom nurses know and work with every day as well as the mass media and general public, and the "what you know" as being the experiential knowledge of nurses. While it is critically important for nurses to communicate through the mass media, we also believe there are many other "publics" nurses must educate. The techniques a nurse uses in talking with a patient, a family member, a neighbor, or a friend about her work are vitally important, and they are transferable. A nurse who can talk comfortably about nursing with family or friends can also talk effectively on the radio or television or to a reporter. So we start the communication process by describing how to communicate with people nurses encounter in everyday life. This chapter also examines fears and internal obstacles nurses have told us they confront. Many of these inhibitions can be understood and managed by exploring their sources and by testing them in the real world.

Chapter 5 offers instruction on how to create compelling stories and anecdotes about nursing. The public needs help understanding just what nurses do and why it is consequential. The importance of nursing work can only become known when nurses tell stories that concretely illustrate how the routine activities of daily practice make a difference to patients. We offer storytelling guidelines and present makeovers of stories that nurses have told us. These makeovers transform rough drafts of nurses' descriptions of their work into short, polished illustrations of nursing work—ready for prime time, as it were. Nurses can use these examples to create their own compelling stories to make arguments for nursing from their own experiences and practice.

Because the mass media are so powerful in shaping people's views of reality, and because they reflect the visibility of a profession, the second half of this book concentrates on mass communication and the media. It is clear that the media have too often neglected nursing or even promoted unfortunate stereotypes of the profession. But a careful examination also reveals that when nurses have engaged in outreach and exerted pressure, the results have been promising.

In this part readers will learn how to write a news release—the basic tool for communicating with the media; how to assemble other press materials; and how to develop media strategies to achieve specific goals. We also show how nursing groups have organized special events and media campaigns to publicize their programs and further their program goals.

This part devotes a chapter to publicizing nursing research, one of the most promising ways of acquainting the public with nursing expertise in health care. But communicating the knowledge that goes into nursing is not the exclusive province of nurses who are scholars, researchers, or organizational leaders. This is why we have included a chapter on how to write letters to the editor and op-ed essays. We demonstrate the elements of these forms so that every nurse can present her or his experience, insights, innovations, and policy proposals.

The elements of communication are similar whether they are used in print, on the Internet, or on radio and television. All communication depends on organizing messages to get across the most important points. We devote a chapter to communication techniques for radio and television because they are the most highly used media in our society.

Some nurses berate themselves because they feel they don't have good public communication skills. They assume that knowledge in this field is instinctual, when, in fact, it is learned. Most nurses went to school to learn how to take care of patients not how to speak about nursing on television.

Effective public communication depends on writing and speaking skills. These skills are learned, practiced, and constantly refined. Successful communicators in every field become effective through instruction and practice. So can nurses. But nurses don't have to be expert in every aspect of public communication. They can call on the assistance of public relations specialists, whose work we also describe in this part.

We'd like to explain our choice of certain language in *From Silence to Voice*. Most of the time, for expediency, we use "we" in recounting situations involving one or the other or both of us. We refer to ourselves by name when it is necessary for clarity. As journalists, we have conducted interviews with many people for this book. Whenever a quotation appears without a reference, it means that the material comes from one of our interviews with the source.

Although we talk a great deal about women's culture and its influence on nursing, our intention is not to exclude men who are nurses. Our purpose is to explore the legacy of women's socialization and gender stereotypes on nursing. Men in nursing are affected by these influences as well as women. Because the vast majority of nurses are women, the feminine pronoun is given preference.

Throughout this book, we avoid, whenever possible, the use of the word "consumer" or "customer" to describe the people nurses care for. This is a deliberate choice. The word *consumer,* as defined by the dictionary, has two meanings. One meaning is someone who consumes, spends, wastes, or destroys. The second meaning, "a person who uses goods and services to satisfy his needs," pertains to economics. The first definition is negative, and the second is an extremely narrow marketplace definition of human beings in relationship to health care. We believe it seriously miscasts the relationship between clinicians and the people who seek their care and services.

Even though we understand the term's appeal in avoiding paternalistic language, replacing the word "patient" with a market term like "consumer" (or "customer") puts clinicians on shaky ground. For the clinician, the moral injunction to do no harm can too easily be hijacked by the market ethic of caveat emptor, "Let the buyer beware." From the public communication perspective, talking about nurses in relation to consumers shifts attention from the hospital, home, clinic, or hospice to the shopping mall. It suggests that human beings can choose health the way they choose a new toaster and can, therefore, exercise control even when they are the least able to. We prefer to use the words "human being," "individual," "people," "patient," and "family."

We are American journalists. But we recognize that the problem of silence in nursing is an international one. In fact, this book itself is representative of an international approach to increasing the visibility of nursing. Written by American authors, this edition contains material from the United States, Canada, Australia, New Zealand, the United Kingdom, Europe, and Japan. We hope this book will further the conversation about this topic among nurses throughout the world.

Like everyone else in journalism, and much of the public, we started out knowing nothing about nursing. No doubt, without realizing it, we accepted many of the traditional stereotypes. Our views have been revolutionized. Nurses were our teachers. They have explained their work to us and expressed their insights about health and illness. We are profoundly in their debt. If we could be educated in this way, so can others.

PART I
Silent No More

Chapter 1

Ending the Silence

Envision how things would be if the voice and visibility of nursing were commensurate with the size and importance of the nursing profession.

The typical health care journalist's address book would contain contact information for a broad spectrum of nursing sources. These sources would include not only nursing organizations, nursing schools, and unions but also names of individual nurses with various kinds of expertise. The journalist would have many names of nurse researchers, public health nurses, nurse administrators, staff nurses, nurses with clinical subspecialties, nursing scholars, home-care nurses, nurse practitioners, and hospice nurses, among others.

Journalists would routinely contact nurses when they have questions about health care topics, and, as a result, nurses would frequently appear as expert sources in news reports. Nurses would be quoted on all health topics in newspapers and magazines, on radio and television, and on health Web sites. Nurses would be regular guests on influential news and analysis programs as well as on local news and talk shows.

No longer would medical research be perceived as the only scientific endeavor leading to health improvements. Health experts, journalists, policy makers, and the public would know about nursing research and would see it as a dynamic, evolving field that expands our knowledge about health care and the human condition. In fact, public support would lead to vastly increased governmental and private funding for nursing research.

The visibility of nurses in the mass media would reflect the expanded participation of nursing in the ongoing public discussion about health care. Nurses would be key participants in all health care forums whether they occur at community centers, town meetings, state capitals, provincial legislatures, churches, schools, universities, consumers' and patients' organizations, economic conferences, national legislatures, or international assemblies.

Physicians' responses to health coverage would no longer dominate the letters-to-the-editor sections of influential newspapers and news Web sites. Nursing perspectives expressed in letters, opinion pieces, and on the Internet would expand the knowledge and point of view of journalists and the public. Articles and essays by nurses in various media would include personal and ethical reflections, anecdotal accounts of their care of the sick and vulnerable, descriptions of innovations in clinical practice, analyses of major health care issues, and recommendations addressing treatment, preventive practices, and health care system issues.

Nurses would not just sit at the tables of power where top-echelon governmental, corporate, or academic experts make policy, they would be full-fledged vocal and assertive decision makers who would talk and be listened to and respected for their knowledge.

Because nurses would educate patients and their families, friends, relatives, neighbors, and community members about nursing work, patients would be fully cognizant that nurses are key to their survival and recovery. Just as people recognize that it takes someone with education and expertise to perform brain surgery, they would know that it takes someone with education and expertise to care for a patient who has just had brain surgery.

When faced with medical treatments or procedures, patients would do more than inquire about the details of the procedures and their physician's qualifications to perform them. They would seek information about the qualifications of the nurses who would care for them during and after their treatments. They would want to know the nurse-to-patient ratio in the hospital unit to which they would be admitted. They would recognize that nurses are critical to outpatient surgery and would inquire about the availability of nursing at such centers and about the extent and type of nursing services available to them in their homes or in other community settings.

Prospective nursing home residents and their families would investigate the extent of nursing services in the facilities they are considering and the qualifications of the nursing staff. Similarly, families would be well aware of the need for and the importance of the health services provided by school nurses, public health nurses, and home-care nurses in their communities. People would understand that many nurses, like physicians, have specialized expertise. They would readily accept and often seek the services of nurse practitioners, mental health nurses, nurse midwives, nurse anesthetists, and hospice nurses.

Health care administrators and public officials would be under pressure to provide funds for the actual cost of nursing care. Hospitals could no longer afford to treat nurses as a cheap, disposable labor force or as interchangeable cogs in an industrial machine. Because the public would understand the critical role of nursing in health care, hospitals could no longer

rely on paring nursing staffs as their strategy for dealing with budget problems. Attempts to cut nursing staff, substitute aides for registered nurses
(RNs), and stretch staff through floating and mandatory overtime would
produce public outcry. To the public, floating a nurse from, for example, an
oncology to a pediatric unit would be in the same league as asking a medical
oncologist to take over for a pediatrician.

Nursing salaries would more accurately reflect the expertise and responsibilities of nurses. This greater investment in nursing would mean that full-
time jobs, with predictable schedules, would be readily available.

A more complex and accurate image of the nurse would replace dated or
distorted stereotypes such as physician handmaid, self-sacrificing angel of
mercy, lewd sex object, and vituperative harridan.

Everyone would know that nursing requires education and training, not
just niceness. It would be common knowledge that nurses are educated not
born. This understanding would translate into widespread public support
for nursing education at the undergraduate, graduate, and postgraduate levels. Nursing education would be fully integrated into higher education systems. Schools of nursing would be viewed as major contributors to the academic enterprise at universities. Politicians and academic administrators
who tried to eliminate nursing programs or create courses of instruction designed to replace nurses with some form of generic health care worker
would be roundly opposed.

The public would understand that medical interns and residents are not
the only learners, and physicians are not the only teachers, in teaching hospitals and other health care institutions. It would be generally known that
hospitals are educational institutions for nurses and that, in them, nurses
teach physicians as well as nurses-in-training. Institutional budgets would
reflect this fact by allocating money for in-house nursing education. It
would be accepted that veteran nurses, like physicians, need to keep up with
the latest treatments as well as with methods of disease prevention and
health promotion. Health care facilities would be amply staffed so that RNs
could participate in the planning and management of services during their
workdays and could take time away from the job for continuing education.
Budgets would include resources for clinical education and extramural educational programs.

Respect for nursing would mean that young women and men who show
an interest in nursing careers would be strongly encouraged, not grilled
about why they aren't planning to go to medical school. With the challenges
and rewards of nursing more fully appreciated, many intelligent women,
with a full range of professional options, would choose nursing. Nursing
would be an increasingly attractive career choice for men. Just as female enrollment in medical schools steadily increased after it became more accept-

able for women to be physicians, the percentage of men who would enroll in nursing schools would also rise.

Nurses would receive the three *R*s that foster professional satisfaction—recognition, respect, and reward. Indeed, nursing shortages would not be tolerated because it would be understood that human health and well-being depend not only on medically necessary care but on *necessary nursing care.*

Does this vision of the future seem like science fiction?

It's not. Elements of this scenario are attainable through sustained action and effective public communication. All areas of nursing—clinical practice, education, research, and policy—depend on public understanding of how and why nursing is indispensable to health care. Nursing is not practiced in a vacuum. Nurses require significant social and economic resources to do their work, including physical space, equipment, staff, research, and education. If the public doesn't understand the significance of nurses' work and the context in which it takes place, it will be difficult to correct conditions that drive nurses out of the clinical setting and even out of the profession. Similarly, it will be hard to attract the best and the brightest young people into the profession and keep them in it. If the public and opinion makers are to allocate adequate financial resources to support nursing, they must have a good idea of what nurses really do. If the work of contemporary nurses is unknown or misunderstood, then nurses cannot be appreciated or supported and cannot exert appropriate influence in health care. And if they can't do that, nurses will have difficulty delivering appropriate, high-quality care.

Missing in Action

Being unseen and unknown has been a perpetual problem for nursing. Studies of the visibility of nursing in the news media at the beginning of the 1990s and at the end of the decade found remarkably similar results—the largest health care profession is still underrepresented.[1,2] One way this plays out is that nursing is simply overlooked, even in its most obvious and familiar form—hospital nursing.

A disturbing, but not isolated, example was an article in the *New York Times* about the Greater New York Hospital Association contesting the refusal of managed care and insurance companies to reimburse for patient days during which no surgeries, diagnostic tests, or other medical procedures occurred.[3] Did the Hospital Association tell the insurers that patients are in the hospital not just for medical procedures but for nursing care, and that the success of many procedures depends on the nursing care patients receive before, during, and after them? Apparently not, because there was no mention of nursing in the article. So the reader was left with the erroneous view that patients are in hospitals only to undergo procedures that doctors perform.

This article is a textbook case of how patient care is misrepresented when nursing is omitted. If the public is deprived of information showing that nursing is essential to patient care, particularly from a newspaper as influential as the *New York Times,* then how can the public support the funding of nursing care? When omissions like this occur, nurses must always respond with letters and phone calls that correct the public record and the misconceptions of journalists. In so doing, they are educating the media and participating in the creation of an accurate picture of their work.

Friendliness versus Accuracy

To respond appropriately to the media, nurses need to know what they should expect from press coverage. We've heard complaints that the media are not "nurse friendly" and that they pick on nurses. The media, some nurses point out, seem quick to broadcast stories that paint nurses in an uncomplimentary light. There are stories about killer nurses, incompetent nurses, poorly trained nurses, and, of course, the entertainment media have their "naughty" nurses.

Some nursing groups have said or implied that problems of nursing image could be remedied if the media were somehow more friendly to nurses. "We feel that there has been little nurse-friendly media to date," says the Center for Nursing Advocacy on its Web site. The Center, which monitors and maintains an electronic archive of media depictions of nursing, also suggests that "nurse-friendly language" is needed to refute stereotypes and misconceptions about nursing.[4]

Other nursing groups say they want "positive" coverage. But how is "friendly" or "positive" or "negative" defined? There is little clarity on this score.

The final report of the Woodhull Study on Nursing and the Media, for example, gave examples of what it categorized as positive or negative references or quotations about nurses in the news media. It categorized as negative a report in *USA Today* that said that 1,200 nurses picketed a Kaiser hospital in California protesting changes to telephone triage lines that could cut many nursing jobs. It was not clear from the Woodhull report whether the story was negative because it cast or miscast the protest as being about nursing jobs, or whether the student researchers from the University of Rochester School of Nursing regarded coverage of protest itself as negative.

A *St. Petersburg Times* story about an RN who stopped her car and delivered CPR to an injured child was categorized as "mixed." What was wrong with this story? "Was it necessary to mention that [the nurse] was on her way to traffic court?" the study report asked. "That aspect added a negative tone to an otherwise positive reference."

The researchers found the following to be positive references or quotations about nursing: "They are truly angels of mercy" (a quote in the *Rochester Democrat and Chronicle* referring to nurses at a Rochester hospital); "In the future your doctor may be a nurse" (a quote from an American Nurses Association [ANA] spokesperson about nurse practitioners that appeared in the *New York Times*).

Many of the examples in the Woodhull report could be easily classified as positive or negative, such as this one from the *St. Petersburg Times*: ". . . Martin lost a large amount of blood because his nurse was distracted by a telephone call to discuss her breakfast plans" (pp. 24–25).[2]

But are the two we cited above so clear? One could argue that coverage of the nurses' picket line showed that nurses are strong advocates who are willing to take risks when they feel that changes to a triage system will endanger their patients or will deprive them of jobs.

As for the nurse who was on her way to traffic court when she stopped to save a child's life, it is unrealistic to think a reporter would withhold that bit of information about any rescuer be it physician, plumber, or priest. To suggest that it shouldn't be in a story about a nurse smacks of special pleading and raises the question as to whether the researchers think that nurses belong to a unique class that should get special (kinder, friendlier) treatment than others. That argument is grounded in the notion that nurses have to be more virtuous than other people.

Similarly, casting nurses as "angels of mercy" reinforces a sentimental cliché that offers a stereotype in place of an accurate description of nurses. Referring to nurse practitioners as substitute doctors and competitors for doctors' practices does not advance the public understanding of what NPs know and do.

Positive/negative classifications are notorious in mass media research for being too simplistic to produce meaningful information. Nurses do not need a template that makes them feel that they need "media-friendliness" to get a fair shake.

In fact, the media are not particularly unfriendly toward nursing. A lot of journalists, like many members of the broader public, feel very friendly toward nurses. The problem is they aren't particularly interested in reporting on nurses because they don't know much about what nurses do. That may well have been why the *Times* reporter, or her editor, while preparing the story on insurance reimbursement to hospitals, apparently didn't ask, "Hey, aren't patients in the hospital because they need nursing care?" Just raising that question would imply some grasp of nursing practice.

The media could be said to be more indifferent or inattentive to nursing than hostile or unfriendly. Most journalists don't know enough about nursing to know they could find interesting stories to write about nurses. If they have bought into the idea that nursing is fluffy, hand-holding TLC done by self-sacrificing angels of mercy, few will understand that nursing is as interesting and important as what physicians do, and they won't be inclined to test this perception.

This is why longing for a kinder, gentler press should be jettisoned in favor of a quest for attentive and accurate coverage. The media are likely to be attentive if they think something newsworthy is going on in nursing. And accurate reporting on nursing—warts and all—would be an indication that nursing is being taken seriously.

An accurate picture of nursing will emerge only when nurses and their organizations tell journalists not who nurses are and how virtuous they can be, but what they do and why it is so important.

Personal Image/Professional Practice

At the moment, nurses are seen more, and may be appreciated more, for who they are rather than what they do, for their virtues rather than their knowledge and action.

Surveys in many countries seem to bear this out. Nurses perennially are at the top or rank very high in listings of occupations whose members are seen as being trustworthy, honest, and ethical.[5] In fact, nurses rank higher than physicians. However, these surveys don't tell us if the public ranks the *work* of nurses highly, or even if the public knows anything about the knowledge, judgment, and expertise that goes into it. This is a key question when the public is told that other, cheaper substitutes can do the work of nurses. Moreover, at least one of these studies found that although members of the public say they believe nurses are ethical and honest, they would not ask nurses questions about major health issues like sexually transmitted diseases, drug and alcohol use, abortion, birth control, menopause, or osteoporosis.[6]

If a public image of nursing that is centered on the personal attributes of those who go into the profession hasn't convinced patients to consult nurses about critical health issues, it is not likely to convince governments or insurers to pay what it costs for nursing care. Only a professional image based on the work, skills, and knowledge of nursing can do that.

Many nurses have told us they believe that it is too hard to communicate

> *"Most people know they can't get into a hospital without a doctor. What they don't know is that they won't get out of one— at least not alive—without a nurse."*
>
> —*Nursing historian Joan Lynaugh*[7]

the "essence of nursing" because nursing is too diverse and varied. Just because nurses do widely varied work does not mean that nursing work cannot be communicated. Medical practice is also diverse, but physicians have created a strong professional image. Most people believe they know what physicians do. Even if they have qualms about physicians, most people do not regard physician care as optional. Doctors are considered to have the kind of knowledge and skills that make them irreplaceable. Some people even think that the definition of being really sick is that you have to go to the doctor!

To explain nursing, nurses don't need to describe what every nurse does nor do they have to describe the indescribable—the essence of nursing. What they have to do is explain what they as individuals do. They need to describe the problems they deal with, why they are important, how they deal with them, and how that makes a difference.

Constructing a Credible Professional Image

To construct an image of nursing that explains how nurses rescue patients from harm does not mean repudiating caring. It does mean that nurses must be careful not to depict caring as simple intuition or as something commonplace. When nurses focus on the caring aspects of their work, they can deepen the public comprehension of caring by explaining that caring is complex and skilled work that is essential to patient care. Creating a credible public image also means being careful not to omit or repudiate the medical, technical, and bodily aspects of nursing in favor of an idealized image. The gap in the public's understanding of nursing can effectively be filled through depictions of what nurses do, how they do it, and why nurses do what they do.

Of course some people do have a favorable and accurate impression of nursing based on firsthand experience. Many people who have experienced nursing care as patients understand how critical nurses are to their survival and well-being. But patient experiences do not automatically translate into broad public support for nursing. Some patients who experience good nursing practice have only a simplistic idea of its content and don't grasp the skill and knowledge of the nurse. Some believe that nurses do what they do solely out of kindness—"she stopped by to chat with me," "she told me more than the doctor,"—but don't understand that the nurse has engaged in purposeful actions that may have saved their lives or prevented potentially lethal complications. Still others may attribute nurses' skill and knowledge to physician guidance. Many patients will praise their nurses yet not express public concern when nursing is threatened. Unless nurses help patients and the public understand the complexity of nursing care and relate nursing to the larger health care picture, they are likely to regard their nursing care as a private transaction whose sufficient reward is privately expressed gratitude. They may even thank the doctor for having trained his or her nurses so well.

Those in a position to influence legislation, policy making, and funding must know that nursing-rich health care environments save lives and reduce serious complications whereas understaffed settings put patients at risk. They need to be aware of the incipient tragedies awaiting patients when nurses are not available to prevent falls, complications, and errors in treatment and care, or to "rescue" patients in need.[8-11]

Just as doctors have created a strong public image based on physician centrality to life and death, nurses—both as individual and within organizations—can illuminate the consequential nature of their work.

This is not to say that doctors haven't been concerned with their personal image. In the days when patients were presumed ignorant about their bodies and diseases and were encouraged to trust their doctors to make decisions for them, the character and caring of the doctor were emphasized. But the key to this trust was always that doctors had the knowledge, skill, and competence to make such decisions and to execute them.

The kindly village doc has all but disappeared from popular culture, and the all-around good guy seems to have been replaced, at least on TV, by the guy or gal medico with interesting foibles. Even so, doctors remain dominant in health care by emphasizing their special knowledge, technical skill, and participation in lifesaving medical advances. And on TV shows like *ER* and *Grey's Anatomy,* doctors often save lives in spite of who they are. The paradigm is much less about who the doctor is than what the doctor can do for you.

Nurses' public image and recruitment campaigns have shown some ambivalence on that score, particularly in connection with how prominent "care" and "caring" should be. As we write this, in the midst of a serious nursing shortage in many parts of the world, there seems to be a revival of sentimentalized images of nurses in which "caring" is seen either as an inherent attribute of the nurse or, in simplistic form, as the totality of nursing.

This swing of the pendulum contrasts significantly with a U.S. recruitment campaign in 1990 (during *that* nursing shortage) to appeal to potential recruits by punching up the high-tech aspects of nursing work. One kinetic television ad showed nurses racing around with equipment and ended with this slogan: "If caring were enough, anyone could be a nurse."[12] The implied message was that since anyone can "care," there is nothing special—or skillful—about nurses' "caring."

That depiction of nursing could be interpreted as an over-correction to a problem identified in a survey commissioned in 1989 to assist planning for a nurse recruitment campaign. The survey, by Peter Hart, found that the public had a limited professional concept of nursing: "When people think of nurses, they are significantly more inclined to dwell on either their care giving and comforting aspect or their customary role (such as in a hospital) than they are to focus on nurses' professionalism or qualifications" (p. 15).[13]

Hart's report asserted that successful recruitment and the willingness of the public to entrust nurses with more sophisticated duties "lies in elevating the stature of and professional respect accorded to RNs. The [public relations recruitment] campaign must increase people's awareness of nurses' professionalism and trustworthiness by highlighting RNs' health care training, experience, skills, and expertise" (p. 15).

Notably, the report did not advocate diminishing or jettisoning the caring and comforting aspects of nursing in any campaign. In fact, caring and comforting was the basis for what the Hart report called "the impressive goodwill nurses enjoy." The report suggested that in communicating with the public, nurses should *build on* the high regard they already had.[13]

However, in the rush at that time to promote advance practice nursing, "caring" was sometimes viewed as antithetical, and even embarrassing, to professionalism. Some advisers seemed to think that the very word "nurse" was tainted. Bernice Buresh was present when Kathleen Hall Jamieson, a leading communication and public policy expert, suggested to trustees of the University of Pennsylvania School of Nursing that "nurse" be dropped from the title "nurse practitioner" in favor of something new that might sound "more professional." Some nurses suggest that getting rid of the title "nurse" will solve nursing's image problem.

The fatal flaw in such a strategy is that it strips nurses of an image that the public relates to without adding a more compelling *nursing* component to it. It tears down, rather than builds on, nursing's foundation in caregiving work. If nurses convey that there is nothing special about the way that nurses care for and comfort patients, then those activities—as well as a lot of other so-called routine tasks—can be turned over to assistants or dropped altogether. If nurses project an image of themselves doing work like that of psychologists, social workers, or chaplains, the danger is that they may be replaced by psychologists or social workers, who have more training in patient communication and emotional processes than most nurses. Similarly, if the professional advancement of nurses relies on nurses taking over responsibilities traditionally associated with physicians, or physicians' assistants, then nurses are vulnerable to being cast as junior or cheaper doctors, or, once again, as assistants to doctors.

Ending the Silence

Today every profession must speak for itself and justify its existence. The public needs to know that nursing care is *consequential*—as much so as medical treatment.

How can nurses end the silence about nursing and tell a credible compelling story about their work?

1. Nurses must inform the public about nursing.
2. Every nurse must make public communication and education about nursing an integral part of her or his nursing work.
3. Nurses must communicate in ways that highlight nurses' knowledge rather than their virtues.

Not every nurse has to be seen or heard in the mass media to be a successful public communicator. Nor does a nurse who would like to be a more effective public communicator need to go back to school to get a degree in public relations.

However, day in and day out, every nurse could take advantage of the openings that occur in professional and social settings to communicate more about nursing. If nursing is to acquire public *significance* commensurate with its role in health care, then many more individual nurses and nursing organizations must be actively reaching out to influential and broad publics. They need to talk in clear, everyday language to illustrate just how nurses save lives, alleviate suffering, and even keep down health care costs.

There is untapped power in nursing's numbers. In most industrialized countries, nursing is the largest health care profession, with nurses often outnumbering physicians by more than three to one. Let's say that only 10 percent of nurses and nursing students try to bring nursing and nursing issues to the larger public by participating in a rally, calling up a legislator, telephoning a radio or television talk show, writing a letter to the editor, talking to a television producer about doing a nursing feature, meeting with the editorial board of a newspaper, sending out news releases on timely research in nursing journals, testifying at a hearing on health care delivery, speaking to a journalist about a nursing innovation, or engaging in outreach in any of the myriad ways that lead to public recognition. In the United States alone, this would mean conscious activism by more than a quarter of a million nurses.

By using their numbers, nurses could succeed without huge budgets. It only takes a few callers to get the attention of most editors. A legislator or chief nurse or health minister who gets twenty calls, faxes, or e-mails (or sometimes only five or ten) on an issue is likely to pay attention. In some circumstances, one hundred calls would constitute a landslide.

One might reasonably ask why so many individual nurses are required to take on this role. Isn't that the job of organizations?

Yes, it is the responsibility of nursing associations, unions, and research and academic institutions. Without deprecating what they have accomplished, they can and must do much more. Every nursing group must treat public communication as an inseparable part of its core mission. However, not even assertive spokespeople for professional organizations and institutions can be substitutes for the authentic voices of nurses in the field. Organized attempts to promote nursing are often defeated when nurses are afraid to participate in public discussions of even noncontroversial health care topics. If rank-and-file nurses don't tell the public what it is they do, their work will remain hidden.

To educate the public about their work, nurses—all nurses, whether they are at the bedside, in homes, in managerial roles, in clinical specialties, in the colleges and universities as educators and researchers, or studying nursing as students—must make nursing more visible and voluble.

Public Communication

Some basic concepts are helpful in moving nurses toward the goal of being effective public communicators. The phrase "public communication," contains two words, both of which we define broadly.

The *public* is not a singular mass. There are many "publics," or audiences, that nurses need to communicate with. These publics include patients and family members, doctors and other nurses, managers and administrators, a nurse's own family and friends, members of community and religious organizations and social groups, marketing and public relations professionals in hospitals, professional organizations and colleges and universities, regulators and legislators, and journalists and other media professionals.

Putting it simply, a public or audience is anyone a nurse is in contact with or can reach via the media.

Similarly *communication* is multidimensional. There is more than one way to communicate. Verbal communication can be oral or written, and some forms of communication are nonverbal.

The fact is that we all communicate in various ways with many publics everyday. A great deal is being communicated about *nursing* whenever a nurse introduces her- or himself to a patient, whenever a nurse calls a doctor, whenever a nurse talks to a patient about his or her treatment, whenever a nurse makes a complaint to managers or administrators, whenever a nurse tells stories about nursing, and even whenever a nurse remains mute. Similarly, what a nurse wears to work and the body language that a nurse employs speak volumes.

The question is, do these communications convey what nurses want them to? Do they contribute to a strong professional identity, or are they, at times, at cross-purposes to that goal?

Three Tiers of Communication

In this book we focus on three tiers or modes of communication that can educate the public about nursing:

1. Public communication through professional self-presentation.
2. Public communication through anecdotal descriptions of nursing work.
3. Public communication through the mass media.

Every nurse is already sending messages about nursing via at least one and, most likely, two of these modes. The intention of this book is to show how to make those messages purposeful and effective and to encourage many more nurses to increase their communication skills in order to educate various publics about nursing.

Chapter 3, for example, covers the first mode—self-presentation—and shows how nurses can heighten their professional identity through the way they present themselves. Chapter 5 gives concrete instructions for creating anecdotes about nursing and arguments for nursing. Several chapters concentrate on the media, and chapter 9 examines in detail communication and action campaigns designed for specific goals. Throughout the text, we point out opportunities that exist or can be created to increase public communication in every mode.

While communication skills are important, willingness to communicate about nursing is even more important.

Within nursing there is a big push toward improving nurses' communication with non-nursing audiences. But there is also an ambivalence about, and even resistance toward, public communication that winds up inhibiting and frustrating efforts in this area. When it comes to setting up and sustaining communication programs and activities, at times it looks as though nursing has one foot on the gas pedal and the other on the brake. In this text we address specific fears that nurses have told us tend to silence them.

We believe that by developing what we call a "voice and persona of agency," more nurses can comfortably communicate about their work. This "voice of agency" can help strengthen bonds between nurses so that individual advocates will be supported by a culture of collaborative and collective advocacy. In such a culture, nursing will be far more likely to develop supports outside of nursing. It can lead to nurses finally getting the recognition, respect, and rewards they have so long deserved.

Chapter 2

Creating a
Voice of Agency

As we lecture to nurses all over the world, we encourage them to talk more about their work in a variety of settings—at home, in the workplace, in the community, at social events, in professional settings, and at meetings on health care attended by opinion makers such as politicians and journalists. Our presentations and workshops suggest specific ways that nurses might be more visible and vocal both as individuals and as members of organizations. While most nurses respond enthusiastically to the suggestion that they develop the skills needed to be better public communicators, some express reservations about the merits of increasing nurses' public visibility. They are resistant to the idea that they, as individuals, should talk about their own work.

"Patients know what we do," a Boston nursing student insists. "We don't need to talk about it."

"I don't need adoration and admiration from the world or my patients," a new nursing graduate in Perth, Australia, contends. "I just do my work and that's enough for me."

In Coimbra, Portugal, a veteran nurse forcefully addresses our entire audience. "*My* patients know and appreciate what *I* do. *I* don't need to tell them about my work."

In Japan a nursing professor admonishes nurses to avoid anything that would call attention to themselves: "No me, me, me," she says, agitatedly pointing her finger at herself.

Sadly, some nurses take these admonitions to heart. Eventually, they may lament that even the people closest to them don't know about or understand their work. "My son always asks me what I do, but I never know what to tell him," a surgical nurse confesses.

"I worked all day and when I came home I had to take care of my family," one nurse told us. "I made dinner, did the laundry, and cleaned. I did the same thing on weekends. It seems like I never had time to talk to my family about my work. Now my kids are grown up." She paused and asked, "Is it too late?"

How will people know what nurses do and understand the complexity of their work if nurses don't tell them?" we ask audiences. Some nurses respond, "People know that naturally, just from watching what we're doing."

Really?

What many people "naturally" assume about nurses' work is that doctors order every one of their interventions and stand behind every nursing action.

Consider a typical incident. A nurse on the oncology floor at a major teaching hospital spends hours trying to get a medical intern to write an order for a narcotic for a patient suffering from pancreatic cancer. The nurse has informed the intern that the patient is in excruciating pain. Far more familiar with cancer patients and their pain management than the intern, she recommends a course of intravenous (IV) morphine.

The intern refuses to order the narcotic. He simply will not listen to the nurse. Over a period of several hours, she repeatedly engages with him, trying, to no avail, to teach him about cancer pain management. Finally, she corners a more senior resident who agrees with her and directs the intern to write the order. In the patient's chart—the contemporary and historical record of the case—the nurse's struggle with the young doctor is absent. Reading the chart, one would never know that the nurse was responsible for easing the patient's pain and that the intern resisted her attempts to provide appropriate care. In this chart the new physician is "credited" with taking the action that reduced the patient's suffering.

Not surprisingly, the patient and her family believe the doctor was her savior. Several days later, the patient wrote letters thanking her caregivers. She expressed her heartfelt gratitude to her attending physician who, during her hospitalization, rarely saw her when she was awake. She specifically thanked the intern whom she thought brought her relief. She did not thank her primary and associate nurses by name. She included only a general thank you to "the nurses."

Some nurses do not respond well to the suggestion that they take credit for their work and insist it doesn't matter whether anyone writes a letter acknowledging what they did. They recoil at the idea of explicitly explaining their work to patients and families in a way that highlights the *nurse's,* rather than others' clinical knowledge and judgment.

For example, Suzanne Gordon's purpose as a guest on a National Public Radio talk show was to explain the importance of nursing and explore why our society does not sufficiently acknowledge, respect, and reward nurses' work. She argued that nurses need societal respect and recognition if they are to get the resources they need to deliver quality care.

A hospital staff nurse called in and angrily refuted these assertions. "I don't need credit for my work," she said. "Working with patients is reward enough."

She continued with heated remarks that diverted attention from nurses to physicians. She told the audience that physicians are hard-working, highly educated, and intelligent. Her statements diminished nursing, reinforced the stereotypical notion that the nurse exists to support the physician, and legitimized the traditional allocation of resources to medicine.

Although, it would be a positive step if patients did write letters thanking specific nurses for their fine work, we are not arguing that thank you notes to and about individual nurses constitute the solution to nursing's visibility problem. Nor do we believe that patients and the public should express adoration for nurses. What is necessary, however, is realistic recognition by patients, doctors, family members, and the broader public of what nurses know and do. The intern in the example above lacked an understanding that the nurse was a clinical ally and teammate who had something professionally valuable to offer him. If he had, he would have listened to her and she wouldn't have had to seek out the resident who, hours later and to the detriment of the patient who suffered needless pain in the interim, told the intern the same thing she did.

There is a direct connection between the three Rs—recognition, respect, and reward—and quality patient care.[1] Nurses like the one who called in, however, construe recognition as personal rather than professional. Their discomfort and elaborate rationales for remaining hidden suggest, at the very least, confusion about whether increased visibility would be personal or professional. Their concern is well-founded because, to this day, many of nursing's forays into the public spotlight are based on promoting the goodness of the nurse as a person whose work is an outgrowth of idealized character traits. So any suggestion that individual nurses should act to attract public attention is bound to stir up uneasiness about who or what might be exposed.

Let us be clear where we stand. We come down solidly on the side of *professional* visibility and voice, which is not to say that the nurse herself or himself is effaced. Quite the contrary. The individual nurse who talks about her or his work is present front and center, but the attributes of the nurse that should get public attention are those that pertain to the work of the nurse such as clinical judgment, caring, and skill.

The three Rs are essential in this professional framework if our societies are going to have necessary nursing care. The three Rs are sequential. The various publics with whom nurses work and upon whose support nursing depends must first *recognize* what nurses do. People must perceive what goes on in nursing in order to *respect* the work and *reward* it. By reward we do not mean token acknowledgment in the form of cheery, sentimental Nurses' Week celebrations complete with trinkets, door prizes, and a cash bar. We do mean, in addition to appropriate pay levels, institutional supports that provide nurses with appropriate caseloads, time with patients, authority and autonomy in their workplaces, and continuing education.

Despite some nurses' insistence that virtue will be its own reward and that they need no more than the gratitude in a patient's eyes, the reality demonstrated in the current nursing shortage is that nurses who are poorly paid, poorly treated, and professionally unrecognized end up burnt out, injured, demoralized, and uncaring toward their patients. Some even flee the profession. The people punished then are the patients who are unable to get adequate nursing care.[1]

The process of gaining recognition is conventionally seen as being the job of nursing organizations and "leaders." Some nurses have told us that their business is to do their nursing job, not to promote nursing. The problem with this notion is that "nursing" cannot become visible while the individual nurses remain anonymous. "Nursing" cannot speak. It is a category. It has no voice if individual nurses don't give it one. While it is important for nursing to have credible spokespeople, if nurses who are involved in the direct care of patients don't talk about their work, it is unlikely that the realities of everyday nursing practice will be made visible to the public.

Agency versus Well-Being

The appropriate use of voice is, therefore, not a threat either to nurses or nursing. Silence is the threat to nursing. Nursing recognition hinges on individual nurses employing what we call a "voice of agency" that accurately represents the experience of illness as well as the experience of those who care for the sick and vulnerable.

What do we mean by a "voice of agency?" The word "agency" stems from the Latin verb *agere* meaning to act or to do. *Agency* is the capacity for acting or the condition of acting or exerting power. An *agent* is a person who is instrumental, "through whom power is exerted." "Agent" can denote someone who is acting on behalf of someone else, like an agent for a movie star. But we are concurring with what Nobel Prize–winning economist Amartya Sen describes as "its older—and 'grander'—sense as someone who acts and brings about change, and whose achievements can be judged in terms of her own values and objectives, whether or not we assess them in terms of some external criteria as well" (p. 19).[2]

In writing about the social, economic, educational, and employment inequities that women suffer in a number of countries, Sen applauds the increasing emphasis on "the active role of women's *agency*," as contrasted with the state of women's "*well-being*." Well-being, according to Sen, offers "a very restricted view of the personhood of women," whereas "the agency role is . . . central to recognizing people as responsible persons [who] can choose to act one way rather than another." This shift of emphasis is especially significant in developing countries, Sen writes, where women, "[n]o longer the passive recipients of welfare-enhancing help . . . are increasingly seen, by men as well as women, as active agents of change: the dynamic promoters of social transformations that can alter the lives of *both* women and men" as well as the entire society (pp. 189–192).[2]

For nurses, developing a sense of agency depends on *recognizing* the importance of nursing work *and* their own importance in carrying out this work.

> *The voice of agency is the voice that says: "I helped the patient to walk after surgery so that she wouldn't get blood clots in her legs." "I taught the patient how to take his medications so that they would be effective and produce fewer side effects." "I listened to the patient's fears about the surgery and I was able to give her some information that reassured her."*
>
> *The voice of agency is the voice that conveys the message, "I'm here. I am doing something important."*

To speak with a voice of agency is to admit the incontrovertible fact that the 79-year-old patient did not teach himself how to take his diabetes medication, that the 61-year-old stroke patient did not read her own EKG, and that the demented man did not assess his own skin, discover the beginning of a decubitus ulcer, and act to prevent further skin breakdown. Most patients do not monitor and evaluate their own conditions themselves. When they are most vulnerable, they do not have the ability or the responsibility for preventing catastrophes or educating themselves about their conditions, treatments, and medication regimens. Nor can patients always effectively negotiate the complexities of the system and advocate for themselves. This is what nurses do for them through their professional agency.

All the classic definitions of nursing incorporate the idea of agency in the sense that they emphasize the importance of the nurse making her or his own observations and acting on them. In nursing theory, mastery is seen as developing from the nurse's own informed experiences. It is not present just because one is a "good" woman. Mastery is active, not passive, and thus leads to agency.

Without using the term, Florence Nightingale saw agency as essential to nursing and derided the trivialization of qualifications needed for nursing. In *Notes on Nursing* she wrote:

> It seems a commonly received idea among men and even some women themselves that it requires nothing but a disappointment in love, the want of an object, a general disgust, or incapacity for other things to turn a woman into a good nurse. This reminds one of the parish where a stupid old man was set to be schoolmaster because he was 'past keeping the pigs' . . .
>
> The everyday management of a large ward, let alone of a hospital—the knowing what are the laws of life and death for men, and what the laws of health for wards—(and wards are healthy or unhealthy, mainly according to the knowledge or ignorance of the nurse)—are not these matters of sufficient importance and difficulty to require learning by experience and careful inquiry, just as much as any other art? They do not come by inspiration to the lady disappointed in love, nor to the poor workhouse drudge hard up for a livelihood. (Pp. 133–134)[3]

Patricia Benner's more recent analysis of nursing practice in *From Novice to Expert* is grounded in the daily reality of agency. One can't possibility move from novice to expert without being an agent. Even such seemingly passive nursing work as "being with the patient" and "maximizing the patient's participation in his or her recovery," according to Benner's analysis, requires skill, knowledge, and action.[4]

Yet, while leading nurse theorists emphasize agency as the heart of nursing work, nurses seem to have been taught to deny the agency involved in their work. "We were taught in nursing school that nurses are 'facilitators,'" a nurse interjected when the concept of agency was brought up at one of our workshops. "We facilitate healing and we help people to get better, but we don't do it for them."

To facilitate means to make something easier. The word connotes agency, but in a diluted form. Interestingly, the nurses at the workshop saw the act of facilitating as counterposed to agency and were wary about embracing agency lest it take them beyond the acceptable bounds of nursing.

Nurses sometimes say they are "behind-the-scenes" players. Marion Phipps, a clinical nurse specialist in Boston, described herself this way in a narrative she wrote for a writing class Suzanne Gordon taught for nurses. Over several pages, Phipps described how she had helped a patient to die in peace and with dignity, and how she worked with his family so that they could cope with his dying process.

In the final paragraph, however, Nurse Phipps got stage fright. Instead of summing up her accomplishments, she undercut her actions by arguing that it was the family that did everything worthwhile.

Gordon pointed out that by retreating into the background at the end, Phipps erased the point of her story, which was to show the important work *nurses* do. Why did she drag the nurse from the center of the action to the periphery, Gordon asked Phipps.

"My role as a clinical nurse specialist is to support the primary nurse, and to do that, I tend to pull back," she explained. "I feel very good about my work, but I don't talk much about it. I see my work as supporting others. I'm a sort of a behind-the-scenes person. There are many people in the hospital like this. We're the ones who hold the place together but we don't stay very much in the forefront."

An oncology nurse we'll call Ruth Jones similarly placed herself in the background in her description of her work with a cancer patient. Nurse Jones had cared for a young woman with breast cancer for several years. During this time, the woman not only had to grapple with cancer and chemotherapy but contend with beatings from her abusive husband. As her nurse, Jones administered, monitored, and managed the many side effects of the young woman's chemotherapy and also helped the patient to bring an end to the abuse.

When Nurse Jones told us about her work with this patient, she added that the patient had filed for divorce. "Terrific," we said. "You helped her get away from a person who was harming her."

Rather than acknowledge her accomplishment, she demurred. "Oh no, I didn't really do that much," Jones protested. "The patient's doctor helped a lot."

When we suggested that the doctor's contribution sounded minimal, she agreed. But then she attributed the pivotal role to others—the social worker, the patient, the patient's family. After a full ten minutes of discussion, this nurse finally owned up to her essential work. Then she described in detail exactly what she did and how she did it.

Why would nurses diminish their agency?

Why would nurses believe that backstage players should not be allowed to come to center stage and take a bow?

Why would nurses resist taking credit for their accomplishments even when the credit is given to them?

To answer these questions, it is useful to look at the religious and secular influences that shaped nursing and left their mark.

The Virtue Script

For centuries in the Western world, nursing as an organized institutional intervention was delivered through Christian religious institutions. Most nurses were monks or nuns. They belonged to and obeyed the rules of Christian religious orders and adapted to what feminist scholar Isabel Marcus has called a strict "moral script."[5] As nursing historian Sioban Nelson and Suzanne Gordon have argued, this "virtue script" framed nursing in particular ways.[6] While religious nurses had great technical and even, for their day, medical mastery, their work was cloaked in a veil of deference, submission, obedience, self-abnegation, and anonymity. Religious nurses were taught to view themselves as God's agents, to attribute their own skills and accomplishment to the divine.

Most important for the purposes of this discussion, they were taught to be self-effacing. Religious nurses were devoted to the performance of good deeds through which souls were saved—their own as well as their patients. To talk about a good deed, to hint at one's own accomplishments, was to be guilty of the sin of pride, which turned the good deed into a sinful one.

When nursing was professionalized and feminized in the nineteenth century (men were literally kicked out by not being allowed to register as nurses), reformers did not rebel against this religious virtue script. Instead, Nelson and Gordon posit, they used the religious template to help women navigate the treacherous passage from the domestic to public sphere, from unpaid work within the family to paid work outside the home.[6] "Respectable" women who entered this first large profession for women were moving into dangerous moral territory. They were taking care of strangers' bodies—many of which were male. In this context, nursing could be practiced by women only if it were desexualized. The calling to do God's work provided the proper context. The cloak of God's agency allowed nurses to develop their own agency, but not to claim it as their own.

Another force that encouraged nurses to deny their agency was the entrance of physicians into positions of power in hospitals. When medicine (perhaps the quintessential patriarchal profession) and nursing met on the "contested terrain"[7] of the hospital in the nineteenth century, medical men were not at all eager to allow a cadre of edu-

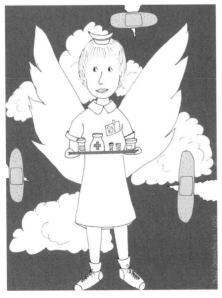

Sonia Oppenheim, www.familycomic.com

cated women (either as nurses or as physicians) to have authority or auton-omy within the hospital. Many favored the idea of a better-trained nurse, but only if that nurse was conceptualized as the physician's servant, or handmaid. To function in the hospital, nurses thus had to negotiate a deal with medicine, one that gave doctors a dominant role over nursing as well as medical practice. Just as nurses had, for centuries, deferred to the divine, they now would learn to defer to the doctor and view themselves as fulfilling his medical mission.

If the modern doctors' authority stemmed from education and unique knowledge, and if they would cast their profession as singular in that regard, then what could nurses claim as their own province that would not provoke competition with physicians? The answer was already in the culture—women's moral superiority and natural caregiving abilities. As Susan M. Re-verby has noted, nursing's very mission then depended on "women's self-sacrificing service to others."[8]

Patriarchal culture places women's work under the control of men and conceptualizes it as an extension of male agency. Women have been, and in some countries still are, seen as being men's possessions. In patriarchal cul-ture, when the man leaves the home, he temporarily assigns his agency to his wife, but reclaims it when he returns. Exciting, dynamic work is reserved for men. In such a culture, caregiving is defined not as an opportunity for self-assertion or self-fulfillment but as self-sacrifice. Nineteenth century nursing thus established a template that endures to this day: Nursing is self-sacrificing, altruistic, devotional, poorly paid, anonymous, silent work. The idea that women are "naturally" caring and that caring is instinctual or hor-monal also lives on and conceals both the complexity of caregiving and the agency of the caregiver. "Women's work" is said to rely on instinct rather than knowledge, intelligence, or judgment. The complex caregiving that is de-scribed by such feminist scholars as Sara Ruddick,[9] Laurel Thatcher Ulrich,[10] and Patricia Benner[11] is missing from the patriarchal conceptualization of "women's work." Most important, the traditional definitions of "women's work" deny women belief in their own agency. The female caregiver isn't an actor, she is the container for the genetic engine that drives her actions.

What is remarkable today, given nursing's educational and scientific ad-vances and its claims to professionalism, is not only that the virtue script re-mains powerful but that it has morphed into an ideology that undercuts nurses' claims to professional standing and regard today.

How does the virtue script do this? First, it reinforces stereotypes that discourage nurses from claiming credit for their own work and accomplish-ments. Second, it deploys an iconography that calls into question both the agency and the *maturity* of the nurse.

When members of the public (journalists, politicians, policymakers, and

CAUTION

A Singular Strength: For Nurse Lake, Caring Is Instinctual

—Headline on article honoring
Nurse Practitioner Nancy Lake in
"Salute to Nurses" advertising supplement,
Boston Globe, *May 2005*

regulators, as well as patients) walk into hospitals and other health care settings in North America, what do they see? Often they see nurses wearing teddy bear or angel scrubs adorned with angel pins or smiley faces. When they look at promotional campaigns by hospitals—or by nursing organizations—they are more likely to see pictures of nurses smiling at the camera or the "patient" (who is usually the picture of health) rather than concentrating intently on the work that they are doing. Journalists and other members of the public see nurses with pens decorated with hearts writing on notepads emblazoned with endearing slogans, like this one at St. Mary's (Magnet) Hospital in Madison, Wisconsin: "With love we wrap you in our quilt of caring." Or they see celebratory posters for Nurses' Week, like the one produced in 2002 by Ohio-Health Systems:

> People believe there are beings
> That come to you in your darkest hour—
> Guide you when your life hangs in the balance,
> Cradle you,
> Calm you,
> Protect you.
> Some people call them guardian angels;
> We call them nurses.

A highly gendered promotion like this, while superficially complimentary to nurses who indeed do come to patients in their darkest hours, trivializes the education and skills that *human* nurses need to protect and comfort vulnerable patients by casting them as maternal and angelic.

Yet many nurses embrace these attitudes and images. That was the case with a short Nurses' Day composition e-mailed by a student nurse to her family and friends, and then enthusiastically passed on to friends of friends, and eventually to us.

"Being a nurse isn't about grades. It's about being who we are. No book can teach you how to cry with a patient. No class can teach you how to tell a family that their parents have died or are dying. No professor can teach you how to find dignity in giving someone a bed bath. A nurse isn't about the pills, the IV's, and the charting. It's about being able to love people when they are at their weakest moments and being able to forgive them for all their wrongs and make a difference in their lives today. No one can make you a nurse . . . you just are."

—A NURSING STUDENT IN HONOR OF NURSES' WEEK 2004

Lest anyone think this is a minority view of nursing, its sentiments were applauded by almost every member of a graduate-level nursing class at a major nursing school where Bernice Buresh distributed it, and also by more than half of the working nurses at a large workshop she conducted at a midwestern hospital, who wrote testimonials about it like, "This is absolutely true!"

Is it? It's not surprising that a student nurse might, in a roundabout way, reveal a lack of confidence in her clinical skills. But this composition says learning and clinical activities aren't important, and that nursing professors and scholars don't have much to offer. What is important is the natural moral superiority of the nurse.

Consider the irony. Some of the same nurses who expressed their concern about nurses becoming self-aggrandizing if they talked about their work found the hubris in a student nurse's claim that she could "forgive" patients "for all their wrongs" acceptable.

Human beings need to be valued. If nurses don't get recognition and feel they can't claim recognition for their real contributions, then the need might mutate into a plea or demand for recognition based on something else, like personal goodness, moral superiority, or even the ability to cloak the need for recognition in inoffensive or juvenile imagery.

Possibly the worst thing a journalist or policymaker could do in terms of how they might perceive nurses is peruse a catalog or Web site, like Nurses Station, that peddles assorted products and trinkets to nurses. There they would find such dignity-challenged items as the "Florence Bearingale Plush Nurse," a teddy bear dressed like a nurse (only twenty-eight dollars on sale!) described as "a sweet addition to your doll collection and a great gift for a colleague or yourself."

Whether true or not, the product copy for this item asserts that adult nurses (A) collect dolls and (B) would be thrilled to have a child's toy that reduces the determination and effectiveness of Florence Nightingale to cuteness.

For small sums of money, nurses can deck themselves out with amulets like guardian angel pins, nurse angel key rings, and even angel shoe charms that one should "attach to shoelace, or zipper pull of purse or clothing." A number of outlets offer scrubs imprinted with hearts, teddy bears, or "endearing angels with messages of love, unity and peace."

Many of the dolls, figurines, stuffed animals, and T-shirts sold through these catalogs, doled out by pharmaceutical and medical equipment companies at nursing conventions, and given as door prizes for Nurses' Week cast the nurse not as a grown-up person but as an adorable child-angel. Nurses Station even sells a figurine that depicts the nurse as a baby with tiny wings and a stethoscope. These are interesting images in that children have limited agency and babies none. It's hard to think of any other profession that would find acceptable—or even tolerate—images that cast the practitioner as being as helpless as a very young child.

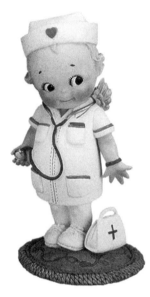

Baby nurse-angel figurine

Some nurses might like these images, and others might find them annoying. But because these images are in such wide circulation, they are not private sentiments but public statements about how health care's largest profession sees itself. Even the International Council of Nurses distributed a Nurses' Day 2000 poster with paintings of nurses as juvenile figures.[12]

Pictures and objects that repeatedly show the nurse as a juvenile raise another serious question: Who needs care more, the patient or the nurse? For example, a homemade "nurse survival kit" sold at a conference that we attended included a "bandage, to mend hurt feelings; a crayon, to color everyday cheerful and bright; and a cotton ball, to help soften disappointments"—not for the patient but for the nurse. Undoubtedly, given the difficult and stressful work they do, nurses need decent working conditions and need to take care of themselves and each other. That is not the issue. The issue is what these childlike symbols and messages communicate, intentionally or not, to the public. Patients' lives depend on the maturity and clinical mastery of nurses. Nurses make this claim rhetorically but contradict it iconographically.

It is no wonder then that the media have such difficulty putting a face (quite literally) on contemporary nursing that they often wind up using vintage pictures of anonymous nurses lined up in full regalia or graphics in which the nurse has no identity. Stories on the nursing shortage are routinely illustrated by an empty nurse's uniform with a cap floating above it.[13] When the *New York Times* printed excerpts from essays written a century apart that commented on public perceptions of nursing in 1900 and in 2000, a drawing of three faceless nurse mannequins was used to illustrate it.[14]

Pictures of Florence Nightingale or of uniformed nurses have advantages. They clearly symbolize "nurse," and, although dated, are at least dignified and professional in tone.

Physicians are more often shown in contemporary settings because they provide the press and the public with mature, consequential images. Whether or not they believe the old saw that MD stands for minor deity, physicians have been acculturated to claim not only their own agency but proprietorship over all of health care. Either implicitly or explicitly they often give the impression that they are the only health care participants with respectable knowledge and intelligence. Some still insist that nurses are the physicians' agents and not consequential players.

This view so pervades our culture that the media often pass it on as a given. In his book *Health against Wealth, Wall Street Journal* reporter George Anders quotes a cardiac surgeon talking about her elderly postoperative patients. "Most of them are scared to go home after four days," she says. "But they end up doing fine when they go home. There's nothing else we really do for them at that stage of recovery. It's just babysitting and helping them walk up and down the hall a few times" (p. 102).[15]

This statement articulates a common medical view that the challenging work of helping an elderly postoperative cardiac patient perform the activities of daily living, and of monitoring, evaluating, and educating the patient, is akin to babysitting. Although there is a lot more to babysitting than the term implies, it is used to diminish the requirements of the caregiver as well as the needs of the one cared for.

Physicians like the one quoted in Anders's book, seem willing, even eager, to cede "unimportant" activities, such as walking a patient after surgery, to nurses. However, when physicians think the work requires education and knowledge, or when it is lucrative or enhances the image of doctors, then physicians assert their superiority. They will insist that these are "medical" activities. If nurses are permitted to execute them, they must do so under medical supervision.

Like the father in the home, the doctor can temporarily assign his or her agency to the nurse. But he reclaims it when he returns. When the doctor finds certain patient populations unprofitable or unappealing, the nurse can become a permanent agent *in situ*. When doctors have good working relationships with RNs, they may also bend the rules stipulated in medical and nurse practice acts by allowing nurses to make "medical decisions" that they ratify after the fact. The unstated agreement between physicians and nurses is that nurses' performance of "medical" tasks remain publicly unacknowledged.

Denial of nurses' agency is also expressed in organizational rhetoric. In numerous practice and policy papers, the American Medical Association categorizes nurses as "mid-level professionals," "physician-extenders," and "non-physician providers." Informally doctors often describe nurses as "their eyes and ears." They compliment nurses by telling them they are so smart, they "could be doctors."

The public echoes these sentiments. Over and over nurses tell us that they are "put in their place" not only by doctors and administrators, but by friends, acquaintances, and even strangers.

"My friends say to me, 'You mean you can do anything, like be a doctor, and you want to be a nurse?'" a first-year master's student at McGill University reported with dismay. She had left a well-paid career in business to do something she felt was useful. She had hoped to receive support for her choice. Instead she encountered only shock.

Another nursing student with a background in biochemistry told us a similar story. "When I told a family friend I was going to nursing school, he said: 'Don't worry, the world is your oyster. When you finish nursing school you can still go to medical school.'"

Continuing devaluation of nursing is costly in this post-feminist era when women have more choices about their careers. When women's options were limited to nursing, teaching, social work, and secretarial work, choosing nursing didn't signal a lack of intelligence or ambition. But today it may seem an inexplicable choice to some when a woman can have higher-paying, higher-status jobs.

The same attitude plagues nurses who become doctors—doctors of nursing that is. Nurses pursuing doctorates in nursing and related disciplines say they are sometimes quizzed by friends and relatives about why they aren't going to medical school to become "real doctors." The questioners don't understand that advanced education enhances *nursing*. They can't grasp that getting a PhD is as difficult, if not more so, than getting an MD.

These attitudes have seeped into nursing. Student nurses we talk to are shocked when veteran nurses reinforce the public denigration of nursing. Young women and men say *nurses* ask: "Why are you becoming a nurse?" or "You could be anything and you're choosing nursing?" Nurses at times actively discourage them with remarks like, "Oh my God, don't become a nurse."

All of this has a marked effect on the confidence of nurses and nursing students. "I feel inferior to them," a nursing student said of her fellow students in science courses.

"When they ask me why I'm becoming a nurse not a doctor," another confessed, "I tell them I'm becoming an advanced-practice nurse not a regular nurse."

"You begin to wonder, is everybody really right? Are doctors really smarter than we are?" another student asked her classmates during a discussion of public attitudes toward nursing. We learned that this student later dropped out of nursing school.

Rifts among nurses often stem from these early and repeated experiences. As they come up against persistent denigration of their work, some nurses may seek positions in administration or academia that offer more autonomy or that seem more insulated from such disrespect. These factors may be part of the motivation to move into nursing roles that look more "medical." As funding pressures destabilize health care systems, managerial models seem to offer relief from both the realities of the workplace and from traditional societal stereotyping. The professional identity of the nurse is supposed to be enhanced if she is a "manager of care" who supervises those who give direct care.

Devaluation is what makes oppressive systems oppressive. Autocratic systems rely on physical coercion and economic blackmail to prevail. Additionally they undermine agency and create doubt about whether one's work is important and one's choices wise. Doubt leads to confusion about who one is, what one deserves, and how one should regard others who have made the same "wrong choices."

Devaluation and oppressive work conditions are the royal road to frustration and anger. But those who study anger point out that nurses tend to express their anger over their powerlessness in the workplace in extremely unhealthy ways. Two such expressions are self-disparagement, which produces hypercritical attitudes and perfectionism, and disparagement of others in the form of back-biting, fault-finding, name-calling, and subtle sabotage of colleagues and superiors. This kind of behavior not only silences the self, it effectively discourages voice in others.

Nurses' way out of this conundrum is "claiming [our] power and using it," writes to Sandra P. Thomas in *Transforming Nurses' Stress and Anger*

Your Turn

The following quotation from an orthopedics nurse appeared in an article about the nursing shortage and was intended to show the pivotal role of nurses in health care:

> "We, as nurses, are the ones who are advocating for our patients. We can make recommendations and communicate to them what the recommendations for their recovery have been. We're teaching them, and they're teaching us."

Does this statement show the agency of nurses, or does it convey the idea that nurses merely transfer information? Does it establish that nurses' have clinical expertise, or does it imply that nurses and patients have the same level of knowledge in the health care setting? Rewrite it to strengthen the nurse's voice of agency.

(p. 233).[16] This means nurses taking the risk of standing up for themselves, each other, and for the nursing work they know is important by describing what they do and by demanding resources to support it. Nurses will more readily do this when they understand and believe in their own agency. If the identity of nurses is linked too closely to angelic or saintly stereotypes, then nurses are hobbled in trying to expand their own agency and risk public displeasure when they act "out of character" by taking assertive public action.

How does the voice of agency sound? The following article by Nurse Jeannie Chaisson is an example.[17] When you read it, you can decide if Nurse Chaisson is trying to shine a spotlight on herself personally or is attempting to articulate the essence of expert nursing care.

Article

Asking the Right Questions

BY JEANNIE CHAISSON

Published in *Technology Review,* October 1992

As an experienced nurse, I am often called upon to assess a person's ability to function. Last year, a woman I'll call "Mrs. A" was denied Social Security disability benefits, and her attorney asked me to review her appeal. When I agreed, I received a file of paperwork that told me almost nothing. Mrs. A was in her early 60s, an immigrant who spoke little English and had found a job in a cafeteria. For several years she had worked diligently, but she had been fired when a new manager refused to let her co-workers assist her with the heavy lifting inherent in the job. The application for benefits, filled out by an intake worker who did not speak Mrs. A's language, stated that she did not fit into the bureaucratic pigeonholes defining disability. Letters from physicians detailing her currently stable medical condition did little to bolster her cause. They said her breast cancer, for which she had undergone surgery, showed no signs of recurrence.

With physicians as the lens and disease as the definition of the field, fragments of a life were examined. The questions asked had little relevance to her ability to function. Would it be possible for me to meet this woman and do a brief nursing assessment? I asked the lawyer.

Two days later, I met Mrs. A and her son, who served as translator. She was small and slim, smiling anxiously as she shook my hand. Her son, a man in his early 30s, was a graduate student at a local college and spoke English well. I explained that I was a nurse, and that my questions might be different than those she had already answered. Addressing me in hesitant English, or in rapid-fire phrases to her son, she talked for over an hour.

I learned that Mrs. A's comfortable, middle-class life had been blown apart by revolution in her native country. One son had been killed, and she had managed to escape with the other. In the United States, her lack of English had disqualified her from the managerial work she had formerly done. And she had been happy to take any job. Only when her pain had become intolerable had she asked her fellow kitchen workers to help her with lifting. They had agreed willingly, but her boss had quickly intervened.

I asked her to tell me about the pain: How severe was it? Where was it located? What made it worse? What could she do to help make it better?

Mrs. A's pain, which so many others had dismissed, turned out to be a relic of 11 operations for breast cancer that she had undergone before coming to this country. One by one, each new lump and node had been removed, and each time the cancer had reappeared. Terrified to permit the doctors to cut her chest muscles out and "take everything," she had lost both breasts bit by bit. A disfigured body and horrible pain that started in her scarified chest tissue and knifed its way up through her right arm and shoulder was her reward. Nothing could banish this pain—not heat, cold, or medications.

Any activity was difficult. Moving the right arm, or even moving the hand to write or turn the pages of a book, was excruciating. She couldn't lie on that side at all. She had some pain in her other arm, and sometimes her knees hurt from arthritis, but it was the pain in her right arm and chest that cut her off from life. She said that she didn't blame her boss for firing her. After all, she admitted sadly, she had been able to do less and less of her work.

Mrs. A went on to recount a "typical day," and I saw that the feints and parries of a few years ago, when she had gone to work, to English classes, and to doctors for help, had given way to total defeat. She could achieve an uneasy truce with her pain only by giving up her job, her intellectual pursuits, her relationships with others. As my questions uncovered this tale of overwhelming loss, she became animated, then tearful. "Nobody has ever asked her about these things before," her son explained. "Nobody has cared what it is like for her."

I filed my report, and three weeks later, when Mrs. A's attorney informed me that she had been granted disability benefits, I could only wonder at the "health" of a health care system that had provided regular scrutiny of her body for recurrent disease yet had utterly failed to listen to the story of her illness, to bear witness to her pain. Other health care professionals had talked about her disease; I had asked about her life.

> *Jeannie Chaisson is a nurse who works in hospice and home care in the Boston area. At the time the article was originally printed, she was a nurse at Beth Israel Hospital in Boston.*

Chapter 3

Presenting Yourself as a Nurse

Not so long ago everyone knew who was a nurse. First, the nurse was a woman in a world of male medical doctors. She wore a starched white dress, white hosiery, white shoes, and a stiff white cap bearing her nursing school insignia. Her appearance left no doubt about her professional identity. Nor did her title, "Nurse," or "Miss," or more rarely "Mrs." Nurses' roles and responsibilities were limited, but their dress and etiquette emphasized professionalism.

Today nurses claim that their work is more complex and far more autonomous, but contemporary self-presentation and dress tend to downplay professionalism, blur the identity of nurses, and make the "place" of nursing in health care more ambiguous. Now patients and staff alike are not always sure who is a nurse, what nurses do, or how nurses should be treated. Without a protocol to provide clarity, it is up to individual nurses to convey that information through their appearance, language, and behavior.

Professional Self-Presentation

Nurses have choices about how they present themselves to patients and families, physicians, other clinicians and health care workers, administrators, and the general public.

They can present themselves and insist on naming practices that assert their professional identity. Or they can appear as part of an undifferentiated mass.

They can highlight their clinical knowledge and competence. Or they can conceal it.

They can affirm their professional independence. Or they can appear to be institutional property.

They can present themselves as mature adults. Or they can infantilize themselves and their colleagues.

They can convey a sense of stature that elicits respect. Or they can present themselves as porous and vulnerable.

Each day in the workplace, nurses perform as public communicators and educators. While caring for patients and families and interacting with other nurses, physicians, social workers, administrators, and health care workers, nurses convey messages to these "publics" about nursing's status and importance. Some of the messages are explicit. Others are more implicit—delivered through presentation, body language, tone of voice, and conversational style. These communications can convey precisely the right—or the wrong—thing about nursing.

For example, if a nurse thinks it is advisable to speak to a patient's physician, she can inform the patient by saying, "I'll *consult* with the doctor about this." This language indicates that she has clinical knowledge and judgment herself and sees herself as a colleague of the physician. Or she can establish herself as both ignorant and a supplicant by saying: "I don't know. I have to ask the doctor."

When a nurse like the oncology nurse described in the last chapter diagnoses a patient's pain and suggests the remedy, she can hide her actions or reveal them. As she administers the medication, she has a choice. She can say, "The doctor has ordered your pain medication." Or she can say, "I recommended that the doctor give you pain medication, and he agreed. I will now administer it and make sure it's effective."

When she calls the physician, the nurse can establish collegiality by beginning the conversation: "Hello Dr. Richards, this is Joan Adams (or preferably, Nurse Adams), Mrs. Smith's nurse. She is experiencing some pain and I think . . ." Or she can place the physician above the nurse by starting: "This is Joan, Mrs. Smith's nurse. I'm sorry to bother you . . ."

When a nurse is talking to a doctor about what's happening to the patient and what should be done, she can say, "The patient is experiencing frequent urination and pain. What do *you* want to do about it?" Or she can include herself in the action by saying, "Here's what I think. . . . What should *we* do about it?"

Nurses can be conscious of the impression they are making without being self-conscious or artificial. Since the health of patients depends on nursing as much as on medicine, nurses can reaffirm this important fact by presenting themselves as experts and equals in the health care setting.

The most immediate way to educate the public about your work is to begin with those members of the public—patients, families, and colleagues—with whom you are in the closest daily contact.

Introducing Yourself

Your introduction to the patient and to his or her family is an important moment that has lasting consequences for you as an individual professional and for nursing as a whole.

You can give a firm handshake, introduce yourself with your first and last name, inform the patient or family member that you are a registered

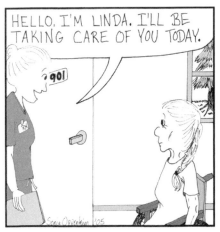

nurse, and explain your role in the patient's care. Or you can say: "Hello, my name is Joan," and leave it at that.

Many patients meeting you for the first time have few visual cues as to your identity and role. Your introduction is your best opportunity to let people know that you are a nurse—a serious professional with important clinical knowledge. Being serious and professional is not synonymous with being distant and aloof. It simply means presenting yourself as a knowledgeable, expert caregiver. This is a presentation that tends to reassure patients rather than alienate them.

Sonia Oppenheim, www.familycomic.com

What's in a Name?

Many nurses complain that other workers are passing themselves off as nurses and that patients often confuse other health care workers with nurses. That may be true. But what's also true is that not enough nurses are asserting their professional identity. The confusion starts right in their introduction to their patients. The convention in many countries is for nurses to introduce themselves with *only* a first name. They might say: "Hi, I'm Sally. I'm your nurse."

Sometimes the *N* word might not get mentioned at all, as in, "Hello, I'm Sally. I'll be taking care of you today," or "Hello, this is Jane from the VNA." In the United States and Canada, "I'll be taking care of you today," may be perceived by nurses as code for "I am a nurse." (In Australia and in the United Kingdom, the code is "I'm looking after you today.") Unfortunately, the patients may not be in on the code, and are thus at a loss to identify who is who in the clinical setting.

Sometimes it seems that when a nurse graduates from nursing school, she substitutes a blank space for where her last name should be. The assignment board in a hospital might list the patient as "Mrs. Smith," "Mary

Smith," or "Smith;" the physician as "Dr. Jones," or "Jones," and the nurse as "Pat." A name badge might bear only a first name and sometimes not even an "RN." Or it might have a first name and last name initial.

When nurses answer the phone or call patients, they might introduce themselves as "Mary from Four South," "Jim from the Emergency Department," or "Pat from General Pediatrics." In this way, nurses present themselves as institutional property rather than as either individuals or professionals. Some nurses construct an image of themselves as physicians' personal property by introducing themselves, "Janet, Dr. Wilson's nurse."

Lack of parity in the workplace is reinforced when nurses allow or encourage physicians to call them by their first names while they routinely address physicians by title and last name.[1] Some nurses and physicians communicate with each other on a first-name basis. Usually, however, that happens when patients are not present. When the doctor and nurse enter the exam room, the physician who was "Jim" in the hallway becomes "Dr. Smith." The nurse remains "Sally." The physician in such a situation may think that the nurse prefers it this way.

It's true that naming practices have changed as our society has become more informal. Nurses have told us that as recently as thirty years ago, many institutions did not permit them to use their first names with patients. It was strictly "Miss Jones," or "Mrs. Jones." Today the tables have turned completely. Some younger physicians avoid using the title "Dr." and introduce themselves with their first and last names. However, in this situation, the patient understands through various other cues that the person presenting him- or herself is a physician. We've noticed that even physicians who present themselves informally rarely leave patients confused about their professional role. So, if one profession insists on clear identification of its function in front of patients—usually by use of title and last name—and another profession in the same setting uses only first names and no identification of function, then there is a status imbalance between the professions. If nurses uphold and reinforce these identification practices, it means that nurses, as well as physicians and patients, regard physicians as special in the health care environment.

This kind of deferential behavior reinforces what sociolinguists call asymmetrical power relationships in which one group is clearly subordinate to another, and its subordination is maintained by modes of address. Thus, the subordination of nursing is constantly reintroduced and reinforced when doctors call nurses by their first name and nurses call doctors by their last name and title. This is the equivalent of a German, French, or Spanish speaker calling a child or servant by his or her first name and addressing them in the informal, rather than the polite version of "you." Nonreciprocal naming practices come from and reinforce social hierarchies.

> *"Patients don't want a friend, they want a nurse with knowledge and skill. A really good nurse will establish the context for a relationship. She or he will communicate to a patient: 'This is what I do. This is what you do. This is what I know. I will make sure everything is all right for you.'"*
>
> *—Nursing historian*
> *Joan Lynaugh*

Reaffirming nursing's subordination to medicine may not be the intention of nurses who use only their first names. "When nurses use their first names, they are doing it in the hope of showing the patient that they are on their side, that they are equals, on a par with, in the same shoes as the patient," says nursing historian Joan Lynaugh. "Nurses generally are not seeking 'respect' from their patients, but some kind of identification with them. Indeed nurses are often taught to do that." The problem is that this practice conceals what patients need and want most from nurses—competence.

A nurse can quickly establish context by introducing her- or himself with *both* a first and last name, explicitly stating that she or he is a registered nurse, and briefly explaining her or his role in the patient's care.

This sort of opening: "Hello, this is Ruth Smith, the nurse practitioner with urgent care. I understand you are running a fever. Can you tell me what your temperature is and when you began to feel ill?" would establish that context more than this: "Hello, this is Ruth from the health center. You called about wanting to talk to someone about how you feel."

Similarly, "I am Janet Jones, a registered nurse who works with Dr. Wilson," conveys a different message than "I'm Dr. Wilson's nurse."

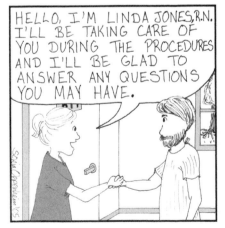

Sonia Oppenheim, www.familycomic.com

Resurrecting "Nurse" as a Title

Nurses say that one obstacle to parity with physicians is that they don't have a title like "Dr." But nurses do have a title. It is "Nurse." To us, it's a word that could and should be used to reassert nurses' professional identity.

Nurses could ask those physicians who prefer to be addressed as "Dr. (Last Name)" in front of patients, to please address them as "Nurse (Last Name)" in the same setting. Similarly, when nurses refer to each other as "Nurse (Last Name)" they show professional respect for each other and indicate to physicians and patients that they expect such respect.

Use of the title, "Nurse," does not have to be stilted, nor need it jeopardize nurses' sense of closeness with their patients. Once the precedent has been set, you can move to first-name communication with a patient or a physician if you choose. Just as a physician might be "Dr. Jones" in one situation and "Joe" in another, nurses can be flexible according to the situation. At the moment, the conventions of many workplaces give nurses no flexibility at all—only a first name. This is why, as nursing educator Elizabeth M. Grady puts it, nurses must insist on symmetrical titles and naming practices with physicians.[1]

A Canadian nurse who described how she approached a resident for pain medication illustrates how the absence of such an identity sets nurses up for failure.

The nurse said she began the phone conversation with the resident by saying: "This is Seven North. I need an order of . . ." The resident responded angrily to being bothered while he was busy with another patient. He asked for the nurse's name. Diffidently she said her full name. He got her name wrong. She did not correct him. He said he'd get to her request later. She did not try to establish a time frame. He never did write the order. She never called him back.

This physician may well have been a difficult case. But the nurse, on the other hand, did not make a professional presentation or stand up for herself or for her patient who needed her care. She did not give her name and title. She did not specifically state her patient's condition and what she needed. The nurse became so intimidated she could not negotiate an agreement with the doctor to attend to her patient's need in a reasonable amount of time. She did not, as nurse Crystal Lindaman advises, "Set a tone that assumes that compliance is inevitable."[2] She did not persist. She did, however, instruct this young physician that he need not accord nurses professional courtesy.

In workshops, we have sparked some vehement opposition when we've urged nurses to use both their first and last names and to adopt the title "Nurse." Some nurses assert that nurses should use *only* their first names for these reasons:

1. First names make patients feel that nurses are more approachable than physicians. Patients want nurses who are on "the same level" as they are.
2. Patients don't want to know nurses' last names. In fact, it's too much to ask patients to remember the last names of their nurses.
3. Patients don't need to know nurses' last names to respect nurses and value what nurses do for them.

4. "Nurse Adams" makes people think of "Nurse Ratched."

5. It's dangerous for nurses to have their last names known.

6. It's an invasion of privacy if patients and families know nurses' last names.

7. Even if it is a good idea to use last names and a title, it is too difficult to change established cultural practices within an institution.

Are these assumptions correct? Let's examine them.

1. First names make patients feel that nurses are approachable. Nurses have good reason to try to counter the distancing or brusqueness that characterizes some physician-patient encounters. Many nurses initiate reciprocal first-name interactions with patients to ease patients' fears, lower their defenses, and facilitate communication. This ability to establish closeness within a professional context is one of the great qualities that nurses bring to patient care. As patients ourselves, we have noted the rapport and ease we usually feel talking with nurses compared with the apprehension and stiffness that accompanies conversation with some physicians.

Indeed nurses might believe that the use of first names helps to create and protect one area where they can claim superiority in any doctor-nurse comparison—the ability to establish intimacy with patients. Nurses might feel that in their struggle for recognition they can't win the knowledge (number of years in school) competition with physicians, and they can't win the status competition, but they can easily win the intimacy competition. They might fear that a more formal self-presentation will erode their greatest strength.

But does connection really depend on a first-name introduction? Do patients respond more candidly to nurses because they use their first names? Or do they respond to nurses and trust them because nurses spend more time with them than doctors; because nurses really listen to their concerns without frequently interrupting and respond effectively to these concerns; and because nurses know how to *be with* patients as well as *do things* to them?

In other words, does connection reside in the lack of a name and title, or does it reside in reside in genuine affect, attentiveness, and empathy?

Physicians' use of their last name and title is not the primary way they distance themselves from patients. Those that distance themselves do it by failing to listen, by interrupting what Arthur Kleinman calls patients' "illness narratives"[3] by focusing on diseases to the exclusion of the human beings who bear them, and by abandoning patients when their illnesses can no longer be cured.

A common rationale for using only first names is that this introduction puts nurses "at the same level" as their patients. While it is laudable that nurses do not want to patronize or disempower their patients, the belief that the proper nurse-patient relationship is one in which nurse and patient are "at the same level" is problematic. It assumes that patients want nurses to be equals rather than experts. But think about it. To be at the same level as the patient is to be frightened, anxious, and even ignorant about the care and treatment the patient needs. Is this what patients really want from nurses?

The literature shows that it's the expertise of nurses that makes it possible for nurses to do one of their primary jobs, which is to rescue patients—from falls, urinary tract infections, medication errors, bedsores, or other mishaps.[4,5] Even the health maintenance and disease promotion work that nurses engage in is a form of rescue—rescuing patients from potential harm. How can nurses do this if they don't have knowledge and insights that their patients lack?

2. *Patients don't want to know nurses' last names; patients can't be expected to remember the last names of nurses.* Maybe, maybe not. Some patients might be interested in and capable of remembering a nurse's full name. Others may not care a whit. By the same token, many patients may not be especially interested in, or capable of, remembering the last names of doctors they encounter in a busy health care setting. Nonetheless, it is important for nurses to make the point that they have a last name and, like physicians, are individuals rather than part of an undifferentiated mass. Even the patient or family member who cannot remember the last name will register that their nurse has one.

The sociologist Erving Goffman noted that institutions enforce obedience and conformity by ritually stripping inmates or initiates of the clothes, hairstyles, and private possessions that give them a sense of identity. "The most significant of these possessions is not physical at all. [It's] one's full name." More than any other, Goffman asserted, that loss forces the inmate to suffer "a great curtailment of the self" (pp. 12–13).[6] Historically nurses have been at risk for exactly this kind of institutional depersonalization.

Just as physicians are usually known to nurses by their full names, nurses should be distinguished as individuals by their names, and not, as one physician put it, as "Maureen in the yellow angora sweater." Besides,

Your Turn

Think about the encounters you have in your personal life. If someone calls you at home and says, "Hello, I'm Joan from MCI," what mental compartment do you put them in? The one reserved for consequential people or the one marked "forgettable and disposable"?

there are patients as well as colleagues who do want to know a nurse's identity to be assured that they are speaking to a qualified professional. A friend of ours is adamant on this point.

"When I call the pediatrician's office because my child is sick, and when the nurses call back, it is invariably an infuriating experience," she explains. "The nurses always introduce themselves with, "Hi, I'm Kim," and give the name of the practice. The first few times this happened, I had no idea whom I was speaking with or whether she was even a nurse. When I asked her to tell me who she was and her role, it was like pulling teeth to get a response. How am I supposed to know that this person actually knows something? I care about the kind of knowledge the person has who's going to advise me about my sick child. I want to know from the minute I meet or talk to her that she is a credible professional."

The first-name-only convention also makes it harder for individual nurses to receive credit for their work. We recognize that the way nurses are treated in some workplaces causes them to be defensive and to anticipate being singled out for blame more than for credit. But lack of a last name rarely protects a nurse from the former and may deprive her or him of the latter.

In the world of work, people who receive credit often do so because they make it easy for others to acknowledge their contributions. A businessman we know, whose first name is John, recalled that during his years as an employee in a large company, he made a point of introducing himself with his first and last name when he had occasion to speak with the executive responsible for salaries. "I wanted him to be clear that I was the one who should get the raise, not some other John," he says.

For example, one woman we know was impressed with the performance of the nurses at an outpatient surgery center where her mother had a basal-cell carcinoma removed. The nurses identified a potential heart problem that physicians had overlooked and suggested that her mother make an appointment for a cardiac evaluation. When, three weeks later, the cardiologist described a previously undiagnosed heart condition, the woman was once again impressed by the nurses' clinical astuteness. She wanted to write a letter to the hospital administration to commend their actions. But who were these nurses? They did not introduce themselves with last names. Only their first names appeared on their name badges. The woman felt she could not send a letter with just the first names of these nurses. If she had been inclined to call the hospital personnel office or department of nursing for the last name of the Maureen or Joan who worked at three o'clock last month in the out-patient operating room, she wouldn't have gotten very far because hospitals generally don't give out such information. She could have written a "the-nurses-were-wonderful" letter, but praising the group instead of individuals didn't seem meaningful. So she did nothing and the commendable work of individual nurses went unnoted because of nurses' preference for anonymity.

3. *Patients don't need to know nurses' last names to respect nurses and value what nurses do for them.* "They don't care what my last name is. All they need to know is that I'm Susan and I'm there to help them through their delivery," a labor and delivery nurse insisted.

"It doesn't matter what they call us, patients value us for what we do," a student in an advanced practice nursing program argued.

These comments are illuminating. Hopefully patients do value nurses for their contributions to care and recovery. But patients can value their nurses while simultaneously assigning them a lower status in the health care hierarchy.

If nurses introduce themselves by their first names only, they are asking to be regarded as nonprofessionals because that is the conventional way that nonprofessionals present themselves. Restaurant servers, garage mechanics, and others who introduce themselves with their first names certainly can and should be respected and valued for the work they do. But they do not have the responsibility for defining their work and their place in the work-place in the same way that nurses do.

In most societies, there are conventions that govern how professionals present themselves. When members of the largest health care profession opt out of the standard professional greeting, they risk communicating that they do not regard themselves as professionals or on a par with the other professionals.

4. *Nurse Adams = Nurse Ratched.* In many of the seminars, nurses eventually agree that calling themselves "Nurse (Last Name)" may be a good idea. But then they argue that patients will automatically associate "Nurse Adams" with one of the most heinous literary portraits of a nurse—Ken Kesey's sadistic Nurse Ratched from the book and movie *One Flew over the Cuckoo's Nest*.

Nurse Ratched was a terrible character. But why assume that juxtapos-ing the title "Nurse" with any of the millions of last names nurses have will instantly evoke this evil character?

Many younger people have never even heard of Nurse Ratched. But let's say someone does associate Nurse Adams with Nurse Ratched. So what? A knee-jerk response does not indicate that this is a fixed and total image of any nurse who uses her title. If millions of nurses adopted the title "Nurse," it would quickly become normal. After all, medicine has it share of evil or controversial doctor prototypes such as Dr. Mengele (the death doctor of Auschwitz) or Dr. Kevorkian. But because "Dr. (Last Name)" is such common usage, negative connotations don't prevail.

5. *Potential danger.* "I will not take any more risks," an emergency department nurse declared heatedly when the subject of introductions came up at a workshop. "I'm already in danger. People come in with weapons and sometimes they go berserk and hit us."

"If they know our last names, they might stalk us. They might follow us home," other nurses contend.

Whenever the use of last names is discussed, many nurses argue that the personal safety of nurses depends on concealing their last names.

We do not take the subject of personal safety lightly. We are aware of the vulnerability that women, in particular, could experience in dealing with strangers. Health care workers *are* often verbally or physically attacked. The very nature of nursing work puts nurses in close contact with people who may be violent, mentally disturbed, or who misconstrue caring as a sexual invitation. According to the U.S. Bureau of Labor Statistics, the rate of nonfatal assaults for hospital workers in 1999 was considerably higher than that for all private-sector industries—8.3 per 10,000 for hospital workers compared with 2 per 10,000 for all workers. While anyone in a hospital could become a victim of violence, statistics indicate that those who have the most direct contact with patients, nurses and aides among others, are at higher risk (p. 3).[7]

Because personal safety is so important, it merits a thorough evaluation. Nurses must protect themselves and be protected from physical danger to the greatest degree possible. The question is, does the use of a nurse's last name subject her to additional personal risk?

Emergency nurses point out that attempted or actual physical assaults by patients are not unusual. The emergency nurse quoted above indeed is "already in danger." She works in a hospital with inadequate protections. People carrying weapons are able to enter the facility and the protocols for controlling physically aggressive patients apparently are nonexistent or not implemented.

We asked this nurse whether nurses and physicians are attacked at random in this facility, or whether attackers deliberately single out a particular clinician. She said that physical violence was directed against anyone who was around. She said it made no difference whether the staff member's last name was known or not. Still, she was adamant. She would never use her last name at work because she already was exposed to diseases such as tuberculosis, human immunodeficiency virus (HIV), and hepatitis and to physical attack. Her last name would add one more layer of vulnerability, she insisted.

This nurse was so terrified, she couldn't perceive the illogic of her position. She was hoping for some kind of magic to protect her—if they don't know who I am, maybe I'm safe.

We're concerned that some nurses are relying on an ineffective measure. If a nurse works in a situation in which disclosing her last name to certain persons could be dangerous, of course she must behave accordingly. But nurses and other health care workers must go to the source of the problem when their institutions are failing to provide proper security. They must find out from their professional associations and other groups what systems are effective and require their own institutions to adopt such measures.

One serious question in this debate is whether nurses belong to a special endangered class. When we've discussed this with nurses, several have suggested that it would be easier for a person to harass or stalk a nurse if her last name were known. But just how much safety does last-name anonymity confer? If a patient is disturbed enough to harass or harm a nurse, couldn't he just follow her home after work? If someone is determined to find you, they will.

As female reporters we have covered volatile situations and violent

Minimizing the Chances of Violence in Hospitals

The National Institute for Occupational Safety and Health (NIOSH) makes these recommendations, among others, for minimizing violence in hospitals:

If your workplace is understaffed, raise the issue with management. Point out that understaffed, overcrowded hospital workplaces are at higher risk for violence, particularly during meal times and visiting hours.

Watch for signals that threaten violence, like expressions of anger and frustration, pent-up body language, signs of substance abuse, and presence of a weapon.

Behave in ways that help diffuse anger, such as appearing calm, caring, and unthreatening and acknowledging the other's feelings.

Be alert and vigilant and don't isolate yourself with a potentially violent person.

Make sure you have an exit strategy or possibility.

Remove yourself from the situation.

Call security for help.

Alert management to the problem. Insist on security devices such as cameras, good lighting, escort services, and workplace design that restricts public access to certain areas (pp. 5–8).[7]

people. We've experienced our share of danger. For those who deal with the public, irate customers or clients come with the territory. But lawyers, judges, journalists, stockbrokers, and therapists—a few of whom have been threatened and killed by deranged people—simply do not have the option of jettisoning their last names. As a professional, it's standard practice to use one's whole name.

There are precautions that can be taken to reduce risks. It might be prudent to limit the amount of personal information given to a patient. Having an unlisted home phone number is an option. Employing a firm tone of voice and assertive body language can be effective in setting boundaries. Studies on violence in the workplace suggest that the best preventions are good security systems, instruction to employees on how to identify potentially violent people, and conflict resolution strategies and practices.

In many health care systems, patients and families—and staff—feel stretched to the limit and may respond with abusive language or behavior. In this context, it could be wiser for nurses to use the title "Nurse" and their last name when introducing themselves instead of their first names. This technique can establish distance while the nurse ascertains whether the patient presents a danger to her. If she feels comfortable with the patient, she can move from title/last name (Nurse Smith) to first name whenever she wants, as in, "Please call me Susan."

You can always move from distance to closeness, but it is much harder to move from closeness to distance. Health care workers are at risk for violence because they have so much interaction with the public. But we have found no studies that suggest that nurses are particularly at risk because they are nurses. Except in special cases, the anonymity that comes from using only a first name provides minimal, if any, physical protection, but considerably lessens nurses' agency and status. For nurses, who have long fought for professional legitimacy, demoting themselves to nonprofessional status is a big price to pay for little or no return.

6. *Giving one's last name to patients is a violation of the nurses' right to privacy.* When we suggest that nurses use their last names, some students and working nurses reply that this violates their right to privacy. As one student put it: "If patients know our last name, then they can call us up and ask us questions at home if they want to."

Another nurse cast it in terms of unwanted attention. "We don't want our patients to know our last names. It's not an issue of professionalism, it's a privacy issue. A few years back, we had to wear name tags with our first and last names. Some male patients developed crushes on nurses and looked up their names and addresses in the phone book. There are a lot of creepy people out there and I know several nurses who were called at home for a date or even approached at their front door by an ex-patient."

While this nurse is correct in asserting that "there are a lot of creepy people out there," she is wrong to believe that concealing one's last name is not a professional issue. If nurses are to be accepted as professionals they must fulfill a central tenet of professionalism, which is to be responsible for one's practice and accountable to one's patients. The American Nurses Association Code of Ethics states: "Nurses are accountable for judgments and actions taken in the course of nursing practice, irrespective of health care organizations' policies or providers' directives."[8]

Nurses have a right to privacy but not anonymity. "How can you be held responsible for your practice if patients don't know who you are?" asks medical sociologist Ross Koppel. "When you become a professional you take on responsibility for your practice. You can't be anonymous and be a professional."

To insist on a form of anonymity, Koppel argues, violates the entire process of professional licensure. "A professional is licensed not as Suzy or Bob. A professional is licensed as an identifiable adult—Susan Smith or Robert Jones."

The claim to anonymity also contradicts the patient bills of rights posted in hospitals and other health care institutions that explicitly grant patients the "right" to know who is taking care of them. We find it ironic when nurses argue that they are so vulnerable that patients don't have the "right" to know their last names because the vulnerable party in the nurse-patient transaction is usually the patient. It is also the patients' private lives that are routinely exposed to the nurse. Nurses know patients' first and last names, their addresses, their personal data, sometimes financial information, and embarrassing secrets about them. When nurses insist that they have a right to conceal themselves from patients, we wonder how they can then ask for the patient's trust.

7. *It's just too difficult to change cultural practices within an institution.* It certainly is difficult to change cultural practices if nurses unwittingly reinforce them. That's why it's important to start deconstructing deferential naming practices right now.

If patients do find out your home phone number and call you to request information, why interpret this as a violation of privacy? It may be a compliment. It suggests that you have important information or insights they are seeking. If you don't want to talk to patients at home, you can refer them to the appropriate resource or tell them you would be glad to talk to them during working hours. You could also get an unlisted phone number.

If a patient appears on your doorstep and harasses you, it's imperative that you notify the police and the hospital.

Many nurses say they would like more recognition and egalitarian treatment in the workplace. But they may be habitually enforcing an atmosphere of reverence and subordination to physicians.

Consider the nurse who works at a major teaching hospital, has a master's degree in nursing, and generally behaves in an autonomous and assertive manner—except when it comes to naming practices. Privately she calls her doctor colleagues by their first names, but in front of patients, she always uses Dr. (Last Name). When she talks to nurses in the presence of patients, however, she always calls them by their first names. "Why?" she was asked.

"Well, the patients should respect their doctors," she replied.

If respect resides in a last name and title, then why doesn't she call her colleagues "Ms." or "Nurse (Last Name)." The idea startled her so much she was speechless.[1]

People sometimes defend familiar conventions that really don't do them justice. This is the case when nurses insist they must use the physician's title and last name so that the patients will know that the person treating them is, in fact, a doctor. If the term "Dr." indicates function, then why don't patients need to know that the women and men who are RNs also have a function, as their nurses? The importance of nurse identification seems even more urgent when nurses might be replaced with aides who have little nursing education or training. Patients will know who is a nurse is by hearing the word *nurse* applied repeatedly. They will hear that word if a nurse introduces herself as Nurse (Last Name), if the physician refers to Nurse (Last Name), and if a nurse refers to her colleague as Nurse (Last Name). Workplace conventions will change when nurses ask physicians to address them this way in front of patients.

Decoding and altering naming practices ought to be a part of nursing education so that new nurses will not reinforce the idea that physicians are better than they are.

When we counseled nursing students in Philadelphia to insist on being called "Ms.," "Mrs.," or "Mr." if residents and interns want to be referred to as "Dr." in front of patients one student demurred. "But he's a doctor," she responded, "and I'm just a nursing student."

"So what?" an older African-American student countered. "I do it all the time. I just walk up to them, put out my hand to shake theirs and say, 'I'm Mrs. Smith. How are you?'"

We have noticed that African-American nurses often are more sensitive to naming practices than their white colleagues. There is a reason. It wasn't so long ago that African Americans were purposefully addressed only by first names, by nicknames, or by insulting titles such as "boy" for an adult man or "auntie" for an older woman. This naming system was used to keep an identified population in a subordinate social and economic position. Stopping this practice was one of the goals of the civil rights movement of the 1950s and 1960s. There was great resistance in some areas to adopting a more respectful form of address, namely one that used honorific titles and last names, because the change would prompt and symbolize an elevation in status. We should not forget the courage it took to press this issue and the significance of the change.

To apply these hard-won rights to nurses might not be as daunting as some nurses fear. An older nurse in one seminar explained that she would like to be on a first-name basis with the physicians she worked with, but feared that these young doctors would be offended if she called them by their first names. The instructors suggested that she pretend to arrive at work, and say to the doctor, "Hi, Tom, how are you?" She replied that she was terrified that Tom would chastise her. The instructors countered that if "Tom" responded that way, the nurse should continue to use his title, but ask him to call her "Mrs. (Last Name)."

She rehearsed at home until she felt more confident. One morning she went into work and said, "Hi, Tom, how are you?" Without batting an eye, Tom replied cheerfully, "Fine, how are you?"

The system of deferring to doctors, even when they may not want such treatment, can be quite entrenched. "I keep telling the nurses I work with to call me Emily," one physician we know says. "Some nurses say they can't bring themselves to call me by my first name. So then they call me Dr. Emily."

Nurses are not alone in having to sort through the significance of various forms of address.

We decided some time ago to establish ground rules before participating in panel discussions or radio or television programs. We ask the host or moderator how they will address panel members who may be physicians, PhDs, or nurses. If the interviewers say they will refer to MDs and PhDs as "Dr.," then,

Two nurses in Victoria, British Columbia, attended one of our workshops. One of the nurses thought we were crazy to insist that nurses introduce themselves with their last name and title. The other thought we were right and suggested they give it a try for a day. Both nurses said they liked the results of the experiment. They felt better about their own work and patients seemed to view them with greater respect and asked them more questions.

Their badges, however, read, "Sue–Nursing." They went to an office supply store and ordered badges with their full names and "RN." First the badges were a conversation piece, then they caught on. The manager ordered new badges for the entire unit.

Your Turn

Go around your workplace and note the asymmetrical naming practices. For example, do the appointment secretaries refer to the physicians as Dr. (Last Name) but the clinical nurses and nurse–practitioners as just "Nancy" or "Janice?"

---

we insist, they must refer to us as "Ms." and to the nurses as "Nurse" or "Ms." or "Mr." If the hosts plan to call us by our first names, then, we tell them, they must address and refer to the MDs and PhDs by their first names also. The risk of appearing odd is far outweighed by the benefits. We know that any disparity of address cues listeners to take our knowledge and insights less seriously than another expert, particularly one with a doctor title. We feel that our messages about caregiving are too important to be overshadowed by traditional messages about status and hierarchy.

Looking like a Nurse

Even though we write about current health care issues and contemporary nursing, we've learned the hard way that editors might illustrate our articles with an image of Florence Nightingale, with or without her lamp, or an old hospital-school photo of student nurses in their aprons and caps. Now we inquire about the illustrations well in advance of publication.

Both the lay public and nurses seem to find nostalgic images compelling. And why not? These images are the icons of nursing. Images of contemporary nurses at work usually require a caption to identify the subject as nursing.

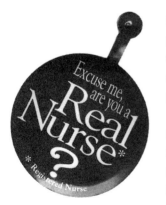

Courtesy of New York State Nurses Association

Now freed from the laborious upkeep of starched uniforms, nurses must provide new visual cues to their identity to deal with the familiar patient lament: You can't tell whether the person coming into the room is a nurse, an aide, a housekeeper, a technician or what. Because of the confusion, you also can't tell if a hospital unit is understaffed.

When patients express these concerns, you can be sure that they want to know who the nurses are, and that what they consider to be an un-nurselike appearance makes them anxious. An elderly couple we know wrote a letter to the administrator of a Boston teaching hospital complaining that there was no way to identify the nurses because everybody in the institution looked "slovenly."

Perhaps this couple had antiquated expectations about how nurses should look. Nonetheless, the issue is serious. Patients in our increasingly informal society find it unnerving not to know the professional or occupational identity of the myriad people who saunter into and out of their rooms. The formality of the traditional uniform had the effect of making hospital nurses—who often were very young—look older and more professional. In contrast, much of the clothing being marketed for today's nurses—many of whom are middle aged—is very informal, even girlish, in tone.

Pediatric nurses might consciously choose teddy bear smocks to put their young patients at ease. But what impression does this clothing convey in a setting where maturity (irrespective of one's age) is an essential qualification? A nurse in this garb may believe she is telling a patient to not be afraid of her, but she is also suggesting that the patients and her colleagues should not take her seriously.

There is a big debate within nursing about what would be an appropriate nurses' uniform today. A celebrity designer, commissioned by a New Jersey hospital, found it was harder than she thought to come up with affordable, stylish, functional apparel for male and female hospital staff. As amusingly recounted in the *New Yorker* magazine, the stuff that one nurse took out of her scrub pockets—pen, notepad, tissues, scissors, adhesive tape, beeper, phone, and stethoscope—wouldn't fit into the "horizontal pockets, which were crucial to the line of the coat" that the designer came up with.[9] Standardization of dress is another hot topic. There is considerable debate about whether nurses should adopt standardized dress at all apart from what a uniform might look like. But to us, that is not the issue. More important is the need to adopt a *style* of dress that assists nurses' efforts to be treated more professionally. Some nurses feel that lab coats and solid-color scrubs fit the bill. A badge or pin that gives the wearer's full name—minus the hearts and smiley faces—and that clearly identifies her or him as an RN is essential.

Who's a Girl?

There are other words and phrases that tend to undercut the agency of nurses and place them in a juvenile category. The most common in everyday interactions is "girl."

The son of an elderly patient tells the nurse manager that his mother needs help. She wants to assure him that a staff nurse will soon be there by saying, "I'll get one of the girls to help her." Through her word choice, she is undercutting the professional standing of nurses.

The word *girl* has various meanings and connotations. Sociolinguist Deborah Tannen, author of the best-selling book, *You Just Don't Understand: Women and Men in Conversation,* told us that "girl" (or "lady") has traditionally been used as a euphemism for "woman" because the latter term, in some cultures, carries the unacceptable suggestion of sexuality and/or age.

So your eighty-year-old grandmother might tell you that she is having lunch with the girls and mean it as a compliment. We might refer to our best friends as "girlfriends." An African-American woman might say to her friend, "Girl, let me tell you . . ." A husband might say to his wife, "How's my girl?" In these settings, the word conveys closeness and affection.

However, in the workplace, the word "girl" connotes standard dictionary definitions: a female child; an immature or inexperienced woman; a daughter; a female servant; a female sweetheart.[10]

Do patients want a child to take care of them when they are sick? Do nurses want to be thought of as maidservants or sweethearts or young unmarried women? Just as forms of address were a major focus of the civil rights movement, one of the goals of the women's movement was to stop the routine use of the term "girl" to describe grown women.

Some might argue that men use parallel terminology. In fact, they don't. According to what Tannen told us, men use "boy" in a stylized way, as in "old boys' network" (which emphasizes the power of older males) or "night out with the boys" (which conveys the idea that men will temporarily put aside their adult responsibilities). Men don't use the term in a generalized way or in a professional setting. Has anyone ever heard a physician tell a patient, "I'll get one of the boys to come in for a neuro-consult"?

Today a male physician probably wouldn't dare call a female physician a "girl." Nor would a female physician refer to another female physician as a "girl."

When "boy" is used in a professional setting, it is overtly demeaning. Similarly, if a nurse uses "girl" to refer to nurses aides or other health care workers—some of whom may be people of color—they risk sounding not just condescending but racist.

For all of these reasons it is essential that nurses in the workplace cease using the word *girl* to refer to other nurses or to other adult workers. Instead, when referring to an RN colleague, one could simply say, "I'll ask my colleague for help," or, "I'll ask another nurse for help." And when referring to an aide or other health care worker, "I'll ask one of the aides to help you."

Body Language and "Presence"

Just as seemingly innocuous words and phrases can communicate volumes about nursing, so too can gestures, postures, physical arrangements, and actions.

Consider the following examples:

1. In one HMO, the physicians, male and female, usually shake hands with patients when they greet them. The nurses rarely do.

2. Nurses at one East Coast medical center point with pride to their strong nursing department and their collaborative relationships with physician colleagues. At this hospital, nurses round with physicians each morning and insist that they communicate their concerns as equal members of the health care team. Professionals from other facilities frequently visit to examine this collaborative model in action. We notice on one unit, however, that nurses and physicians arrange themselves in a stratified way to discuss cases. The interns perch on an air conditioner ledge in front of the windows. The resident stands a little to the side facing them. The nurses fan out behind the resident. With her back to the nurses, the resident speaks to the interns, and they direct responses to her. When the nurses provide information about patients, they tend to speak in deferential tones, and the resident barely turns her head.

3. A nurse needs to talk with a physician about a patient. She finds the physician in the waiting room engaged in a conversation with another physician. The nurse stands quietly next to them. The physicians continue to talk without acknowledging her presence. Eventually the nurse shrugs and walks off, muttering that she'll catch the physician later. About an hour later, one of the physicians comes up to the nurses' station where the same nurse is talking with several of her colleagues. Without apologizing, the doctor interrupts the nurses with a question. They immediately stop their conversation and the nurse responds politely.

4. A physician does a thoracentesis on an elderly woman with lung cancer while her daughter holds her hand. When the physician finishes, he starts to pick up the debris from the procedure. "Oh, let me do that," the nurse who is assisting says, reaching past him and commandeering the clean-up job.

What do these scenarios communicate? What do they teach physicians, nurses, and the public about the status and roles of RNs and MDs?

1. By opting out of the traditional handshake, the nurses are communicating that their role is not as significant as that of the physicians. No matter what the nurses say about themselves in the introduction, their failure to assert their individual presence through physical contact suggests that they prefer to be more in the background.

A firm but cordial handshake is an essential part of a professional introduction and provides the opening for nurses to state their names and credentials. When meeting a patient, a nurse can simply extend her or his hand, shake the patient's hand firmly, make eye contact, and say, "I'm Bill Jones, RN" or "I'm Nurse Jones," or "I'm Bill Jones, a registered nurse."

2. Nurses claim to be equal collaborators in patient care. But by standing behind the resident, the nurses collaborate in entirely another way. They construct a configuration that makes them look like spectators. The physicians have arranged themselves so that they converse with each other. When a nurse tries to contribute to the conversation, her hesitant speech conveys what she seems to feel, that she does not have a rightful place in this discussion, a point that is reinforced by her physical location.

Nurses on rounds could intersperse themselves among the physicians (rather than positioning themselves in the background) and speak up with authority when they have something to say. (When we pointed this behavior out to the nurse manager on the unit, she told us that she hadn't noticed it. She observed the nurses' placement at morning rounds. Yes, she agreed, we were right. From then on she made sure that nurses arranged themselves among the interns with some in front of rather than behind the resident.)

3. Nurses are undermined in their assertion that what they have to say to physicians about patients is as important as what physicians share with each other. In this case, the physicians' communication not only took precedence but also shut out the nurse. As in the second example, nursing is positioned outside the circle of influence. The nurse assents to this interpretation by shrugging and walking away. And, when the physician interrupts her and her colleagues an hour later, by answering immediately she reaffirms that what the physician needs to know is much more important than what she and her colleagues are discussing.

The nurse could politely interrupt the physicians and state her business. And when the physician barged in on their conversation, the nurses could politely but firmly ask him to wait a moment until they finished consulting about a patient.

4. This scenario goes to the heart of the stereotype of nurses as handmaids to physicians. In this case, the physician, by cleaning up after himself and the nurse, communicates that he does not see the nurse as a maid. But the nurse becomes anxious about collegial treatment and rushes to reaffirm the traditional definition of the nurse—even though she might well have protested, or at least complained later to her peers, if the physician had ordered her to clean up. By taking over the cleanup, this nurse is communicating a stereotypical job description of nursing to the doctor, patient, and family member.

In this last case, the nurse could let the physician clean up after himself (as he had started to do).

Workplace encounters such as these are both "private" interactions and "public" communications that convey information about the status and agency of nurses. As sociologist Erving Goffman noted in exploring this issue, how one presents oneself contributes to the construction of social and professional reality. "When an individual plays a part," he wrote in *The Presentation of Self in Everyday Life,* "he implicitly requests his observers to take seriously the impression that is fostered before them" (p. 17).[11]

Paying attention to self-presentation does not require a personality transplant and definitely does not mean that nurses have to turn themselves into unapproachable authoritarian figures. As British sociologist Celia Davies suggests, the choice need not be limited to either the authoritarian male professional model or the passive/dependent female role. She recommends "reconstructing" a model of professionalism appropriate to both the needs of the sick and of the largely female nurses who care for them. This new model of professionalism could be constructed around the concept of "meaningful distance" that "acknowledges that there will be a commitment and emotional response, but seeks to avoid over-identification on the one hand and under-involvement on the other" (p. 150).[12]

In other words, by asserting their agency in their self-presentation, nurses need not worry that projecting a professional image will make them seem distant or feel self-conscious, false, or stilted. Instead, nurses will be presenting a strong image of themselves, one that calls forth responses that are respectful of them as nurses and as human beings.

Chapter 4

Tell the World What You Do

A medical-surgical nurse who had participated in a major nursing conference called the hotel bellman for help in getting her bags to the airport shuttle bus. As the nurse and bellman were walking to the elevator, the young man turned to her and remarked, "The people here aren't ordinary nurses, are they?"

Intrigued by the question, the nurse asked what he meant. "Well," he said, "I've been walking through the exhibit area and there are all these fancy medical machines and equipment. 'Ordinary' nurses don't use such complicated equipment," he stated confidently. "This must be a conference for chiefs."

Without skipping a beat, the nurse replied: "This *is* a conference for ordinary nurses. We use all kinds of sophisticated medical equipment and medications when we take care of you. Ordinary nurses *are* the chiefs of patient care in hospitals."

Another nurse told us about an incident that occurred when she flew into Rochester, Minnesota, for a conference at the Mayo Clinic. On the way into town, her cab driver proudly boasted about Rochester's medical reputation. "We have some of the best medical care in the world," he said. "The best doctors and researchers are here. People come here from all over the globe just to see them."

She listened and then gently reminded him that he forgot an important part of the health care team. "All of these great doctors," she told him, "wouldn't succeed without great nurses. You must remember to tell your next passenger about that too."

Life presents nurses with countless conversational openings to talk about nursing. These openings occur at cocktail parties, backyard barbecues, relatives' weddings, school events, church programs, and, most important, in patients' rooms. Not every nurse will be called by a reporter from the

New York Times, but nurses constantly speak with small publics—relatives, friends, neighbors, patients, teachers, or guidance counselors who ask what they do or who make a comment about nursing. Sometimes these comments contain erroneous information that needs to be corrected. Other times, the comment may give you an opportunity to advance someone's knowledge about your profession.

Describing Your Work

Most nurses, of course, mobilize communication techniques when they take care of patients. As they elicit information about patients' problems and provide information to the patient and family, nurses are also imparting information about themselves as professionals and about nursing's work and status. You can consciously influence what people know about nursing in this setting.

In conversations with patients and others, you can educate people about the scope of nursing by being more specific about the kind of nursing you do. Instead of saying generally that you're a nurse, you might say a bit more, such as, "I'm an oncology nurse, I work with children with cancer," or "I'm a psychiatric nurse, I work with patients with mental illness."

When the opportunity presents itself, you can also describe in more detail what you are doing and why you are doing it. Say you are taking care of a patient who has just had a stroke. His daughter comes to visit while you are feeding the patient. You can do your work silently. Or, while you are feeding the patient, you can explain to him and to his daughter the significant aspects of what you are doing. It isn't necessary to deliver a dissertation on the four phases of swallowing. But it may be useful to explain that you are assessing the patient's gag reflex and why that is important. In describing all this, you are teaching the patient and his daughter not only how to eat safely but also that nurses have special, life-saving knowledge.

To many people, the more domestic activities of nursing seem simple or trivial. They may even wonder why it takes an educated person to do it. This is an opportunity to enlighten them. Explain why activities such as feeding, bathing, toileting, walking, or turning patients can be some of the most important things a nurse does.

You might assume that a patient and family understand your work— even its most high-tech aspects—just because they see you do it. Like the bellman we introduced you to at the beginning of this chapter, they might think that what you do as a nurse is the exception not the rule. "You're an extraordinary nurse," they might think, not an "ordinary" nurse doing extraordinary things. That is why when you are caring for a patient using high-tech devices, teaching the patient how to master drug regimens at home and answering questions about the patient's disease, or helping educate the patient about health promotion, it is necessary to point out what you're doing and why you're doing it.

Many people confuse complex nursing activities with kindness or niceness. For example, the mother of an artist we know had a brain tumor and underwent surgery to remove it. Her daughter explained that the nurses were so "nice." They were very attentive, talked kindly to her mother, and took advantage of every opportunity to "chat with her." She was surprised to learn that the nurses were doing much more than she or her mother imagined, such as tracking her mother's intracranial pressure, making sure she didn't develop an internal bleed, checking her temperature to make sure she didn't have a wound infection and myriad other life-saving activities. "I had no idea," she said.

In the course of a patient's treatment, nurses need to convey information about their skilled activities. This does not mean that the nurse should be lecturing sick patients. It does mean that nurses shouldn't do their work in silence. They can listen to a patient's chest and say, "I hear some congestion, I will keep an eye on that," instead of simply coming into the room and listening to the patient's chest. They can say they are monitoring the patient for any signs of infection.

Making the Agency of Nurses Known

Nurses are too seldom given credit for relying on their own knowledge and judgment. Many people believe that everyone in health care follows the doctor's orders as though an invisible line runs from the doctor's brain to nurses', conveying his knowledge. That's why many patients thank their doctor for the good work that nurses have done.

Perhaps the most public example of this tendency to attribute nurses' activities to doctor's knowledge and judgment appeared in the late actor Christopher Reeve's book, *Nothing Is Impossible*. Listen to how Reeve described his care on the ICU at the University of Virginia Hospital. "The critical care," he wrote, "was nothing short of miraculous. Dr. John Jane—arguably one of the best neurosurgeons in the world—achieved the nearly impossible feat of reattaching the base of my skull to my spinal column with wire, titanium, and bone grafted from my hip. Under his watchful eye, a team of internists and pulmonologists cured me of ulcers and pneumonia" (pp. 60–61).[1]

Reeve overlooked intensive care nurses' contribution to his cure and recovery. This is hardly surprising. Most people are programmed to view their cure and recovery as a doctor-only activity. When, as in a case like Reeve's, re-covery involves major surgery, this tendency is heightened—particularly when a world-famous doctor is treating a world-famous celebrity. Which is why nurses have to be mindful not to reinforce this conventional way of viewing medical action. When nurses repeat slogans like "Doctors cure and nurses care" and "Doctors pay attention to diseases and nurses pay attention to the people who have them," they may believe that they are efficiently and effectively explaining nursing, but these catch phrases do little to educate the public and instead reinforce conventional views of medical treatment and cure.

Nurses need to communicate that often there would be no cure or re-covery without highly skilled nursing, as was surely the case with Christo-pher Reeve. Without nurses, would he have survived and gone on to have nine productive years? When cure and care are dichotomized, cure is always going to be more significant because patients would prefer to be "cured" than cared for. If nursing does not claim its actual contribution to the "cure," it will be marginalized or obscured.

Depict Your Agency, Not the Doctor's

To convey the content of nursing, nurses must describe the complexity of the care *they* give and the clinical judgments *they* use. They must be careful not to depict themselves as extensions of the doctor's agency in their discus-sions with patients and families, the broader public, the media, and political representatives.

In a seminar we conducted in Canada, a nurse reported with some dis-may an experience she had had with a hospitalized diabetic patient. She had worked long and hard with this patient to teach him his complicated drug regimen. She thought they had a good rapport and was sure he trusted her expertise. As she was walking past his room, however, she overhead a conver-sation between the patient and his doctor that she found disheartening. The patient was checking up on the information she had just given him. "The nurse said this. Was she right?" was the gist of the conversation.

Why was he verifying the information she'd just given him? she asked sadly.

The group asked her how she had presented the information to the pa-tient. "I told him the doctor wanted him to take this medicine, and the doc-tor wanted him to follow this diet," she responded.

"Ah," her fellow nurses commented. "No wonder he's checking up on you." The group explained that she had presented herself as a handmaid to the doctor—a kind of human medical tape recorder repeating his instruc-tions—rather than as a partner in care. The other nurses thought it was perfectly rational, indeed even wise, for a patient to ask the proverbial horse if the horse's mouth got it right.

What would have happened, they speculated, if the nurse had spoken from her own agency, covering points like the following:

"Let's review what diabetes is about. Here is what has happened to you. Here's what makes your blood sugar go up. Here's what makes it come down. What diabetes means is that your body no longer corrects for these things. And here's what the medication does to prevent damage. Here's how you need to take the medicine. Here's the diet you need to follow."

The oncology nurse we described in Chapter 2 faced a similar problem. Her patient and the patient's family should know her role in getting much-needed pain medication. Telling the patient that the doctor "ordered" her morphine would conceal the nurse's contribution. She couldn't tell the patient she'd fought with the doctor to get the morphine, but she could have negotiated the dilemma by saying: "I've consulted with the doctor, and he agreed with my recommendation to give you IV morphine. I will make sure it's effective."

Even innocuous remarks offer an opportunity to present your agency. One nurse told us that after she'd given excellent care to a patient, he remarked that she knew so much about medicine, she could have become a doctor. This was a golden opportunity to say something about what would happen to patients without intelligent and knowledgeable nurses.

If the patient is healthy enough to comment on your choice of profession, they're healthy enough to reflect on the contradiction involved in suggesting that a good nurse stop doing nursing and start doing doctoring.

Dealing with the Fear of Making Doctors Angry

Many RNs report that they don't voice their opinions or talk about their work because they are worried that if they do doctors will become angry with them. Sometimes doctors act aggressively to silence nurses and put them in their place. We believe nurses should discuss with physicians the aspects of their behavior that are related to gender, hierarchy, patient care, collegiality, and etiquette.

The Institute of Medicine reports that disrespect by physicians or others in the workplace poses a danger to patients.[2] In 2005, the American Association of Critical-Care Nurses (AACN) published a set of standards "for establishing and sustaining healthy work environments" and distributed them widely with a call for "individuals, units, organizations and systems" to use the standards as a framework for improving interpersonal relationships in the workplace. The AACN report gave examples, like the following, to show just how destructive abuse and disrespect can be to nursing practice and to patient outcomes:

> At 3:30 A.M. in a busy ICU, a nurse prepares to give insulin to a patient with an elevated blood sugar level. The sliding scale doses of insulin on the medication sheet are unclear and the physician's order sheet is difficult to read. From past experience, the nurse knows how late-night calls to this physician often result in verbal outbursts and demeaning slurs, no matter how valid the inquiry.
>
> Needing to act but not wanting another harassing encounter with the physician, she makes a judgment of the appropriate dose and administers the insulin. Two hours later, she finds the patient completely unresponsive. To treat the critically low blood sugar level, she administers concentrated injections of glucose and calls for additional emergency help. Despite all attempts to restore the patient's brain to consciousness, he never awakens and his brain never functions normally again.[3]

As this example demonstrates, there is no benefit to tolerating abuse and intimidation from physicians. Nurses who make public such abuse might be surprised at the social support they receive. Today this kind of behavior is not socially or legally sanctioned and is a major public health care concern.

Unfortunately some doctors' behavior toward nurses elicits an expectation that all doctors might behave negatively when nurses express their opinions or talk about their work. Nurses may thus silence themselves even when doctors might not complain or might be supportive.

Nurses have often told us that talking about their own work might "demean" doctors. For example, an officer of a major nursing organization who was practicing speaking on camera during a media training session, told an anecdote contrasting the amount of time that nurses and doctors spend with patients. "Physicians see patients for only a few minutes a day," she noted. Then she gasped and clapped her hands over her mouth. Everyone in the room, including her, laughed at her dramatic gesture. She explained that her gut reaction was not that she had stated a fact but that she had disclosed something bad about doctors and that they would be angry.

An even more significant problem—and silencer—is nurses' desire to find something that is truly theirs that physicians do not own or participate in. For example, a cancer nurse said he felt that much of his work belonged to doctors because it had been initiated by their orders. So in trying to differentiate their work from that of physicians', nurses might omit their medical and technical expertise and focus only on the emotional, psy-

---

Your Turn

Rewrite the following statement to give *equal* play to the medical, technical, caring, and educational components of this nurse's work.

"People may think the most important part of being an oncology nurse is inserting an IV, accessing a port-a-catheter, administering anti-nausea medication, or infusing chemotherapy. This is not true. The part of my job that makes the greatest impact is teaching patients how to take care of themselves safely and efficiently at home."

---

chosocial, or educational aspects of their work. In this way, nurses disown their own expertise and the medical and technical contributions they make to patient care.

Disowning one's medical and technical expertise in a futile effort to find some corner that doctors don't influence, leads nurses, in our opinion, down a problematic path. When nurses don't claim their ownership or participation in the process of diagnosis, treatment, and prescription, this allows the public to believe that the physician is an army of one. Nothing could be further from the truth, as Margarete Sandelowski establishes in her history of nursing and medical technology.[4] In fact, doctors' reputation for scientific and technical mastery is often dependent on nurses' work, knowledge, skill, and competence. Rather than disclaiming this, nurses should make it visible and reclaim it.

Learn to Accept Thanks

Nurses have the opportunity to explain their work when a patient expresses gratitude for excellent nursing care. Think about the last time a patient thanked you. How did you respond? Did you accept their acknowledgment? Or did you say, "Oh, it was nothing," "I didn't do very much," or "It was just my job."

A lot of us rely on this conversational tack when we are complimented. But for nurses it has consequences.

When nurses say, "Oh, it was nothing," the danger is that people will believe them. And if "it"—nursing work—is "just a job" or "not very much of anything," the logical conclusion one draws is that nurses are nothing special. Why then should the public worry about replacing nurses with aides, or, as so frequently happens today, with untrained family members who are expected to act as surrogate professional nurses in the home? If nurses do

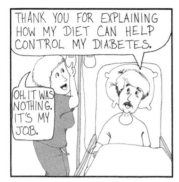 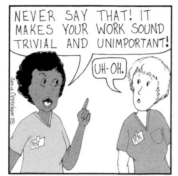 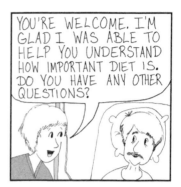

Sonia Oppenheim, www.familycomic.com

little or nothing, why should the public support additional resources for nursing staffing, education, and research?

An alternative response to gratitude can highlight the content of nursing care. A woman tells you: "You were so great. You helped my husband to cope with his diabetes." This is your opportunity to respond: "Thank you. I was pleased to take care of your husband, to teach him how to take his medication, and to help him learn how to alter his diet. If you have any further questions or needs please talk to me about them."

We talked with oncology nurses in Rhode Island about the tendency of nurses to trivialize their own work. Phoebe Fernald, an oncology clinical nurse specialist, approached us afterward. She said nurses' difficulty in saying, "Thank you," and "You're welcome" in response to compliments and thanks struck a chord with her. "It's scary how automatically pat answers come out of our mouths," she said.

Fernald gave an illustration. She had recently helped family friends navigate their father's illness and death from cancer. At the calling hours before the funeral, the family thanked her and told her how much they appreciated what she had done. And what did she say? "Oh, I didn't do very much at all."

"But when I think about it," Fernald told us, "I did a lot. I took time to listen to them. They needed to talk about their pain and hurt. They needed to talk about their concerns—whether they were doing the right thing, choosing the right treatments, and, when he no longer wanted more treatment, they needed to know that was okay too. They needed confirmation that they were making the right choices. And they needed it from someone who was an expert. [Fernald initially said, "From someone who they perceived to be an expert," but changed her wording when we reminded her that she is one.] When patients thank us, they are thanking us for our expertise and our skill in caring. When we say 'Oh, it was nothing,' we're denying that expertise and skill."

When we suggested that Fernald could have said, "You're welcome. It was a privilege to be able to help you," she responded, "That would not be a dishonest answer. It was a privilege."

Be Prepared to Take Advantage of Openings

If you were asked to do a presentation on nursing at your church or to go on a local television show and talk about health care, you would take time to prepare your remarks. The more spontaneous communication opportunities that regularly come your way also require preparation. Although they don't come in the form of an invitation, these openings are nevertheless quite predictable.

For example, someone at a party asks you what you do. You respond, "I'm a nurse." The other person doesn't know what to say. "Oh, how nice," she mutters politely and then goes on to a different subject.

Or, upon hearing that you are a pediatric nurse, an oncology nurse, or a hospice nurse, an acquaintance responds: "That must be so depressing. How can you stand working with sick children—cancer patients—dying people?" To someone outside health care, anything that has to do with sickness, vulnerability, and death may appear to be draining and unbearably depressing rather than enriching and rewarding.

Other conversational openings may come in the form of jibes that seem to overtly devalue nursing. One nurse recounted that she was talking to a businessman about her work as a nurse practitioner. "So you've gotten out of the bedpan business," he retorted.

Another told of a man at a cocktail party who asked: "Why did you become a nurse when someone as obviously intelligent as you could have been a doctor?"

An Australian nurse was the only RN at a dinner party with a number of professional men and women. At the dinner table, one of the guests turned to her and said condescendingly, "So why are you doing nursing? To do a nice bit of caring?" The nurse in question was infuriated, but she said she felt so disarmed she didn't know what to say in response.

A student nurse told us she often goes out with a group of friends that includes medical students. Over dinner, those friends who are in business or law address their questions or comments to the medical students and never ask her questions about what she's learning and doing in nursing school. "What about me?" she wonders. "What about nursing?"

Such experiences are demoralizing. Their frequency can leave nurses speechless, so angry they want to scream or, worse, so inured to it that they just shrug.

Being prepared to respond constructively is a better approach. To be prepared, you must be willing to acknowledge that situations like this are not going to miraculously disappear. Indeed, you can be really effective if you embrace even the most negative comments as educational opportunities. Be glad that someone has mentioned nursing. Consider your friends, relatives, or acquaintances as people requiring instruction and try to evince sympathy for people who are ill informed. Even the most disheartening comments about nursing usually stem from ignorance rather than malice.

This interpretation allows you to prepare yourself to take on the challenge of educating the public about nursing. Remember, if, like the Australian nurse, you don't correct this misimpression with an assertive comment, then the person who denigrates nursing will, literally, have had the final word on the subject.

Responding

When someone says to you, "God, how depressing it must be to deal with sick children or dying patients all the time," you can respond: "Sometimes it's sad, but it's not depressing. Let me tell you what I did yesterday so you'll understand." Then you can describe your work and the difference it made to those who benefited from your care.

If someone makes a crack about bedpans, you can respond the way one nurse practitioner did: "Let me tell you about bedpans . . ." she said and described what the contents of a bedpan can reveal about a patient's condition.

When a nursing student told us that his friends commonly react to his choice of career with, "So now you're going to be a butt wiper," we asked him how he responded. "Oh, I tell them we have other people to do that now." We suggested that this way of dealing with the derogatory comment actually validated the notion that cleaning a patient who has soiled himself is beneath the dignity of a nurse with a university degree.

Why not tell your friends, we suggested, that cleaning up after someone can be one of the most important things a nurse could do? Tell them there might come a day when they will need a nurse who's educated enough to know that cleaning someone is a way to prevent all sorts of potentially catastrophic complications and who will do it without humiliating the patient. Tell them, "If you're ever flat on your back in the hospital, you better hope someone as smart as I am is there to wipe your butt."

Perhaps the most infuriating question you'll get is: "Why did someone as intelligent as you become a nurse?" Or for students: "Why aren't you in medical school instead of nursing school?"

We have thought a lot about this question. We used to advise nurses to explain their choice and illuminate how nursing differs from medicine. We still believe that is an essential part of any response. Now we feel that the erroneous assumptions embedded in the question must themselves be challenged.

The question "Why did you become a nurse, why didn't you become a doctor" is simply illegitimate. When we tell people we're journalists, no one asks us why we didn't become poets. When doctors tell people what they do, no one asks them why they didn't go into bioengineering instead. They ask them what their work is like. When a bright young man says he is in medical school, he's asked what he wants to specialize in, not why isn't he going into a different health profession altogether. Today, when a woman announces her decision to become a doctor, she's viewed as a representative of the advancement of women.

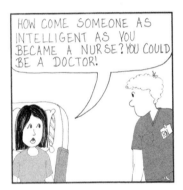 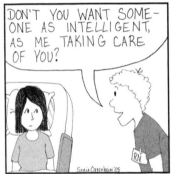 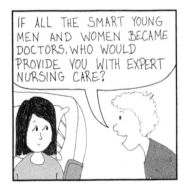

Sonia Oppenheim, www.familycomic.com

Not so with nurses. An interesting social disconnect takes place when an intelligent woman or man is a nurse, or announces an intention to become one. Rather than being viewed as pioneers expanding the definition of masculinity, male nurses or nursing students are often viewed as peculiar, while female nurses or nursing students might be regarded as having made the wrong choice. Nurses can change such attitudes by the way they respond to comments and questions.

Instead of telling people "I became a nurse because I want to care for people," you might calmly reply: "You know, if you asked me what I do as a nurse, and let me describe it to you, then you would understand why I didn't become a doctor."

Or, if you're a student, you might say brightly: "Why don't you ask me what I want to do as a nurse, then you'll understand why I'm going to nursing school and not medical school. I plan to work with geriatric patients and help them stay independent longer."

In social situations, when people find out you're a nurse and say nothing or "Oh how nice," that is an opening. You can direct the conversation with a few engaging questions and comments like: "Do you know much about nursing? Today, with a looming nursing shortage, public awareness of the profession is really important."

The Australian nurse could have said to the condescending dinner guest, "I certainly hope that if, God forbid, you ever have cancer, an experienced oncology nurse will be there to give you that bit of caring that might save your life."

Don't Suppress Your Enthusiasm

As every nurse knows, affect is important in establishing a connection with patients. It is no less so when talking with members of the public. Don't be afraid of appearing engaged or emotional when you tell your stories. Let your eagerness, enthusiasm, and commitment to nursing be reflected in your voice and body language. When nurses speak with passion and conviction—rather than in cautious, passive, and neutral tones—they convince the public that nurses are important professionals who cannot easily be replaced.

When you are discussing changes in the health care system that cause harm, don't be afraid to express your moral outrage. As long as you're not shrill or out of control, expressing profound concern is appropriate and justified. Similarly, don't be afraid to show your sorrow or grief. If you are telling a story about patient care that brings tears to your eyes and a catch in your throat, don't be embarrassed. As long as you don't give the impression that your work overwhelms you with grief and sadness, those who listen to you will be impressed with the depth of your feelings and your commitment to your work and patients.

Respecting Patient Confidentiality

When nurses are encouraged to talk about their work, they often worry that to do so will violate patient confidentiality. This is an utmost concern in school and the workplace. The importance of patient confidentiality is clearly stated in the International Council of Nurses (ICN) Code for Nurses: "The nurse holds in confidence personal information and uses judgment in sharing this information."[5]

Legally and ethically, clinicians and other health care workers may not reveal any patient information without the patient's consent. Family members and friends can't ask for and get these details, nor can other groups or individuals. While it is essential for nurses to respect patient confidentiality, it's also critical for nurses to understand that the injunction to maintain confidentiality does not mean they cannot talk about their work with patients at all. One labor and delivery nurse, for example, said, "I can't go home and tell my husband and children that I just helped a thirty-five-year-old woman deliver a healthy baby. That would violate patient confidentiality."

Do you think that's true?

It's not.

Respecting patient confidentiality does *not* mean you cannot talk about your patients. It means you can't identify a patient, use their name, or reveal details about their care. It is possible to respect patient confidentiality while talking about your work. The rightful concern for patient confidentiality need not silence nurses, as it did in the following example.

A nurse at an East Coast hospital had been interviewed for a Sunday magazine article about the emergency room. A photographer from the magazine called to arrange a photo shoot. The photographer had permission from the administration to do the shoot and wanted the nurse to appear in the article with patients. The nurse's manager told the photographer that the nurse would have to ask the patients if they would agree to be photographed.

But the manager didn't leave it at that. She kept harping on the need to prevent any violation of patient confidentiality. The photographer said the manager made the nurse so nervous that he didn't even want to approach patients to ask their permission. Finally, after much prodding from the photographer, the nurse asked several patients. Like many people, they were delighted that they might have their picture in the magazine and instantly agreed. By this time, however, the nurse had become so anxious about the photo shoot he stiffened every time the camera clicked. None of the pictures was usable. The photographer was frustrated. She said she had never had such a bad experience on a photo shoot. Much to the chagrin of the hospital administrators who were courting good publicity, this hospital and the people in it did not appear in the article.

Nurses can make their work with patients public without violating patient privacy and confidentiality by changing details that might reveal the identity of patients or by talking about a generic patient.

When you describe a particular case as an example of your work, you can explain that you've altered some facts to protect your patient's privacy but that the essence of the story remains. In many instances, patients have similar problems and experiences, and unless you give specific identifying details, there will be no way that anyone could determine who your patients are. Your listeners aren't concerned with the name, age, or address of a particular patient. They're interested in your experience.

When Nurses Break Their Silence

When nurses break their silence, it can lead to great personal and professional satisfaction. We saw this phenomenon play out in Japan.

This anecdote begins in 2002 when Suzanne Gordon did a "Silence to Voice" presentation in Tokyo. Shigeko Takayama, a professor of nursing then at Fukui University, was in the audience and realized that she had never told her family anything about her work. She went home determined to open her working life to her family.

A year later, Bernice Buresh arrived at the Tohoku University College of Nursing for the first of several presentations in Japan. Masako Hayano, who translated *From Silence to Voice* into Japanese and who interpreted for us in Japan, showed Buresh a letter written by Professor Takayama's daughter, Masumi. In it, Masumi described how her views about nursing changed over the last year since her mother began sharing her professional experiences with her. Hayano suggested that the letter be read at the end of each presentation to Japanese nurses. Buresh agreed.

It could not have been more pertinent. During the initial presentation at Tohoku University, a first-year nursing student stood up and complained that two members of her family were nurses, but they never tell her anything about their work. She said her professors never share stories from their nursing careers with the students. She lamented that here she was in nursing school and she still didn't know what was involved in nursing.

Members of the faculty who responded said that there were strong cultural restraints in Japan against nurses telling personal stories. But they said that they believed these societal conventions were not helpful to nursing and that it was time to change them, starting with their own willingness to talk about their work.

That point was driven home by a reading of Masumi Takayama's letter, excerpts of which (translated by Masako Hayano) follow:

When I was a child I asked my mother, "What is your job?"

She said, "I teach nursing in a college."

To tell the truth I didn't understand exactly what she meant. My biggest question was, what does she mean she teaches nursing? Is nursing something you have to teach? I don't mean to offend those who are engaged in nursing work, but I thought that anyone could become a nurse and that it didn't require a special education.

Up until recently, I thought nursing was not consequential for patients. I thought that nurses are physician's assistants and that they are not involved in important decision making such as diagnosing and treatment planning. That's

(continued)

why I thought nurses didn't need professional knowledge or skills. I thought the most important factor in being a nurse was the person's character and personal qualities such as gentleness, thoughtfulness, and capacity for empathy rather than intelligence.

Now I am a college student. Recently I've had opportunities to listen to my mother talk about what she does and to read her dissertation. Let me tell you that what I had thought about my mother's job and nursing has changed since my mother started talking to me about her work. The biggest change is my awareness of the significance of nursing.

I know that nursing is not something that you learn overnight and that it is worth spending your whole life on. I realize that it takes hard work to achieve the knowledge and psychological preparation required for nursing.

After reading my mother's research paper, I learned that nurses have direct contact with patients over a long time and that nursing is consequential to patients because of the central role that nurses have in patient care. I see why nurses need accurate knowledge, skill, and intelligence to care for patients in addition to personal traits.

Now I can talk to other people about my mother's work more clearly, and with pride. I don't think that my career will be in nursing, but I would still like to know more about nursing to deepen my knowledge.

Later that week, Masumi's letter was read again at a forum sponsored by the Fukui Chapter of the Japanese Nursing Association. Professor Takayama was there and received resounding applause when she described episodes from her work and urged her colleagues to share their stories with their families and the greater public.

Some nurses fear that talking about their work might mean that they're exploiting their patients. Nothing could be further from the truth. You don't just owe it to yourself to tell your stories. It's a contribution to better health care to talk about nursing.

Dealing with Your Fears

Many nurses have told us they are afraid that they will make mistakes if they talk about their work. They say they fear being misinterpreted or getting an angry response. Some are worried about generating conflict or controversy, being fired, or being viewed as disloyal to their institutions. Perhaps nurses' worst fear is that nobody will care.

These are serious concerns. Despite good efforts to be knowledgeable, we are all vulnerable to making mistakes when we speak or write. When using facts and statistics, it is important to ensure they are correct. If you are concerned about an argument or tone, run it by a trusted colleague who is knowledgeable about the issue.

At the same time, be realistic. Many mistakes can be rectified. Some points may be debatable rather than right or wrong. Indeed, much of the information about nursing that you might convey to individuals and groups will represent your perspective as a nurse. Others nurses will have different perspectives, but it doesn't mean that yours is "wrong" or "mistaken." Your experiences and ideas are just as valid as anyone else's.

It is also important to recognize that no matter how much you learn, no one ever has perfect knowledge. Try as you might, you can never reach a point where it is guaranteed that you won't make a mistake. If you are waiting for that day before you speak up, you will be silent forever.

Worrying about how others will respond to one's comments is normal. But none of us can control the responses of others. The moment one opens one's mouth to tell a story, share a feeling, or express an opinion, one loses control over how it will be received. The more people you speak to, the more you can be sure that someone will misunderstand, misinterpret, misconstrue, disagree, feel betrayed, or just tune out. This is a fact of life. Just as it does not deter most of us from talking to our friends, acquaintances, or coworkers, neither should it deter us from speaking to a wider audience in person or through the media.

Your remarks might generate conflict and controversy. That may be difficult for some nurses to cope with. After all, for decades, the mandate of nurses has been to conceal conflict within health care institutions, or to try to manage and smooth over conflict with patients and families. This is reflected in the comments nurses have made at our workshops. "I'm afraid of getting into a situation of 'one side against the other,'" one nurse said. One nurse wrote a note that indicated just how dangerous she believes conflict is: "I'm afraid of causing conflict/chaos."

Seeing controversy and conflict solely as stations on the road to chaos obliterates the constructive role of disagreement. Reluctance to risk disagreement hampers intellectual and professional development, not only for individuals but for a whole profession. One editor of a nursing journal feels that "conflict phobia" among nurses is curtailing rigorous intellectual debate about nursing. She says that she solicits critiques of articles in her journal to enlarge the discussion of important issues. But instead of critiques, she mostly receives innocuous commentary that fails to engage the issues.

"I think even highly educated nurses are too afraid that they might offend someone," she says. "So they just give a very tame response."

The oft-stated yearning that nurses should "speak with one voice," can be interpreted as a wish for total safety. In one voice there is no disagreement, thus no risk, and ultimately no story. Waiting for all 2.7 million U.S. nurses and the millions of other nurses throughout the world to speak with one voice is the perfect recipe for self-silencing.

Self-silencing also stems from fear that exposing unpleasant facts will cost nurses their jobs. This fear has some basis. But it is important to do a reality check and find out what kind of public speaking or advocacy might cost a nurse her job. Even if an institution would prefer that nurses be seen and not heard, RNs can and should talk about their practice and the important work that they do. This is unlikely to result in the termination of employment.

However, to minimize the risks, find out about state, provincial, or federal labor laws and recognize that you're on a much stronger legal footing if you act in concert with others rather than alone. In the United States, for example, labor law protects only workers who act in a group (i.e., with two or more fellow workers) to discuss conditions of work. To receive protection under the National Labor Relations Act, nurses concerned about patient care must relate their concerns to working conditions. Before taking action, therefore, it's important to document concerns and try to raise them within the institution involved. If nurses are not represented by a union, they can try to consult with the staff of a local or national union that represents nurses, or they may want to consult with an attorney who specializes in employment law.

Canadian union leader Kathleen Connors advises nurses to work together to expose system problems. "The fear of being fired is a fear that's expressed everyday by nurses who are in unions as well as those who aren't," she says. "The first thing people have to realize is that they're showing the highest regard for their professional nursing judgment by indicating when situations need to be changed and steps need to be taken. If nurses are afraid to do this on their own, they are supported and protected by their union if they have one. And hopefully by fellow nurses."

"In situations where a union is not present," Connors told us, "nurses should make sure they document their case or concerns and have accurate information. Depending on the situation they can enlist the help of nursing colleagues, management, or perhaps physicians. I've said to doctors: 'Are you guys satisfied with this? If you're not, let's get together so we can talk about this.' And we have. It takes a lot of courage and trust in your own professional judgment to do this."

Some nurses are afraid to expose system problems not because they fear job loss but because they do not want to be disloyal to their institution. Nurses have told us they don't want to publicly discuss serious problems because they don't want to harm an institution whose mission, if not its ac-

tions, is a worthy one. They worry that public exposure will rupture relationships in their workplace, a community they value, and harm their hospital or clinic.

Claire Fagin, Dean Emerita of the University of Pennsylvania School of
Nursing, is sympathetic to this dilemma. Fagin and others point out that institutions tend to be far more resilient than nurses may believe and that exposing serious problems may strengthen institutions rather than weaken
them. "I always advise nurses to go through channels before they expose any
serious system problems," Fagin says. "But if you get absolutely nowhere,
it's important to determine your bottom line. Is your bottom line loyalty to
your institution or is it to protect patients? The bottom line has to be to
protect patients."

When courageous nurses take controversial positions to protect their
patients and the public, this sends a powerful message about the value of
professional nursing.

Perhaps nurses' worst fear is that no one will pay attention or care what
they say.

"I'm afraid people won't listen," one nurse told us.

"People are not interested in what we do," another nurse said. "They say
it's too depressing. They don't want to hear about illness."

"It can be very frustrating talking with people who are not in nursing as
they don't really understand what you are experiencing. Unless you are a
nurse, you can never really know what it means to be a nurse," another offered.

When nurses express these feelings, we're always surprised. We are not
nurses. What we know about nursing we have learned from nurses. We have
found that when nurses talk about their experiences with confidence and
conviction, it can be stimulating, sad, moving, anxiety provoking, funny, terrible, informative—anything but uninteresting. Other people *can* understand what it's like and what it means to be a nurse—if you are willing to tell
them.

Chapter 5

Creating Anecdotes
and Arguments

People can begin to understand the nature of nursing and the agency of the nurse through anecdotes that nurses tell about their work or the arguments they make to explain their role in the health care system. To begin constructing your anecdotes or arguments, think of an incident from your work that would help someone else understand nursing. To construct an anecdote:

- Describe your specialty or area of expertise.
- Describe the health condition or the situation you're addressing.
- Who is the patient? Why is the patient there?
- How prevalent is the problem you're dealing with?
- What are its consequences?
- What did you do? What do nurses do?
- What clinical knowledge and judgment did you or nurses bring to the encounter or to the issue?
- Why did you do what you did? How did it make a difference?

You can advance public understanding by explaining how the concrete, routine activities that you or other nurses perform in your/their daily work make a difference to patients, their families, and the public. Silence any internal voice that expresses doubt about the value of nursing such as, "Oh, no one would be interested in hearing about this," or "They would think it's ordinary." What is ordinary to you may be extraordinary to the listener. It's your job to show why these ostensibly ordinary actions are so important.

Three Anecdotes or Arguments

We urge every nurse to have at least three anecdotes or arguments ready to use when openings occur. These aren't designed to make you feel better about your work or to share your experience with your closest colleagues. They are intended for an external audience. They should address the concerns that ordinary people—or policy makers, politicians, journalists, or business people—have about health care or the health care system. They should show how the work of nurses makes a difference to patients.

What health care issues do people worry about? Research and news coverage suggest that people are worried about medication errors and injuries. They don't want to leave the hospital or clinic sicker than when they came in. They don't want a wrong limb or organ removed. They don't want the wrong medication or a drug overdose.

They often don't know who is responsible for protecting them. They assume it's the doctor. It would probably be news to them that often it's the nurse. How many people, for example, know that in one study, 86 percent of medication errors that were caught were caught by nurses, not by doctors?[1]

Administrators and policy makers tend to be very concerned about cutting costs and enhancing patient outcomes and satisfaction. If you are addressing this audience, highlight how your work saves money and improves patient outcomes.

Steps for Constructing Anecdotes about Your Work

1. Paint a picture
2. Avoid jargon
3. Include facts and statistics
4. Paint yourself into the picture
5. Paint the whole picture

1. Paint a Picture

Nurses often tell us that their role is to protect patients, but they usually don't explain how they do it. Nurses have a vast array of experience to draw on when they consider the stories they might tell. Pick the ones that most clearly demonstrate the consequential nature of nursing.

Begin by setting the scene. Include the "telling detail" that sparks the layperson's interest and suggests the complexity and tone of what you do and the environment in which you do it. An example:

> I'm a diabetes nurse. I help patients understand how to take their medications, how to change their diet, and I even make sure they are wearing shoes that fit correctly. If their shoes chafe, because of poor circulation, they could develop sores that won't heal. This could lead to amputation.
>
> This work is very important because diabetes mellitus is one of our biggest public health problems and is on the rise in most industrialized societies. Although many people understand the catastrophic health consequences of type I diabetes—the kind due to genetic factors—too few know that type II diabetes—the acquired kind that is often connected to diet—is by no means a minor illness. Unless properly managed, it too can cause blindness, kidney failure, and amputations. Plus, diabetes can increase the risk of having a heart attack or stroke as much as smoking a pack of cigarettes a day.
>
> In the United States, 12,000 to 24,000 people go blind each year because of diabetes. Some 33,000 suffer end-stage kidney disease, 86,000 have feet or limb amputations, and 77,000 die of heart disease. I work to prevent such complications and suffering."[2,3]

Paddy Connelly, an oncology nurse, chose this way to bring us into the world of oncology nursing:

> I am taking care of a twenty-five-year-old breast cancer patient who will have a bone marrow transplant. My patient will lose her breast, will probably lose her hair, and perhaps lose her ability to have a child. When my patient hears all this, she is overwhelmed. She is processing everything and nothing at all. As a nurse, I am aware that I need to be available to her to probe the questions she couldn't ask initially when she was essentially in a state of shock. Over time, I may even have to help her formulate the questions to ask. No one else but a nurse is there to do that.

In telling this story, Nurse Connelly allowed others to see the patient as a human being, not as a case. She did this by using everyday language instead of medical and technical jargon.

Perhaps you are a nurse fighting for safe staffing or better working conditions. You might argue that nurses now routinely take care of ten or twelve patients and leave it at that. Imagine how much more effective this argument would be if you provide salient details about these patients and their problems.

Nurse Janie Storr did just that when she addressed administrators, policy makers, journalists, activists, and clinicians who attended a public meeting at the University of Pennsylvania titled, "The Abandonment of the Patient—The Impact of Profit-Driven Health Care on the Public." She told the audience:

> Let me describe to you what I encountered when I came to work recently.
>
> One of my patients was a seventy-four-year-old woman with a fractured arm who had been found on the floor by neighbors the night before. She was an alcoholic, showing early signs of withdrawal. She had an IV and was alert, but not oriented, and was to go to surgery the next day.
>
> Another woman was eighty-three years old with back pain from a compression fracture in her spine. She was not oriented and was incontinent, unable to move her bowels, had a history of Alzheimer's, and had to be restrained.
>
> Another patient, an eighty-four-year-old woman who had had her leg amputated at the pelvis, had just had a stroke and was paralyzed on one side of her body. She was alert but unable to speak, had tube feeding, had very high blood pressure, and was treated with medication that I had to prepare and deliver through the feeding tube."[4]

As Storr described the remaining patients she cared for, the audience grew more and more astounded that any nurse could be asked to cope with so many complex patients.

Reflecting Clinical Judgment

An anecdote that critical care nurse Judith Donnelly told us illustrates how veteran nurses employ clinical judgment and experience in situations that call for swift action.

Donnelly, who works in a telemetry unit at a New England hospital, was taking care of a heart patient scheduled for surgery the next morning. That night the patient called for the nurse because he was experiencing shortness of breath. As Donnelly checked him, she found what she had expected: He had fluid building up in his lungs and was sitting up to breathe more easily. His condition was stable, but his heart rate was somewhat elevated. Donnelly asked the secretary to get a med order and began preparing the appropriate medication.

Then the patient said urgently: "Can you help me? I have to have a bowel movement."

Donnelly turned to the secretary and said quietly, "Call a code."

"Code?" the secretary replied.

"Now," Donnelly said.

When the code team and the resident arrived, the patient was still "normal." Suddenly his heart rate dropped to thirty, and he began losing consciousness. The code team went to work. After the patient was stabilized, the resident asked Donnelly, "How did you know?"

She told the resident the patient needed to move his bowels.

The resident understood, but we didn't. Donnelly explained that the patient would not have had that urge under the circumstances unless something was happening with the vagus nerve. This nerve affects both the heart rate and stimulates the bowels. The patient's urgency was the tip-off that his heart rate was about to drop.

As an experienced nurse, Donnelly said she acted on her own "gut feeling" about what this patient needed.

Another kind of clinical judgment became apparent in the story a pediatric nurse told us about her work with a three-year-old leukemia patient. She said she watched "Barney" on television with the little girl every morning so that the child would view the nurse as a source of comfort during painful tests and procedures.

Her ability to articulate this last detail was critical. She wasn't just a tender loving person who sat with the child watching TV; she was a clinical expert who recognized that relationship is a powerful therapeutic tool. The

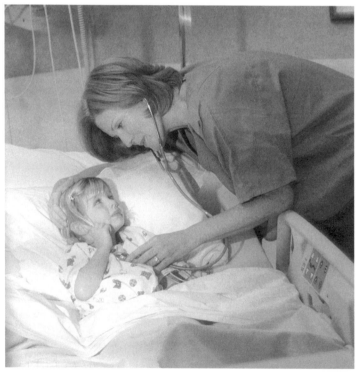

Courtesy of the American Association of Critical-Care Nurses

nurse understood the procedures and treatments the child had to face and knew that if surrounded by strangers, the child would be terrified. She could endure her medical treatment only if a source of comfort and reassurance were available to her.

Many nurses focus on the way they help to reduce the anxiety that patients experience when they are in the alien environment of the hospital. For example, perioperative nurses say that one of their main tasks is to help manage the anxiety of surgical patients. However, they might not explain that anxiety can lead to complications for the surgical patient. For example, it elevates a patient's blood pressure and can cause problems during surgery and recovery. Patients who are calmer have an easier operative and postoperative course and less pain. If you leave out such facts, you risk depicting yourself as a nice person rather than a knowledgeable clinician who does things for specific reasons.

To illuminate your clinical judgment, you need to explain not only what you are doing but also why you are doing it.

Nurses might say "I took the patient's blood pressure, temperature, and listened to his lungs." But this doesn't tell us what the nurse is looking for and why his actions are knowledgeable and consequential. The simplest way to convey this is to use the word "because."

"I took the patient's blood pressure because I wanted to make sure he hadn't developed any internal bleeding after surgery. I checked the patient's temperature because it can indicate the presence of infection. I listened to his lungs to determine whether there were signs of pneumonia."

This helps people to understand why vital signs are considered vital and not trivial.

Depict Your Knowledge as Internalized

In painting a picture of your work, be sure to show that your actions are guided by your own expertise. Sometimes when nurses tell stories, they make it sound like all they are doing is following orders. Starting a sentence with "I had to . . ." gives that impression.

"I had to take his vital signs every four hours."

"I had to call the doctor to get the order for pain medication."

"As J.D.'s assigned nurse, I had to follow the hospital protocol for attempted suicide patients, which included . . ."

Nurses have explained that they must talk like this because their work is dictated by doctors' orders and institutional protocols. This explanation suggests that nurses are in a uniquely subordinate position. In fact, all professionals follow protocols or guidelines. When doctors prescribe a drug or perform a procedure, they are following protocols. When an actor performs in a play, she is required to use the words a playwright wrote and follow the directions of the director. For most professionals, protocols or guidelines become part of the structure in which they do their individual work with their own agency. Neither the actor nor the doctor feels required to say, "I had to do what so and so told me, [or] what the protocol recommended." They are more likely to say, "I did thus and so." When nurses use language that elevates protocols or orders above their actions, they depict themselves as puppets controlled by external sources of knowledge and judgment.

Nurses can counter this impression by simply saying:

"I took his vital signs every four hours."

"I consulted with the physician about the patient's pain medication."

"As J.D.'s nurse, I did what we do to protect all suicidal patients, which included . . ."

Nurses can also depict themselves as more—or less—dependent on physicians. Consider the differing pictures a patient or family member forms from the following answers to a question:

"I have to ask the doctor."

"I will consult with the doctor."

We advise nurses to use the word *consult* or *discuss* when they refer to conversations they have with doctors about patient care issues and concerns. Avoid formulations like, "I don't know, I'll have to ask the doctor." Or, "I have to get the doctor's order." If you have recommended a treatment or medication, make sure your story includes this fact, as in, "I knew my patient was in pain. I consulted with her physician and suggested that she give the patient some pain medication. I administered the medication and made sure the patient was no longer in pain."

2. Avoid Using Jargon

In communicating with the public, distinguish between what one says to other health care professionals and what one says to laypeople. Avoid jargon that makes your story incomprehensible. One type is "medical-speak" in which medical terms and abbreviations are used without translating them into ordinary language or explaining them.

"My patient suffered from a short run of ventricular tachycardia, and my intervention saved him from the ultimate negative patient outcome."

"My patient was admitted from the ED with fulminating pulmonary edema. Opening PA pressures were 58 over 28, with a wedge of 30. O_2 sat was 84 percent and his ABGs showed a PO_2 of 82. He was in sinus tech with frequent runs of multiform PVCs and his SVR was 2400."

Would a non-nurse get it? Any of it? Probably not. A non-nurse would, however, understand the following:

"My patient had an irregular heart rhythm, and my quick action saved him from dying."

"My patient had too much fluid in his lungs. His oxygen levels were low, and he had many irregular heartbeats. He had difficulty breathing and could have died suddenly. So I acted quickly to reduce his fluid volume and gave him morphine to help him relax."

Another version of jargon is "nurse speak." This is academic/nursing theory/caring discourse that creeps out of nursing schools and professional organizations and into ordinary conversation.

We frequently hear it in our communication seminars when we ask nurses to pretend that we are television reporters interviewing them about their work.

"What do you do?" we asked a volunteer in one seminar.

"I'm a nurse practitioner," she said. "I deliver primary health care services. I do skilled assessment. I'm a patient educator and a patient advocate."

On another occasion, an oncology nurse stepped forward. She described

Anecdote Makeover by Nurse Midwife Ruth Johnson of Massachusetts

Gobbledygook version:

"As a nurse midwife, I am the guardian of the birth process and partner with a woman to make sure she has a healthy baby. As wise and understanding professionals, we team with women to help them access supportive networks that will help navigate this important life transition."

Makeover:

"Nurse midwives care for women throughout their pregnancies, deliver babies, and monitor mothers and babies after the birth. Women cared for by nurse midwives are less likely to have a cesarean section, an episiotomy, or a baby admitted to the intensive care nursery than those managed by physicians. In addition to caring for childbearing women, nurse midwives also provide primary health care to women—annual physicals, Pap smears, contraception, testing and treatment for sexually transmitted diseases, hormone management, and treatment of urinary and vaginal infections. Our patients range from young women having their first exam to older women looking for a professional who can help them to negotiate midlife changes."

her work with women on high-dose chemotherapy who experience premature menopause: "I do symptom assessment, I monitor the effect of chemotherapy on ovulatory function, and I do patient education."

Another participant explained: "Unlike physicians, nurses deliver holistic care. As a nurse midwife, I am the guardian of the birth process and partner with a woman to make sure she has a healthy baby."

Other nurses might know what this means. But these descriptions don't show what these nurses do, what problems their patients have, and why nurses' work is consequential.

To kick the jargon habit, remind yourself that you are presenting a picture to someone who is unfamiliar with your workplace, with nursing practice, and with medical and nurse speak.

3. Use Facts and Statistics

A great way to bolster your arguments and descriptions is to use a few choice facts and statistics. These enhance your credibility. When you read useful studies or find relevant statistics in a journal article, news report, or other document, jot them down for future use. If you are preparing for an event or testimony or to speak to a journalist or community group, go online and check out material that will be relevant to your topic.

For information on restructuring and working conditions, two reports by the Institute of Medicine (IOM)—"Keeping Patients Safe: Transforming the Work Environment of Nurses" and "Nursing Staff in Hospitals and Nursing Homes: Is It Adequate?"—are full of useful statistics.[5,6] The IOM reports on medical errors and injuries also have data that nurses can use to tell compelling stories.[1]

Such studies document that in the care of the sick and vulnerable, "small things" can be enormously important. For example, if you're a medical nurse, you could use facts and statistics to show the significance of giving a patient a bed bath. Explain that when you are bathing a patient, you are looking for signs of skin breakdown like a little red spot on the hip or heel that could turn into a bedsore. Explain that it could become a crater-sized decubitus ulcer that goes all the way down to the bone.

According to studies, about 11 percent of hospitalized patients under the age of seventy are at risk for bedsores. When patients are between seventy and eighty-nine years old, the risk jumps to 54 percent. Treatment of bedsores costs from $4,000 to $70,000. Bedsores are largely preventable with good nursing care. If nurses have the time to properly bathe patients, to turn them, to make sure they're well nourished, and to clean them if they are incontinent, this goes a long way toward preventing pressure ulcers. The

United States spends $1.3 billion on pressure ulcers each year.[7,8]

Facts and statistics can be integrated into an anecdote about the role nurses play in preventing deep vein thrombosis (DVT) and pulmonary emboli. The latter is one of the most catastrophic consequences of immobility following surgery or during a hospital stay. When patients don't walk, blood pools and stagnates in the legs, and a clot could develop. A piece of the clot could break off and travel into the lungs where it could lodge in the pulmonary artery, shutting off the supply of blood to the heart and causing instant death.

Without proper prevention and action, 20 percent of patients who have had major surgeries might suffer from DVT and 1 to 2 percent might have a pulmonary embolism. Nurses evaluate which

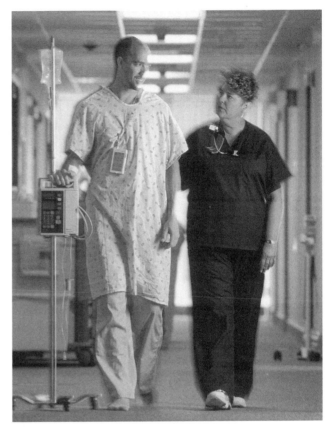

Courtesy of the American Association of Critical-Care Nurses

patients are at risk for DVT, help them to walk or do leg exercises in bed, make sure they have pressure stockings and/or other specialized equipment, and monitor for symptoms of DVT or pulmonary embolism.

In preventing such complications, nurses save money as well as lives. The average cost of treating a three-month episode of DVT is $12,000 for the medications alone.[9]

4. Paint Yourself into the Picture

When nurses tell stories, they tend to highlight the contributions of other health care professionals while often obscuring their own. Although physicians admit that patient care is a collaborative affair, in public they often give the impression that patients' survival or recovery depends on their efforts alone. As nurse and organizational consultant Elizabeth Grady has explained, nurses seem to have difficulty acknowledging the "I" in the "we," whereas physicians more often have trouble finding the "we" in the "I."[13]

Other Useful Statistics Drawn from U. S. Medical and Nursing Studies

- Fifty-eight percent of adverse events that resulted in lengthened hospital stays and disability were due to preventable errors. Drug complications were the most common type of adverse event, followed by wound infections. Most of these adverse events led to disabilities lasting less than six months, but 13.6 percent resulted in death, and 2.6 percent caused permanent disabling injuries.[1]

- Bacteremias (an infection that occurs when bacteria get into the blood stream) account for 10 to 20 percent of hospital-acquired infections. Each episode of bacteremia adds an average of $2,836 to a hospital bill.[10]

- Urinary tract infections (UTIs) account for 40 percent of hospital-acquired infections.[11] Each episode of a UTI adds $676 to the hospital bill.[10]

- Studies show that when nurses work longer than 12-hour shifts, or work more than 40 hours a week, the risk of making an error (most are medication errors) increases significantly.[12]

For example, Susan Sweeney, an emergency nurse at a level-one trauma center in Rhode Island, told us a moving story. A beautiful nineteen-year-old man was brought into the emergency department following a car accident. He was dead on arrival. But the injuries that killed him were all internal. He looked perfect on the outside.

When his mother saw him, she refused to believe he was dead. He was just sleeping, she insisted. See, she said, calling to him to awaken him, his hand is moving. He's in a coma. He'll recover.

Nurse Sweeney and her colleague, a trauma physician, recognized that the woman was in shock and needed a great deal of attention. Sweeney assessed the situation and recommended against medicating the mother because it would only delay what she inevitably had to recognize—her son was dead. Nurse Sweeney spent more than an hour working with the mother to help her deal with her denial and grief.

But when Susan Sweeney initially told us the story, she described the care of the mother solely as a group effort. We asked her to clarify who did what. Did both she and the trauma physician spend an hour with the mother?

No. She explained that early on the physician left to do other work and that she was the one who stayed with the distraught mother.

It was Nurse Sweeney, in fact, who cared for the woman. It was Nurse Sweeney, in fact, who recommended a treatment plan and carried it out. It was Nurse Sweeney who worked with the mother until she was able to be taken home.

Finally, Nurse Sweeney let us see what she did. If she hadn't included herself in the picture, how would we know the important and humane work that nurses do?

5. Paint the Whole Picture

In your anecdotes and arguments, create a full and rich view of nursing practice. Contemporary nurses have a tendency to focus on the psychosocial and emotional aspects of the care they provide to the exclusion of the medical and technical knowledge and skill they employ. This framing of nursing is often taught in nursing school, so much so that many nurses actually put down the medical and technical aspects as they elevate "caring," compassion, or patient education. When nurses eliminate the medical and technical from the picture they are painting, they depict "halfistic" rather than the holistic care that they assert is the heart of nursing, as did this emergency nurse who proudly asserted:

"As ER nurses, people don't value us for our technical wizardry, but for what we give of ourselves to our patients."

It's important for nurses to describe how they monitor medical treatments, how they employ technology, how they help doctors construct medical diagnoses, and how they often recommend medications that should be prescribed. When you construct your anecdote, be sure to show the range of activities you engage in. If you tell us that you're building a trusting relationship with a patient, you can explain that one way you do this is by providing physical care. Medical nurse Jeannie Chaisson talked about how, in caring for a demented patient, she used the bed bath not only to make sure that the patient wasn't developing a bedsore, but also to reassure him. He couldn't understand the words she said, but he responded to a calm voice and reassuring touch.[14]

Make the story both/and, not either/or. In your anecdote, incorporate both the medical/technical aspects of nursing and the caring, compassion, and educational aspects.

The ER nurse could have said: "People really do value us for our technical wizardry when they are in an emergency situation and also appreciate what we give of ourselves to our patients."

Never Put Down Another Nurse

When you're constructing your anecdotes or arguments, be careful not to el-evate your own work or field of nursing at the expense of other nurses. The practice of putting down other nurses has become common within nursing, to the detriment of the nursing profession.

Nurses with baccalaureate or graduate degrees sometimes insist they are "professional" nurses not "technicians" or "technical" nurses. For instance, a nursing director at a major teaching hospital stated that operating room (OR) nurses are "technicians" not "real nurses" in a conversation she had with a medical sociologist. Although she may not have realized it, she was speaking to a "public," and an influential one at that. As it turned out, her views reflected badly on her rather than on the OR nurses.

Such remarks could boomerang because the public has its own percep-tion of what is valuable. Studies indicate that most patients and members of the public value technology and technique, and want a nurse who is compe-tent in these areas. The word "professional" is recognizable code within nursing, but not outside of it.

Labeling has also become a problem as advanced practice nurses (APNs) gain more attention. Nurse practitioners (NPs) and certified nurse-midwives (CNSs), among others, sometimes try to differentiate themselves from staff nurses by insisting that they are APNs, NPs, and CNSs, but not RNs. One nurse practitioner described a NP-operated primary care practice to a *New York Times* reporter as an example of how NPs were "moving nurses into the twenty-first century," inadvertently implying that direct-care nursing is mired in the past.[15]

Nursing has many points of entry into practice, and nurses understand-ably want their particular work and skills to be noticed. You can explain your work without making an inaccurate comparison with other nursing work. It is inaccurate and undermining of nursing to suggest that staff nurses don't use critical thinking, don't make clinical decisions, and aren't capable of handling authority and autonomy.

Rather than insisting "I'm an NP not an RN" (which is factually incor-rect), an NP or other advanced practice nurse will gain more mileage by sim-ply explaining what she does.

If someone asks, "Are you an RN?", the accurate answer is yes, advanced practice nurses are RNs who work in specialized areas.

Similarly, staff nurses should avoid casting aspersions about the au-thenticity of academics and nurse managers. Just as managers should not attack unionized nurses as "unprofessional," unionized nurses should avoid formulations like, "He's not a 'real nurse,'" "She's just one of those 'pumps and pearls nurses,'" or, "She no longer has the 'heart of the nurse.'" There is

a difference between noting that an administrator, manager, or academic researcher no longer engages in clinical practice and making *ad hominem* arguments. Debating positions is a better strategy than questioning who is a
"real nurse."

Makeovers

In constructing your anecdotes, the idea is to first get the basic information
into draft form and then to shape it to make it more effective. One way to
test the anecdote's effectiveness is to tell it to a non-nurse or to a nurse who
isn't familiar with your field. Here are some stories that nurses told us when
they were asked to describe their work. The first versions are often diffuse
and unclear. This is OK because the rough draft is intended just to reveal the
pertinent points. We worked with the nurses to refine the stories. The ones
labeled Version Two are the makeovers.

Anecdote One: Oncology Nurse

Version One

Recently, I took care of a patient in the hospital who was diagnosed with cancer. One of the things I did that was important as a nurse was take the time to
listen to the patient's concerns and needs. I saw him for a period of two days
while I was on my shift. When I went into the room, I would reintroduce myself and take the time to ask how he was and to inquire about his needs. One
of the other things I did was provide a daily bath. The patient was unable to
bathe himself and required full assistance. While I did the bath, I took the
time to make sure his skin wasn't broken down and that he received the care
he needed.

I washed the patient's hair and brushed his teeth. One of the other things
I had to do was provide the patient with medications. He didn't know a lot
about the medications. He didn't know their names; he didn't know why particular pills were being given. He didn't understand why the doctor had
changed his medication. I took the time to explain to my patient that his pain
was being managed by the medication he was receiving and to explain that he
needed to tell me if he wasn't comfortable.

In this anecdote the nurse recounts some aspects of her care. However,
the picture she paints is just a sketch. We don't know what kind of cancer
the patient has or why he is in the hospital. We don't understand the importance and complexity of pain management. We don't see the medical and
technical activities she undertakes to keep the patient safe. We are left with

the impression that the nurse is a well-meaning person who is solicitous of her patient. One might conclude that she could be replaced by someone equally attentive but less educated and skilled, and therefore less expensive.

Version Two

I was taking care of a patient, Mr. R, who had esophageal cancer, cancer of the tube that passes food from the mouth to the stomach. This is a serious diagnosis with an 80 percent mortality rate. Mr. R had surgery two days previously to remove part of his esophagus and reattach the remainder to his stomach. He was in a lot of pain and was very anxious about the chemotherapy he would eventually receive.

One of the things I did was manage his pain. Pain management is a critical nursing activity. Pain is not simply experienced at the emotional level. Unmanaged pain creates changes at the cellular and tissue level. We know that unmanaged pain retards healing, and can even lead to death. Patients who are in pain don't walk and can develop deep vein thrombosis. They don't cough and are at greater risk for pneumonia. Some patients reject pain medication because they think that toughing out pain shows strength of character. When such a patient is asked if he is in pain, nurses know that he might say "no," while the expression on his face or his body language says "yes."

It's important to monitor the effectiveness of a patient's pain medication and stay ahead of the pain. You want to make sure he is always comfortable.

Mr. R was not able to eat. He was being fed intravenously. I monitored his fluid intake and urine output to make sure he wasn't becoming dehydrated or malnourished.

I was also concerned about the risk of pneumonia, so I listened to his chest every four hours for any abnormal sounds. I checked his temperature every four hours for any signs of infection. I checked his respiration and took his blood pressure. One of the risks of this surgery is internal bleeding. I needed to make sure his blood pressure was within the normal range and that he was not bleeding internally, which could lead to cardiac arrest and death.

I listened to his concerns and reassured both him and the family. I didn't just care for him. His wife was at his bedside and was worried about what was coming next in his care.

In version two, the nurse fills in the blanks. We now understand that she is dealing with a very sick patient who has a range of emotional, medical, and technical needs. We understand the intricacies of pain management and why vital signs are so significant. After hearing this nurse describe her work, the listener would understand the complexity of that work and why we need nurses and not nurse substitutes at the bedside.

Anecdote Two: IV Nurses

Members of a nurses union in Pennsylvania discovered that their hospital planned to eliminate its team of IV nurses. At a communication workshop, an IV nurse and her colleague in the ER worked on constructing an anecdote that would show the risks to patients of this clinical change. The nurses wanted to educate the hospital board of directors which, they felt, did not fully appreciate the issues involved. Other potential publics would be journalists, legislators, and policy makers, particularly those interested in hospital restructuring and labor force redesign.

Version One

The ER nurse began telling the story to the others at the workshop:

The board of the directors of our hospital is trying to eliminate the position of IV nurse. The reasons why the IV team is so valuable is that the skill is developed by nurses for patients. They are asking staff nurses to insert and take care of IVs.

But nurses on the floor, who usually have ten to twelve patients, do not have time to assess IV sites so that there is a higher risk of infiltrations, where the medication is infiltrated and amputations increase. For example, someone can have chest pain and be on dopamine, which is very toxic to the vein, and this infiltrates and causes vasoconstriction in the arm and could lead to an arm amputation.

Nurses are now asked to do all kinds of other specialized things. I was trained in a twenty-minute in-service to deal with things like ports so that they could be taken away from the IV team.

Then the IV nurse jumped in:

Bedside nurses don't have the time or specialized knowledge and skill to keep up with this all the time. When the IV team is not in the hospital at night, we're finding that when nurses have to start IVs at night, patients are getting multiple sticks, and by morning whatever has been put in has started to infiltrate. Nurses who don't have the skill will put IVs in hands or in elbows because access is easier there, but every time the patient moves it can infiltrate.

The best person to stick a patient is an IV nurse.

A non-nurse would find it difficult to understand the issues in this fulsome report. There is a lot of medical speak. What does "infiltrate" mean? Vasoconstriction? Why do people have IVs in the first place? Does it have to hurt? How difficult is it to stick a needle in the right place?

The focus of the anecdote should be that IV nurses have specialized skill and expertise and that if they are not there, patients are at risk for complications and pain. It is also better if one nurse, preferably the IV nurse, tells the story.

Version Two: IV Nurse

Most hospital patients have samples of their blood drawn. Many patients in the hospital also have intravenous, or IV, therapy, in which medication is put directly into their circulatory system. Some patients undergoing this therapy have needles in their veins throughout their hospital stay. Certain patients, usually those with cancer or who are in intensive care, have central lines called port-a-catheters that are surgically implanted into a vein in their chest. All of these procedures mean that needles must be inserted into patients.

It requires skill to insert needles into veins. Some patients have small veins or veins that are difficult to see or feel. Some, particularly those who are on long-term therapies, have had so many needle sticks that their veins have been damaged, and it is difficult to find a good spot in which to insert a needle.

Someone who does not have a lot of experience might insert the needle in the wrong place. They might have to do multiple sticks before finding the right spot, which is painful for the patient. An IV that is poorly placed might fail to go into the vein or go all the way through it. In either case, the medication won't be pushed into the vein but will infiltrate—that is, drip into the surrounding tissue. Infiltration is dangerous for two reasons: The medication can't be effective when it doesn't go into the circulatory system and toxic medications inserted into the wrong place can cause burns, which, in extreme cases, require skin grafts.

IV nurses insert needles and monitor for these problems. They teach patients and family members to watch out for signs of trouble such as tingling, redness, or swelling. They also give regular care to patients with porta-catheters who are at increased risk for infections and blood clots. IV nurses keep the lines open by flushing them with anticlotting medication. Even when this is done correctly, the catheter tip can become blocked by a blood clot. An inexperienced person might try to force fluid through the clot and wind up dislodging the clot, which could then travel through the circulatory system to the lungs and cause problems with breathing.

Central lines also require careful monitoring because of the risk of infection. Research has shown that central lines are the most common cause of hospital-acquired bloodstream infections for patients on ICUs. These lead to between 2,400 and 20,000 deaths and cost between $296 million and $2.3 billion annually.[10]

Because the hospital wants to replace the IV team, busy staff nurses, who generally have between ten and twelve patients, are expected to master skills it takes IV nurses years to develop. For example, some nurses have been given a twenty-minute course on how to properly introduce a needle into a port-a-catheter. Staff nurses on the units don't have the time to monitor IVs for infection, infiltration, and other problems. We know this because IV nurses have been eliminated at night, and as bedside RNs assume their responsibilities we are finding a higher incidence of multiple sticks and IV infiltration.

In version two, the IV nurse clarifies what IVs are, why they are important, and what the risks to patients are if they are not skillfully placed and monitored. She does not put down her staff-nurse colleagues by describing the specialized expertise of IV nurses but highlights the demands that increased patient loads impose on staff nurses.

Anecdote Three: Nurse Education

Many nurse educators in the United States believe that a baccalaureate degree should be required for entry into nursing practice. Although a university degree is mandated for nursing in a number of countries, the demand to produce nurses cheaper and faster means this educational standard is often attacked. Nurse educators must effectively explain why nurses need higher education.

Version One

Here is a U.S. nurse educator discussing why nurses should have a four-year degree:

> Nursing is a very complex work. Today, rapidly expanding clinical knowledge and mounting complexities in health care mandate that professional nurses possess educational preparation commensurate with their diverse responsibilities. Nurses are professional not technical workers. Nurses mobilize critical-thinking skills and judgment in their clinical decision-making. They are holistic caregivers who must use this judgment to individualize care to each patient and must also educate and advocate for patients. Any trained monkey can learn to monitor the equipment on an ICU or take a temperature or blood pressure, but only a professional nurse can use her critical thinking and assessment skills to deliver holistic care to a patient.

Here are some of the problems in this argument. It's a grab bag of nurse-speak that fails to show what nurses need to know to do their work. It demeans the activities involved in much of nursing and by extension, the people who do it. Even if some activities are delegated to a less-educated caregiver, do nurses want to suggest that a nurse's aide is less than human?

By using this riveting image, a credible speaker with a PhD has linked the activities of nursing with lesser primates. Try erasing *that* from listeners' minds. On the face of it, it's an inaccurate metaphor because a monkey could not be trained to monitor patients on the ICU and take vitals.

Version Two

Nurses work with complex high-tech equipment, toxic medications, and invasive treatments, and with patients—in hospitals and in other settings—who are sicker than ever before. In urgent situations, they need to make snap decisions that have life-and-death consequences. To rescue patients from preventable complications and to help them survive and thrive, they need to know pharmacology, anatomy, and pathophysiology among other subjects. Because nurses work with vulnerable human beings who are often anxious, frightened, irritable, and sometimes angry, they must have a foundation in psychology and communication. It takes time and financial resources to produce a nurse with the education and skill necessary to take care of today's patients.

Anecdote Four: Nursing Administration

Di Twigg, a nursing administrator in Perth, Australia, wrote the following job description for internal use. A makeover was necessary, however, to communicate with the media, legislators, and the public.

Version One

I am a nurse who is the Director of Nursing. I have professional responsibility for 1445 FTE and a budget of $89.3M. In this role I provide leadership to:
 Ensure excellence in clinical standards. These standards guide nursing practice and benefit the patients we treat.
 Recruit and employ the right number of appropriately skilled nurses. This is essential to provide safe patient care.
 Develop new knowledge by actively supporting the provision of nursing research and education. This is critical because nursing practice is based on the findings of research studies.
 Advocate nursing issues and their importance to improved patient outcomes such as decreased risk of dying, early nursing intervention, detection and minimization of complications, and avoidance of hospital-acquired problems such as pneumonia, pressure ulcers, and falls.
 I make myself available to all nurses so that I am in tune with nurses and their issues so I can:
 Action these concerns at the nursing and hospital executive level.
 Make these concerns known to policy makers and politicians.
 As the Executive Director of Nursing Services, I am also a member of the

Health Service senior executive team. In this role I influence the management and future directions of the hospital and health service.

Version Two

My name is Di Twigg. I am a nurse and the Executive Director of Nursing at an acute 650–bed tertiary teaching hospital, and a member of the system's senior executive team.

I am responsible for more than 1,500 employees and a budget of $89.3 million.

I ensure that there are high-quality clinical standards for nursing practice and that these are maintained as nurses deliver care to patients.

Anecdote Checklist

1. Does your story paint a picture?
   - ☐ Would a non-nurse find your account interesting?
   - ☐ Does your reader or listener see you at work?
   - ☐ Do you include critical details that show the reader or listener what you do and why it is important?
2. Is your story jargon-free?
   - ☐ Do you translate complex terms into lay-language?
   - ☐ Do you decode your work for the listener or reader?
   - ☐ Are you using language appropriate to your audience?
3. Do you bolster your argument with facts and statistics?
4. Do you paint yourself into the picture?
   - ☐ Do you use the voice of agency?
   - ☐ Can the reader or listener see what you are doing and what your role is?
   - ☐ Is your clinical knowledge and judgment evident?
5. Do you paint the whole picture?
   - ☐ Do we see the full range of your nursing activities—medical and technical, emotional and social, and body care?
   - ☐ Do you focus only on the psychosocial?
   - ☐ Do we understand why vital signs are vital?
   - ☐ Is the nurse's intelligence, curiosity, and decision making evident?
   - ☐ Does your anecdote refute traditional stereotypes about nursing, or inadvertently reinforce them?
   - ☐ Does your anecdote help us understand the *significance* and *consequential nature* of nursing work?

I recruit and employ the right number of appropriately skilled nurses to provide safe patient care. I make sure that health care administrators, clinicians, and the public understand that monitoring and early intervention by nurses reduces patient mortality (deaths) and complications such as pneumonia, pressure ulcers, and falls. Because nursing practice is based on research findings, my department actively supports nursing research and education to help nurses deliver safer, better, and more efficient care.

I work closely with the nurses in our institution so that I am aware of the changing realities of the practice setting. This allows me to respond to nurses' needs and provide resources for nursing practice and innovations. I communicate and raise concerns with hospital executives, policy makers, and politicians to influence the management and future directions of the hospital and health service.

Tailoring Your Anecdotes for Various Audiences

Now that you have three all-purpose anecdotes handy, you can tweak them to appeal to specific audiences. To do this, ask yourself: Who are you talking to? What are their concerns and interests? What arguments, facts, or ideas will move them?

For example, if the oncology nurse who told her story in anecdote one were talking to a high school class, she might punch up details about the cutting-edge treatment that she delivers and monitors. At a community meeting, she might emphasize the part about how cancer nurses manage pain and debilitating symptoms. If she were jumping into the debate about end-of-life care, she could discuss how she would help this patient if his treatment were not effective and he faced difficult choices about continued treatment or hospice care. If she were talking to a group of hospital administrators or politicians, she must address their concerns about costs and highlight how her actions save money by preventing complications, readmissions, or expensive futile treatments.

You may be able to reshape one anecdote to address various issues, or you may need several different anecdotes to illuminate aspects of nursing that most people aren't aware of, such as:

- Nurses prevent costly complications and medical errors.
- In teaching hospitals, nurses teach physicians and physicians-in-training.
- Nurses contribute to medical cures and to medical diagnosis and often recommend the medications doctors prescribe.

- Nursing care saves money and lives and lessens suffering.
- Hospitals are nursing institutions. People aren't admitted to hospitals unless they need nursing care.
- Nurses are the first clinicians a patient sees in an emergency department. It's the triage nurse who decides how quickly the patient needs to be seen, where, and by whom.

Hot Topics

When you construct your anecdotes, think of what issues are timely, in the media, or the subject of public conversation. Consult our discussion of "news values" in Chapter 6.

Many hot-button issues are nursing intensive, but the public may not know the role nurses have. Here are some issues that offer an excellent opportunity to make nursing more visible:

- *Death and dying.* Nurses play a vital role in palliative care.
- *Obesity.* Nurses help patients with diet, nutrition, and exercise and are critical to those undergoing new surgeries.
- *Diabetes.* Nurses teach and monitor diabetic patients.
- *Women's health.* Midwives care for women from adolescence through menopause.
- *Geriatric care.* Nurses work in home care, assisted living, and long-term care.
- *Heart disease and stroke.* Nurses educate patients about heart attack and stroke symptoms and the urgency to get to the ER if such symptoms occur.
- *Nursing shortage.* Better pay and working conditions are essential to ending the nursing shortage.

Finally, there are some issues that are not on the media radar that could gain more attention if nurses talked about them.

- *Wound care.* A nurse's choice of an appropriate dressing to apply to a wound can save a limb.
- *Pain management and palliative care.* Nurses are the ones who keep patients comfortable even though they often have to make a greater effort than should be necessary to get appropriate meds for their patients. Intractable pain was an issue in the media when Jack Kevorkian was killing patients. The media focus then shifted

to the illegal use of pain meds. Meanwhile seriously ill patients continue to suffer.

When nurses stop being silent and talk about their work, the public listens. The story of Barry Morley, an Australian critical care nurse, is a dramatic example.

In 2002, Morley, his wife Kate Simpson, a clinical nurse, and their fourteen-year-old daughter Grace, took a vacation trip to Bali. The Morley's twelve-year-old son had died three months earlier, and the family was in mourning.

All three were in their hotel room on October 12 when around 11 P.M. they heard an explosion. A second explosion then blew the roof off their hotel, extinguished the lights, and shattered the windows. They rushed outside. Bloodied and wounded people began streaming down a small lane to the hotel. These were the injured fleeing from the terrorist attack on Bali that killed 202 people and injured more than 400 others.

Morley and Simpson flew into action. They set up, in effect, a field hospital, recruiting guests and the less severely injured to gather supplies and help treat those whose lives were at stake. They were confronted with massive head wounds, traumatic amputations, lung injuries, and severe burns. They bandaged wounds with strips torn from sheets, employed surf boards as stretchers, and wrapped chest wounds with plastic bags to prevent lungs from collapsing. Morley triaged the wounded at the bomb site and saved those he could while Simpson worked at the hotel. Young Grace consoled the dying.

Morley and Simpson were the only health professionals at the bomb site for almost five hours. Their knowledge, expertise, and action saved dozens of people. Yet, hardly anyone knew that Morley and Simpson were at the Bali bombing, much less what they did there. This is because, Morley said, they didn't want to talk about it. They worried about gaining status from other people's suffering. They also worried that other nurses would consider them boastful. When Morley gave a rare newspaper interview, he attributed what he and his wife did to "common sense."

Finally, about a year and a half after the incident, Morley realized that to tell their story was not to brag, but to illuminate the knowledge and skill of nurses. And he began to talk about his and his wife's actions. His nursing colleagues had nothing but appreciation for his decision to break his silence. The broader community responded with equal respect. He and his wife and daughter received the Order of Australia, the country's highest award. A scholarship was founded in the name of their late son Ben for members of the College of Emergency Nursing who are engaged in research and education in emergency preparedness and continuity management.

In an article he wrote, "The World Is Loud but Nurses Remain Silent," Morley entreated his colleagues to speak up. "Any event that affects the health and well-being of a nation or group of people should gain a public comment from the nursing profession," he argued. Failure to do so, he contended, makes the public think "nursing is ill-equipped to offer an opinion." Morley called on his colleagues to "to be more vocal for the benefit of our profession, our society and other societies." He continued:

In this respect, that is being silent, I must confess I am no better. My wife and I were the only health professionals at ground zero when those two massive explosions occurred. My wife and I assisted in the retrieval of victims from those night-clubs, set up a triage point 120 meters away and began front-line management. We personally treated over 55 victims, 25 of whom were critically injured. On our return to Australia we were interviewed and asked how we managed to be so resourceful. The first time I was asked this question, I answered rather poorly saying, "It was all just common sense really." The fact is there was nothing common sense about it at all. Our response was remarkable and life-saving, and reflected years of critical care nursing expertise.

Through trial and error of subsequent interviews we now take the opportunity to express the incredible expertise that one gains over a career in nursing and also feel compelled to express political opinion. It's highly important for us as humans and as nurses to state our belief that violence, whether perpetuated by an individual or a government, is a solution for nothing. We believe that violence merely serves to exacerbate the original problem. I ask you as my peer; is Iraq more stable, is the threat of terrorism now gone, now that our country has participated in the war upon that nation?

It is not correct for nurses to view such events as non-nursing issues and thus, although important, as not a part of the core issues that nurses discuss or upon which we make political comment. Where issues affect the health and well-being of a nation or group it is incumbent upon us to form an opinion and voice it publicly. . . . It is the public voice of nursing that increases our capacity to hold a greater share of power in shaping policy and public opinion.

I am concerned less about the fact your opinion may differ from mine than I am that you and other colleagues have nothing to say at all. Be vocal, express your opinion publicly and within professional journals. Nursing must start to talk before it can expect to be heard."[16]

PART II
Communicating with the Media and the Public

Chapter 6

How the News
Media Work

Look at newspapers, popular magazines, television news, or Internet sites and inevitably you will encounter health information and news. Today people have unprecedented access to research and other materials that used to be available only to health practitioners. Studies suggest that many Americans rely on the media and the Internet as their *primary* sources of health information. As a National Health Council report put it, "The media have become an integral member of America's health care team."[1]

Many cultural, political, and economic factors have contributed to the media's unprecedented power to inform and influence people about their personal health and health care. Nurses cannot afford to ignore or underestimate the role of the traditional and electronic media in shaping the public credibility and prestige of nursing.

A Brief History of Health News

For most of human history, people have been at the mercy of deadly diseases and epidemics. It's not surprising that public health was front-page news in the first North American newspaper—*Publick Occurrences Both Forreign and Domestick*—whose first and only issue appeared on September 25, 1690. "Epidemical Fevers and Agues grow very common, in some parts of the country..." the newspaper reported and followed with another, more reassuring item: "The Small-pox which has been raging in Boston, after a manner very Extraordinary, is now very much abated" (p. 11).[2]

The power of the press to influence health care policy is hardly a recent phenomenon. In 1721, half of Boston's 10,500 inhabitants were infected with "the small pox," and hundreds were dying. Convinced that the theory of immunization was sound, Dr. Zabdiel Boylston began inoculating residents, including his own children. Despite positive results, many citizens, including physicians, were outraged that someone would intentionally infect people who might then become carriers. James Franklin, the brash publisher of the newly launched *New-England Courant,* (whose brother Benjamin worked for him as a printer-apprentice) crusaded against the practice by printing diatribes against the Puritan leaders who supported Boylston. No one will ever know whether Boylston's vaccine would have stopped the smallpox onslaught because the public frenzy Franklin helped to unleash curtailed the experiment (p. 34).[3] It took another seventy-five years before Edward Jenner's development of a safe cowpox-based vaccine in England laid the foundation for widespread immunization.

In recent decades, dramatic medical and surgical breakthroughs such as antibiotics and organ transplants have stimulated media and popular interest in medicine. The first heart transplant surgeons, for example, received so much publicity they became household names. Publishers of medical journals also grew more sophisticated about how to present new medical interventions to the media and the public.

A parallel development fueling health coverage was the rise of the women's movement and its revolt against medical paternalism. It may be hard to believe now, but when the Boston Women's Health Book Collective published its first version of *Our Bodies, Ourselves* in 1969, the book was considered a radical, underground document because it urged women to investigate how their own bodies function. In the 1980s, people with acquired immunodeficiency syndrome (AIDS) proved the power of patient activism when they confronted medical, research, and governmental institutions and demanded information and a greater commitment to fighting the disease. Since then, other health activists, notably those concerned with breast cancer, have learned how to get media attention to further their goals. Even the U.S. government seemed to put its imprimatur on this kind of patient activism when it issued a special stamp to help fund breast cancer research.

The global debate about allocation of health care resources became such a big story in the 1990s that one journalist declared, "Health care has supplanted once-trendy subjects, such as the environment, to become the hot topic for coverage."[4] Conflicts over how to finance health care, problems with access and delivery, shortages of health care personnel, and disputes over the roles of government and business in the health care systems still drive this area of coverage. As physicians and nurses have less time to spend with patients, and as patients question the motives and morale of their health care providers, the public is demanding more health information from media sources. Today, increasing numbers of people are using the Internet to ferret out health information. While it appears that more people are getting information for themselves and relying less on professionals, professionals play a critical role in this information spiral because they are needed as sources and as interpreters of complex reports and data.

Advertisers—not just reporters—are happy to provide extensive information about health issues. But the recent withdrawal of a number of medications from the marketplace because of safety concerns raises the question about the trustworthiness of information supplied by those with a vested interest in selling their products.

Where People Go for Health Information

While television remains the most popular medium for news, the Internet, according to a 2005 report by the Kaiser Family Foundation, is "an increasingly important resource for informing decisions about health and health care options."[5] A survey of older Americans found that less than a third (31 percent) of seniors age sixty-five or older had ever gone online, but that more than two-thirds (70 percent) of those fifty to sixty-four years old had done so. The Internet was fifth on a list of media sources of health information for seniors but first for the baby boomer generation, ranking higher than television or books.[5]

The Internet is a big place. For media companies, it is one more medium for distributing information. But it is also a grab bag of material from unverifiable sources. "Some sites may provide inaccurate or incomplete information, and consumers who fail to consult their providers may endanger their health," the Kaiser Family Foundation warns.[5]

The Broad Scope of Health Care Coverage

In this book we are primarily concerned with the news media and how they report on health care. When we speak of the news media, we are referring to the coverage that results from the practice of journalism. Journalism may be disseminated via any of the traditional or new media including print, electronic, and digital media. However, whether the specific medium of communication is newspapers, magazines, radio, television, or the World Wide Web, the role of the journalist is "to find, gather, organize, explain, interpret, and disseminate the news, ideas and opinions of the day to an ever-increasing audience," and to do so with accuracy and fairness (p. 44).[6] By definition, journalism is a dynamic process. The name itself derives from the old French *journal*, meaning daily. The timeliness of journalism is also captured in the word *news*—something that is "new." Advances in communication technology have sped up the process even further.

Today, competition for audiences is blurring the line between news and entertainment. As media companies merge into giant conglomerates, there are fewer divisions among the various types of media. Print reporters are in TV. TV stations have Web sites. The newspaper has a TV broadcasting station on site. A search engine such as Google compiles reports from various national and international media. Nevertheless, the function of the journalist is to give people the information they need to make informed decisions as citizens and, increasingly, as consumers. Journalists receive an overwhelming amount of material from interested parties. It is up to them along with their editors and producers to decide what is credible and worth passing on to their readers and viewers.

Advertising and public relations communications, on the other hand, are referred to as "controlled" communications because they are under the control of the corporations and organizations that create and pay for them. Their purpose is to influence directly what people buy, do, or believe.

Although advertising and public relations campaigns represent vested interests, they can be helpful to the public. Indeed, in Chapter 8, we urge nurses to be more actively engaged in public relations to benefit both nursing and the public welfare. Keep in mind, though, that the goals of advertising and public relations are different from those of journalism. This is why pharmaceutical companies, despite spending enormous amounts of money on direct advertising, still make a full-fledged effort to get their products mentioned favorably in the news. A news story that talks about the efficacy of a drug carries the imprimatur of truth, while an ad stating the same thing is expected to be taken with a grain of salt.

News Media Coverage of Health Care

Health care reporting has many facets. One reporter might cover health care policy issues out of a national capital, while another reporter might cover health care legislation and regulation that occurs on a state or provincial level. A business and economics writer might track corporate activities or labor actions within the health care industry. Another reporter might focus on a branch of that industry, such as biotechnology or pharmaceuticals. A medical writer is likely to be responsible for reporting on research studies published in medical and other scientific journals. The same writer might also report on problems with patient care. Yet another might do human-interest features on patients' experiences with illness, on health care trends, or on interesting approaches being taken by individual physicians or nurses. A large newspaper is also likely to have an editorial writer who specializes in health care. Columnists with a broad range of interests might write about health care from time to time.

Television is by far the most popular news medium. Even so, it is important to pay attention to newspapers to understand what constitutes health care news. Major daily newspapers cover a broad range of health topics more regularly and in greater detail than most television news programs. Television news staffs often look to local or national newspapers for direction on what stories to pursue. But television coverage veers toward those events that have a strong visual component and away from issues, like health policy, that require in-depth exploration.

Many of the reporters who end up covering stories on health care are not specialists in the field. One of the conventions of journalism is that reporters with no particular expertise in an area are often assigned to take on complex stories and produce them in a very short time. Even reporters who cover a health beat may venture into unfamiliar territory.

A Day in the News

By looking at health coverage on one heavy news day, you can get an idea of what is newsworthy and why. On March 24, 2005, we looked at health care-related stories in two major newspapers, the *Boston Globe* and the *New York Times*. The two newspapers produced a total of sixteen health-related items—six ran in the *Globe* and ten in the *Times*.

Breaking News

On this day there were two breaking health-related stories reported on both newspapers' front pages. The biggest story concerned the case of Terri Schiavo, a woman in a permanent vegetative state who had been on life support for fifteen years after suffering cardiac arrest. This end-of-life case mobilized unprecedented legal and political action in the United States. The story concerned a protracted fight between Schiavo's husband and parents over whether her feeding tube ought to be removed. By jumping into the legal proceedings, the U.S. Congress and religious conservatives made what might have been a private dispute an enormous public issue with significant legal, political, and medical ramifications.

The *Times* ran a front-page article on the parents' appeal to the U.S. Supreme Court to have Schiavo's feeding tube reinserted, and devoted two-and-a-half inside pages to the continuation of the main story and sidebars to additional stories related to the subject. The newspaper also carried five letters to the editor about the Schiavo case from readers. The *Globe* made the appeal its lead story and ran almost a full page of additional material inside the paper.

Ellen Goodman's syndicated column in the *Globe* and Maureen Dowd's column in the *Times* focused on the politics of the case.

The other story that ran on the front page of both papers concerned a troubled teenager who three days earlier had killed five students, a security guard, a teacher, and then himself on the Red Lake Indian reservation. A *Times* headline referred to the mental health issues: "Signs of Danger Were Missed in a Troubled Teenager's Life." The *Globe* reported on mental health, poverty, and other ills on reservations, in a story headed "Reservation Where Ten Died Has Long Known Pain."

Other health-related articles that day were about health care policy and health research. There was one health care business article, and one article we classified as human interest.

Health Care Policy News

As health care costs around the globe escalate—particularly in industrialized countries—private insurers, government health programs, and politicians and policy makers are trying to cope with costs and increasing demand for health services and medications.

On our sample day, both newspapers ran stories about a move by India to amend its 1970 patent act in a way that would make it more difficult for the world's poor to get "low-cost copies of expensive Western medicines" (in the words of the *Boston Globe*). The *Times* featured this story on its front page, and the *Globe* put it inside its first news section.

A journalist would regard the India health care story as newsworthy because it has several of the factors or "news values" that constitute newswor-

---

News Values

Timeliness: something just occurred.

Prominence: an "important" person, corporation, organization, or institution was involved.

Currency: the event is part of a larger continuing debate or discussion.

Impact: the event or issue affects a lot of people.

Conflict: individuals or groups are competing or fighting with each other.

Scandal or wrongdoing: the activities are unethical or illegal.

thiness. These include timeliness (the announcement just occurred), prominence (India is a prominent player in the manufacture of drugs), currency (there was an ongoing political debate about the cost and availability of drugs), impact (millions of poor people around the world would be affected by this action), and conflict (it pits the interests of poor people against corporate profits).

For months the news media had been concentrating on the Bush administration's proposals to privatize a portion of Social Security and, as critics pointed out, ignoring far more sweeping changes in funding for the U.S. Medicare system. On our sample day, the *Times* noted this with its story: "Medicare Outlook Called Direr than Social Security's." The story was based on a report to Congress by the trustees of the Social Security and Medicare programs. Reports from authoritative bodies like this constitute a major news source.

The Business of Health Care

The business sections of newspapers frequently carry reports on companies involved with health care, biotechnology, and medical equipment and products. This section is also where reports on employment disputes between nurses and hospitals or government payers usually appear. Business sections cover the business ramifications of health policy and health care reform proposals. These sections, along with the U.S.'s premier business newspaper, the *Wall Street Journal,* and other business publications, see their main audience as investors and business people.

On our sample news day, the *Globe* ran a front-page business-section story entitled "Partners Chief Issues Call to Cover Uninsured." This story was prompted by an article that had just appeared in the *New England Journal of Medicine* written by the president and the chief executive of the Partners HealthCare System, described as "the state's largest and most influential physician network." According to the *Globe,* the executives "issued a public appeal for higher taxes and mandates on employers to cover millions of uninsured Americans." The *Globe* reporter followed journalistic conventions in writing this story. She sought out and incorporated comments from people knowledgeable about health care or health policy, none of whom was a nurse.

The front page of the *Times* business section also featured a story on employer-based health insurance. The headline was "G.M. to Seek Cuts in Health Benefits." The story told of the car manufacturer's intention to save money by cutting health care benefits to union workers. The piece was substantial in length and carried reactions from union members and corporate sources including the rival automaker, Ford. The *Times* ran a second story inside its business section on the India patent change that emphasized the impact on pharmaceutical companies large and small.

The fortunes of companies can be affected by what is said about them in the news media. This is why corporations make extensive efforts to get positive coverage.

Research News

Much health care news comes from studies published in medical journals. Health care news tends to swell midweek because the biggest medical journals, the *Journal of the American Medical Association (JAMA)* and the *New England Journal of Medicine* (NEJM), publish on Wednesday and Thursday, respectively. The *NEJM* was the source of one story in each newspaper on our sample day.

The *Globe* carried a story titled "Sleep Apnea Kills at Night, Study Says." This was based on a *NEJM* report on a Mayo Clinic College of Medicine study that found that patients with sleep apnea are more likely to die from heart attacks at night while sleeping than during the day.

The *Times* ran a second *NEJM*-prompted story, "A Study Ties Loss of a Child to Mental Ills." It was based on a Danish study that found that parents who have lost a child are at increased risk for hospitalization for depression, schizophrenia, and drug or alcohol abuse. The report said that such problems had been generally unrecognized and that this large and rigorous study would call attention to the needs of grieving parents.

Medical reporters for such newspapers as the *Globe* and *Times* monitor the *NEMJ* and *JAMA* and perhaps other journals such as *Circulation* and *Annals of Internal Medicine* for newsworthy studies. They either subscribe to or receive complimentary copies of the journals.

But reporters usually need more than the studies to do a credible job. The journals, which want coverage, accommodate them by providing additional information and resources on their Web sites. Some of this material, such as advance reports, access to experts, and audio and video packages that can be used for radio and television reports, might be available exclusively to journalists, but a remarkable amount is accessible to the general public.

For example, with debate raging over the Terri Schiavo case, the NEJM posted an "early release" notice on its homepage two days before the publication of its March 24, 2005, issue. Advance material from the issue included a "Perspective" on the Schiavo case written by a noted palliative care expert, Timothy Quill, MD. The piece could be downloaded as a PDF file. It was accompanied by an audio interview with Quill by public radio reporter Rachel Gotbaum. In ordinary language, Quill described what it means for a person to be in a permanent vegetative state, how families might respond,

Hard and Soft News

Reporters traditionally classify news as being either "hard" or "soft." A timely event or breaking story is *hard news.* It has to be covered right away, and if it isn't, it will cease to be news. *Soft news* generally lacks a pressing time component and, therefore, has a much longer shelf life.

These categories are no longer as discrete as they once were. A political campaign, for example, produces news in both categories. Reporters will do hard news stories on who won a political contest and soft news features, perhaps about the candidate's personal history, as sidebars to the main story.

what happens when there are disagreements between family members about what to do for the patient, and what important questions courts need to examine in such a dispute.

In addition to being reported on as breaking news, medical studies are the basis for general or analytical pieces on illnesses, treatments, and preventive health measures. On Tuesdays, the *New York Times* has a science section that covers developments in all aspects of science including biomedical innovation and research. Within the section is a subsection, "Health and Fitness" that focuses more specifically on illnesses and treatments. It contains stories, based on medical studies, on a wide range of health subjects. In the March 22, 2005, issue, for example, one story countered the prevalent notion that diseases are readily spread on airplanes.[7] Another dealt with the implication of genetic testing for breast cancer,[8] and yet another explored "a bizarre and extremely rare psychiatric condition" in which patients with healthy limbs seek amputation.[9] The subsection features essays by physicians about patient care issues or their personal experiences. It also carries Jane E. Brody's popular column, "Personal Health." Reporters like Brody, who write regularly on health issues, "save string" on subjects they think will be newsworthy by keeping a file of journal articles, other materials, and the names of experts in the field.

Human Interest and Features

Feature articles and human-interest pieces that deal with illness, treatment, or the experiences of health professionals appear frequently in newspapers and magazines and on radio and television. Although none appeared on our sample news day, the illnesses of prominent people have become a staple of health care coverage because they provide a peg on which to anchor a news story. It was worldwide news when former President Bill Clinton had heart bypass surgery and when he subsequently returned to the OR to have scar tissue removed. When the late actor Christopher Reeve was injured in a riding accident, the media were filled with stories on spinal cord injuries. Reeve's progress and problems were charted through the remainder of his life. When he died, the media once again discussed the medical challenges of such patients. Although Reeve died from complications of a bedsore—a nursing problem if there ever was one—nurses were not featured prominently in news reports. The medical treatment of victims of sensational crimes—such as the "Central Park jogger," a woman who was brutally attacked and left for dead in Manhattan—can stimulate continuing coverage. Such stories often cast physicians as heroes working to save the lives of these seriously injured patients. The nurses, who care for the patients and also save their lives, are rarely seen.

What Is News?

Journalists don't sit down with a list of news values and refer to it each time they get a phone call or press release. Their training teaches them that some things are "stories" and some aren't. Developing a news sense can help nurses plan successful media strategies.

Say a specialty organization notes that its members are having greater difficulty providing quality care because of staff cuts in hospitals and clinics. But the organization is wary of rocking the boat, scaring people, or turning off corporate sponsors. Nonetheless, they feel they have to do something to assuage their members. So they get together with a media consultant to plan a press conference.

"What's the peg?" the consultant asks.

The organization's leaders proudly pull out a policy statement declaring that every patient has a right to quality care by specialist nurses in their field. But the statement contains no reference to the current problems in the health care system, no specific examples of how patients suffer because of declining care, nor any statements from nurses about their difficulties providing quality care. Although health care financing is a constant concern, the statement doesn't consider how the care it advocates would be financed.

Is the statement news?

The leaders of the organization are dismayed when the consultant says there is no "story" in a policy statement that essentially says the members are nice people in favor of good care.

What might be a story?

1. People Talking about the Problem

The organization could ask working nurses to come and talk about the obstacles to giving good care in institutions more concerned with the bottom line than patient care. The organization could ask patients to come and talk about the suffering and sense of abandonment they experienced due to cuts in nursing care. Outside policy experts could be asked to provide historical background and suggest appropriate policy approaches to the problem.

2. Documentary Evidence

Studies documenting the link between widespread cuts in nursing care and increasing problems for patients would help make the case. If no specific studies had been done, the nurses could use research findings connecting nursing care to better patient outcomes in general. Studies linking adequate staffing and the prevention of decubitus ulcers, falls, and urinary tract infections might be relevant. So would studies demonstrating nurses' ability to help patients cope with the physical and emotional suffering associated with the disease and the side effects of treatment.

A news conference that incorporates these elements would be considered more newsworthy. It would attract attention to the work of the organization's members and give the organization itself a dynamic, courageous, and compassionate image. In Chapter 9, we highlight a number of ways nursing groups used the media to spotlight critical issues and concerns.

Organizations are often fearful that if they expose system problems and take strong positions about them they will alarm and/or alienate the public. But it is also alarming to the public when caregivers don't forcefully advocate for patient care. Moreover, timid approaches like issuing saccharine apple-pie-and-motherhood "policy statements" or weak responses to political initiatives won't attract public attention for nurses.

To determine what is news, you have to weigh whether organizational positions are relevant to the public. Organizations produce reams of instant waste paper, or prompt journalists to hit the delete button on their computers, when they disseminate news releases that say they are for or against something (the President's proposal to insure all uninsured children, an expert's plan to reduce violence against women) with no other news elements. This sort of release doesn't have a prayer of producing coverage.

News releases with no news values are not necessarily benign interventions. They can harm nursing's public image by depicting nursing organizations—and, by extension, nurses—as standing on the sidelines watching events set in motion by others. Press releases larded with phrases like "we applaud this," "we share these concerns," "we have a long-standing commitment to," "this is congruent with our long-standing goals," "we have a long history of advocating on this issue," positions a group as a spectator rather than as an actor, or communicates, "We're just nice nurses."

A news release that articulates a stance on an important and timely issue and suggests or announces that the organization is going to mobilize to do something about it (thus containing the news value of impact) casts your group as a participant with influence or power. For example, in February 2005, the American Nurses Association sent a letter to Secretary of Defense Donald Rumsfeld expressing its concern about the possible role of registered nurses in the Iraqi prisoner abuse scandal and asking for further investigation into any possible unethical actions by health care professionals. It sent a copy of its letter, which cited the "ethical code that requires registered nurses to protect and advocate for all patients," to a selected press list.

Monitoring the News Media

As you read newspapers and magazines, listen to the radio and watch television, go to bookstores and libraries, and visit various Web sites, take notes on who is reporting on health care and the way they do it. Even if you are working with public relations professionals, you still need to be familiar with how health care and nursing are reported and where new opportunities for coverage lie.

Newspapers

A good place to start is with your newspaper's health page or section. What do you see there? Does the section usually lead with a health care feature story? What kinds of health subjects and people are covered? Who writes these stories? Do you see the same bylines repeatedly? The bylines may tell you whether the writers are staff members or freelancers who contribute features. Is there a masthead (usually a small box) in the section that names the reporters who do health reporting? Are their e-mail addresses given?

What other kinds of health items appear in the section? Is there a columnist who specializes in personal health and fitness? Is there a regular column on research findings? Who writes it? What are the sources of the reports? Are most from the *New England Journal* and *JAMA,* or are other sources cited frequently? Are nursing journals ever cited? Does the section carry service items? Is there a calendar of health-related events like lectures, support group meetings, and schedules of health screenings or immunizations?

Keep in mind that a regular newspaper section needs stories to fill it. Yes, there is competition for that space, but there is also a big demand for good stories. This presents nursing with an opportunity.

As you are monitoring the newspaper, look at other features and columns that might reach audiences of specific interest to you. For example, some newspapers, especially those in geographic areas with large older populations, have "age beat" features or columns. These might be the ideal place for stories on home care, preventive care, and research in geriatric nursing. Don't overlook the business section. The *Milwaukee Journal-Sentinel's* Joel Dresang was covering the labor beat in 2003 when he became intrigued with the implications of the nursing shortage. He followed three nurses in a Milwaukee hospital for a two-part newspaper series and related stories and audio interviews for the *Journal-Sentinel's* Web site.[10]

The lifestyle section or Sunday magazine could be a good place for a story on a nurse who is doing interesting, unconventional work, who has written a book, or has had an unusual experience.

Columns or articles in which a clinician presents a perplexing medical mystery and solves it are popular. The *New York Times Sunday Magazine* has such a column entitled "Diagnosis." Are nurses ever in these columns?

Opinion Sections

In major newspapers, the last two pages that face each other in the first section are generally reserved for editorials, letters, and opinion columns. The

Your Turn

Monitor the news sections. The first section of a newspaper usually contains a mix of national, international, and local "breaking" news. What makes these stories news? Are they based on an announcement, the release of a report, a hearing, a press conference, an event? Does the newspaper have a separate regional, metropolitan, or local section? What kinds of health stories appear there? Who writes the health-related news?

Monitor the business page or section for health news. How heavily does it cover the health industries in your area? Is this where stories on nurse staffing or on labor disputes appear? What have you observed that suggests opportunities for nurses to raise their public profile?

editorial page will be found on the left and the op-ed (for opposite editorial) page on the right. Some papers put op-eds, or short opinion essays, on the same page as the editorials. Op-eds may also appear in other parts of the paper such as the business or health sections.

An editorial page typically contains more than one editorial. They are written by editorial writers—staff journalists assigned to the editorial page—or by the editor of the page. Editorials usually have no byline because they are supposed to present the newspaper's opinion and recommendations rather than those of individuals. By concentrating on opinion, the editorial staff has a different function than the reporting staff and is separate from it. On a large newspaper, editorial writers might specialize in certain areas such as health care. Editorial writers have to be alert to breaking news and must understand the elements of complex issues. Their job, after all, is to write timely editorials that both summarize and take stances on these issues.

Newspaper editorials can have an effect in the community, particularly when they are well argued and call for specific policy or regulatory actions to deal with pressing problems. It should be borne in mind, however, that when editorial writers make policy recommendations, they do so in accordance with the editorial page's political philosophy. For example, in the United States, the *Wall Street Journal* is noted for editorials that are among the most conservative in journalism. They differ markedly from those in the *Boston Globe*, which tends to be more liberal. Papers throughout the world take a political stance on their editorial pages.

Most newspapers run letters to the editor, usually on the editorial page. Writing a letter to the editor is one of the quickest and most effective ways to draw attention to nursing expertise (see Chapter 10).

The op-ed page also bears scrutiny. This is the home of the 500- to 850-word essay. The work of local or syndicated columnists addressing political and public issues often appears on this page. But many newspapers also take op-ed submissions from nonjournalists who have a strong point of view. Some newspapers run a "guest" op-ed once a day or several times a week. Although many op-eds are sober considerations of policy, sometimes the form is used for "slice-of-life" pieces in which a person takes you through his or her experience to illuminate a timely topic. (Chapter 10 will show you how to write op-eds.)

Also pay attention to your newspaper's weekend magazine and any health magazine special issues. Feature writers may be open to delving into a particular area of health care. For example, the *Boston Globe's* Paul Hemp followed one pediatric oncology nurse in her work and produced a substantive Sunday magazine piece on this area of nursing.[11]

Some of the most innovative pieces in the media are done by freelancers. An example is Darcy Frey's vivid account of doctors' and nurses' efforts to save a twenty-six-week-old infant at Boston's Brigham and Women's Hospital and his exploration of the ethical and emotional issues involved in such medical care.[12] His *New York Times Magazine* article provoked letters from hundreds of readers.

Don't overlook the work of local or national columnists, some of whom are syndicated nationally and internationally. In the summer of 1999, author Mordecai Richler devoted several of his weekly *Montreal Gazette* columns to supporting the nurses on strike in Quebec. Other columnists, such as Bob Herbert at the *New York Times* and Eileen McNamara at the *Boston Globe,* have built their reputations by writing forcefully about cases of injustice, inequality, or abuse of power. Crusading columnists take sides and often revisit issues that capture their attention. By reading various columnists, you can determine if your project or campaign might pique their interest.

While it is important to monitor your local newspaper, it is also useful to take a look at the national newspapers that influence policy makers and the national news agenda. The two largest newspapers in the United States are the *Wall Street Journal* and *USA Today*. The *Wall Street Journal* is must reading for investors, business people, policy makers, and anyone following major industries such as health care and communications. Large newspapers influence the news chain by selling some of their articles to smaller, understaffed newspapers. Thus, a *New York Times* article might appear in an Oregon paper.

Newsmagazines

The newsmagazines *Time, Newsweek,* and *US News & World Report* in the United States and *Maclean's* in Canada circulate nationally and internationally. All of these cover health care to a greater or lesser extent. *US News,* for example, does an annual cover story on the "best" hospitals in the United States. All of these magazines may do special health issues that attempt to pick up on health care trends.

In 2005, *US News & World Report* published a provocative special health issue, "The New Healers," that featured a picture of an oncology nurse on the cover and the headline, "Who Needs Doctors?" The issue captured health care delivery problems in such articles as "Doctors Vanish From View: Harried by the Bureaucracy of Medicine, Physicians are Pulling Back from Patient Care." It covered the work of individual clinical, advanced practice, and research nurses in a piece titled "Nurses Step to the Front."[13]

In general, weekly newsmagazines place breaking national and international news in the front, business news in the middle, and such subjects as education, science, health or medicine, books, sports, theater, and film in the "back-of-the-book." Stories dealing with health care might appear in more than one section.

Newsmagazines' correspondents operate out of regional bureaus. Look on the masthead that lists these bureaus and see which one is closest to you. Usually a story in your area will be covered by a correspondent from that bureau. These bureaus also keep up with the major industries in their area.

Wire Services

Wire services make it possible for news breaking in one place to travel to news outlets throughout the world. Newspapers, newsmagazines, radio and television stations, and networks all subscribe to one or more of the major wire services such as the Associated Press (AP) and Reuters.

The AP is the biggest wire service in the world. Its reporters and photographers cover the globe and transmit stories to member news organizations. It also receives and sends out articles and photos that originate with its member news organizations.

Thanks to wire services, local coverage does not necessarily remain local. Nursing strikes in Ireland and Poland reached audiences in North America, and coverage of North American nursing strikes was transmitted to other countries via the wire services.

News organizations also get specialized material—such as health care advice columns and features, comic strips, editorial cartoons, and crossword puzzles—from news syndicates.

Audio and video news stories and features also go to television and radio stations via satellite services. Public relations sources supply their materials to the news media via computer, personal outreach, and special public relations "wires."

Television News

Television reports tend to be heavy on health tips and brief interpretations of new studies on popular health subjects like obesity, nutrition, heart disease, and diabetes. They pick up very quickly on any disease or health problem a celebrity has. Policy issues, financing, and in-depth reports on the health industry appear more often on public television—the Canadian Broadcasting Corporation, the British Broadcasting Corporation in the United Kingdom, and the Public Broadcasting System in the United States and local public television stations—than on commercial television, with a few exceptions such as ABC's *Nightline*. Some cable channels are fond of fast-paced reality programs set in emergency and operating rooms and in the offices of cosmetic surgeons.

Television "newsmagazine" shows regularly do mini-dramas based on people's experience with illness and health care. A staple of television morning shows is the weeklong series—how to lose weight, how to manage seasonal allergies, how to keep fit after fifty. When you are watching television news, note the kinds of health stories that are covered and who covers them. Seek out serious news analysis such as that offered by the *Lehrer NewsHour* on U.S. public television.

Television relies heavily on interviews to put the story into perspective. Therefore, at least some of the working nurses and academic nursing experts who want to describe nursing practice or expose problems in health care must be willing to speak on the record. A television staple is the expert who, in a few well-chosen words, can provide a snappy sound bite. Television formats are created with the "flighty" viewer in mind. Faced with distracted channel surfers, television uses tight, dramatic formats to keep the viewer tuned in. When you're trying to make a point for this medium, practice doing it in short, quick, pithy sound bites (see Chapter 11).

Radio and Television Call-In Shows

Radio and television so shape our understanding of public events that they are central to any media strategy. While radio and television offer many opportunities for nurses to be seen and heard, the ubiquitous call-in show has become an essential tool for those who are trying to influence public opinion and public policy.

Up and down the AM and FM radio bands, talk radio is available on

Your Turn

As you watch television, note how visual images dictate the presentation. Simply put, television depends more on pictures than words to convey the news, while newspapers use more words than pictures. A story without many visual possibilities, or one that the local television station has failed to get video on, has less news value to the television news organization than to the newspaper. As Richard Salant, former president of CBS news, said: "You see more fires on local television than you do in the newspapers because fires look better on television" (p. 14).[14]

Think of what images could be utilized to convey your work and to help people visualize what you do.

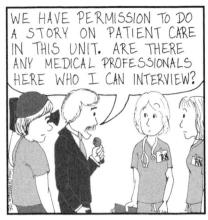

WE HAVE PERMISSION TO DO A STORY ON PATIENT CARE IN THIS UNIT. ARE THERE ANY MEDICAL PROFESSIONALS HERE WHO I CAN INTERVIEW?

Sonia Oppenheim, www.familycomic.com

hundreds of stations in North America. At the same time, the call-in show has emerged as a genre on television, especially on cable stations.

Instead of debating political issues in their town and city halls, most people now turn on the radio or television to sample political discourse. All political candidates use these shows to make their campaigns visible and viable.

Talk radio does have an advantage over television. It can enter workplaces and automobiles more easily than television. Thanks to the cellular phone, commuters stuck in traffic can join the broadcast conversation.

Talk radio and television are especially influential in mobilizing people against something. As Robert Blendon, professor of health policy and management at the Harvard School of Public Health told us, "Talk radio is very important. A large share of people listen to it. And some people who listen to talk radio write letters and take direct action that moves Congress."

When call-in shows deal with health care, nurses ought to be on them both as experts and as callers.

Radio News

Most commercial radio stations offer brief news breaks at the top of the hour from "rip and read" wire copy. "Today news on commercial radio is limited to syndicated headline reports and opinionated talkers," says Lawrence K. Grossman, a former president of the Public Broadcasting System and of NBC News.[15] Still commercial radio offers some opportunities if you're able to do some research and find the people who are interested in intelligent discussion, says publicist Gail Leondar Wright. Those interested in an exploration of the issues should turn to public radio, which, she says, is "the best forum for a respectful exchange of ideas and the most effective medium for sparking public discourse that might fuel social change."

Magazines

There is a magazine for practically every subject on earth. Think creatively as you peruse them. City magazines, for example, frequently do health care service pieces such as naming the "best" physicians in the city, or rating HMOs, hospitals, and other services in the area. (You might ask editors to do stories on the best nurses or nursing services.) Some of the best monthly and quarterly magazines are published by universities for their alumni. They also venture into health issues, particularly if the university has a medical school, a nursing school, and a school of public health. Many publications put out by religious groups also carry features on health care.

Women's and self-help magazines offer almost unlimited potential for stories on health care. Women's magazines have dozens of columns on personal health and fitness. Health and self-help magazines target niche audiences—young men, older men, women between the ages of twenty-five and forty, and, of course, aging baby boomers. There are ample opportunities for nurses to present their perspectives on health and illness in these publications.

Books

Books are critical to informing the public about health care. Every year new books dealing with health care policy, medical practice, specific illnesses and treatments, and other aspects of personal health arrive on the market. Some books that feature heroic medical dramas are written by professional writers. Physicians themselves write others. These are "trade books," meaning they are marketed to large, popular audiences by commercial presses like Simon and Schuster in the United States or McClelland and Stewart in Canada. Increasingly, university presses publish trade books and market and distribute them just like commercial presses.

Physicians have written about their work with particular categories of patients—those with AIDS, cancer, or neurological problems, for example. Doctors who have suddenly discovered what it's like to be a patient themselves have written books on their experiences. One of these, *A Taste of My Own Medicine,* by Ed Rosenbaum was adapted into the film *The Doctor* starring William Hurt. Many physicians have described their personal journeys, as did Rafael Campo in his memoir of his life as a doctor, poet, and homosexual in *The Poetry of Healing.*

As a group, physicians appear to be confident enough about themselves, their profession, and their audience to write about the profession's shortcomings. Books like *The Lost Art of Healing* by cardiologist and Nobel Peace laureate Bernard Lown, Eric Cassell's *The Nature of Suffering,* and Arthur Kleinman's *The Illness Narratives,* among others, take other doctors to task for their failure to listen to patients and for abandoning the humane roots of their profession.

The public learns about new books through reviews and publicity. Reviews appear in newspapers and in general and specialty magazines, on the Internet, and on TV and radio. Publicists send new books to radio and TV news and talk shows hoping to get a mention or even a whole program devoted to the book. Physicians, and the people who write about them, often appear as guest authors, experts, or commentators. Physicians get a lot of mileage out of this kind of public exposure. It reinforces the public perception that medicine is health care.

Books about and by doctors are attractive to publishers because there is a large market for them both in the medical profession itself and among the general public. "When we go to sign up a book, the first thing we try to figure out is how big the guaranteed market for the book is," says Steve Hubbell, a former senior editor at Henry Holt.

The medical profession has helped to create and maintain a physician market for books by running book reviews on all sorts of topics in its major journals. For example, the largest-circulation medical journals in their respective countries, the *New England Journal of Medicine,* the *Journal of the American Medical Association,* and the *Canadian Medical Association Journal,* publish book reviews in every issue. So does the health policy publication *Health Affairs.* These reviews are not limited to books on clinical practice. Physician reviewers and others critique a broad spectrum of books. Memoirs and novels are candidates if they are about health care and medicine. They even review the occasional book about nursing. The *New England Journal* also lists the books it has received that week but could not review.

These journals, knowing that their readers want current information, publish reviews in a timely fashion recognizing that many books have a short time in which to find an audience. Medical journals thus make it possible for publishers to reach the medical market, which, in turn, makes potential books on doctors and medicine more appealing to publishers.

Nursing in North America offers an even larger potential market than medicine. That potential, so far, has not been realized. Too few books by nurses are candidates for publication beyond the nursing press because they are not written for broad audiences even within nursing. When nurses do write books for the mainstream audience—or when other authors write books about nursing or nurses—the nursing profession inadvertently hampers these books from easily reaching the nursing market.

Most nursing journals either do not regularly review books or limit their reviews to books on clinical practice. Few review health policy books, journalistic nonfiction, memoirs, or fiction. Indeed book publicists have told us they have been ignored or rebuffed by editors of nursing publications when they've attempted to bring specific books by or about nurses to their attention. Some nursing journals review books months or sometimes years after their publication. This doesn't help the sales of a worthy book nor deliver timely information to readers.

Nursing journals and other nursing publications rarely run book excerpts, profiles of authors, or interviews with either the author or subject of a book. Publishers trying to reach nurses through nursing publications must buy advertisements. Ads are costly, and these days mainstream publishers try to spend as little money as possible on promotion. All of this makes nursing a difficult-to-reach market.

When considering whether to publish a book by or about a nurse, the first thing a publisher will ask is how many nurses there are. "Any editor would sit up and take notice when an author tells him that a potential market is more than three million nurses in the US and Canada," Hubbell says. "But the question an editor will ask is 'Can we reach that market?' If it's a market of people who don't read, or if it can't be reached, then it's not a good market. It doesn't matter how large a potential readership is if we can't reach those readers."

A difficult-to-reach market of millions has serious consequences for the profession. When nurses don't hear about books of interest to them, they don't buy them. When they don't buy these books, this registers on the sophisticated computer tracking system publishers employ to determine who buys their books, where they buy them, and when. The lack of a viable nursing market means it is difficult for a writer to find a publisher for any project on nurses or nursing. It also means that nurses get stereotyped by publishers as nonreaders.

We believe this problem can be remedied. More nursing publications could create book sections that run timely reviews and excerpts of upcoming books. Journal editors—particularly those of quarterlies—should be aware that publishers will provide them with advance galleys of a book months before its publication date so that they can assign and edit reviews expeditiously. If a book is written by a nurse or about a nurse, interviewing or profiling the authors and subjects will not only make a good human interest story, it will inspire or embolden other nurses to either write themselves or invite journalists to enter and write about their world. This will, in turn, encourage mainstream publishers to pay attention to nursing, to publicize nursing books, and even to solicit nursing manuscripts.

Through the publicity thus generated, the public will learn that nurses are doing exciting work, leading interesting lives, and thinking critically about important issues. All of this will improve not just the income of the nurses or writers who have authored these books, but the image of the profession.

The Internet

Hundreds of millions of people throughout the world now have the capacity to access the Internet. Some use it exclusively to send and receive e-mail. Some use it to monitor breaking news on the Web pages of newspapers and television stations or through the news services carried by Internet providers or search engines. Millions of people use the Web to get health information and to research specific illnesses. Internet chat rooms provide an alternative to radio and television talk shows for discussing current issues.

The Internet is reshaping how news is gathered and disseminated and the interactions between news sources and journalists. The Internet is also a powerful tool for those who want to influence what is on the news agenda and coverage of it.

Increasingly, the Web is a two-way media street. As more news organizations develop Web outlets, the Internet is a choice medium for publishing the news and commentary. It is also a place where journalists go for source material. The Web is a twenty-four–hour billboard. Journalists can get news releases, research papers, and other information from the Web, or via e-mail, and can download this material onto their own computers. Thanks to powerful search engines, reporters can come across sources that they might never have thought of. Thus, the Internet is a resource for finding experts who can speak on a topic or can be the subjects of news coverage. Journalists might locate such experts on university sites where experts are listed by subject category. Or serendipitously they may come across the posting of someone's course curricula. Organizational Web sites also list experts and speakers.

Blog sites are another way news is influenced. Many people now register their opinions, harangues, or newsworthy items in blogs (personal web logs) that are posted on dedicated blog sites or on individual Web sites or on organizational sites that carry blogs, message boards, and chat rooms. While journalists don't have the time to patrol thousands of blog sites, many check certain sites that serve as a weather vane to see what people are talking about and how opinion is moving. They can log on to chat rooms and hear what ordinary people are saying and thinking. As we'll see in the next chapters, reaching out to journalists is also a lot easier because of the Internet.

Because bloggers often trade in opinion, hyperbole, tirades, and rumor, blogs are not considered trustworthy as sources. Some bloggers produce sophisticated online publications in which sources are fully identified and cited. Bloggers are credited with exposing as forgeries documents that CBS news used to question President Bush's national guard service, which resulted in Dan Rather's early retirement and the firing of some staff members. "Blogging does give more and more people their own voice in the news. But the Web makes it harder to distinguish fact from fiction, truth from rumor, and reality from entertainment," says Lawrence Grossman.[15]

What Journalists Need

To get into the news through any of these media, though, nurses must know what journalists need to do their work.

1. Journalists need people who will talk to them. The late Kirk Scharfenberg, editorial page editor of the *Boston Globe,* often pointed out that journalists don't cover disembodied ideas, they cover people and events. They relate even the most complex stories through the voices and images of the human beings involved. Nurses will not get into the media if they do not talk to journalists. On occasion, when sources might lose their jobs or face other penalties, journalists will agree to use their information without naming them. But to do their work, and be credible, journalists require visible sources that can be quoted or put on camera.

When we've interviewed nurses for an article and even for this book, some have asked us, "Is it important for you to use my name?"

The answer is: Absolutely!

2. Journalists need multiple sources of information. Even if some of them are not obvious, most news stories have several sources of information. The story may seem to have one main source or "character," but the writer or producer has undoubtedly talked with other people about it. Sometimes a story will be centered on one person and additional sources are brought in to comment on what the primary source has said or done. Some sources, such as public relations representatives, provide "background" but might never be quoted.

3. Journalists need knowledgeable sources. This doesn't mean that a nurse must have a PhD or be an administrator to be considered knowledgeable. If the story is about the provision of nursing care and you're a caregiver, that makes you an expert. If the story is about research on a particular topic, and you do it, you're in a position to contribute your expertise to coverage.

You can always learn more about issues that concern you. If you are going to approach a reporter or know that a reporter will be talking to you, you can get the information you need to be prepared. You can gather information from nursing organizations, other health care groups, and from the Web. Do you want to know how many people suffer from bedsores in your country? Chances are if you log on to a search engine and type in bedsores, you'll be able to find that out quickly.

The American Association of Critical-Care Nurses is among those organizations that send a regular e-newsletter to members and others that summarizes pertinent research studies and supplies Web links for more information. The Massachusetts Nurses Association puts out a "Tuesday Report" that highlights health issues as well as union activities. Sigma Theta

Tau International e-mails a monthly one-page newsletter on clinical subjects to health care leaders and the media, and the Center for Nursing Advocacy e-mails frequent bulletins about how the news and entertainment media depict nurses.

We suggest that you keep a file on subjects you might want to talk about. Keep in mind that journalists don't expect sources to be omniscient. Don't silence yourself because you might not know every answer to every question that might be posed to you. You can say, "I don't know." You can recommend someone else who might know, or you can offer to find out. Then do it.

4. Journalists need events in order to justify coverage. Something happening at a certain time gives a journalist a peg for an issue. Testimony at hearings is a staple of journalistic coverage because whenever an official body investigates serious allegations, journalists have something to cover. Even the release of a report is an event. Legal and regulatory actions are also events that offer a framework for discussing issues. Journalists also rely on legal actions to tell stories because materials filed with a court may be quoted without fear of libel. Court documents provide a wealth of information about complex transactions. If you know of a relevant court case, bring it to the attention of journalists.

Many groups construct events such as marches, rallies, informational pickets, press briefings and conferences, charitable actions, and supportive statements from celebrities to give the media something to cover.

5. Journalists need sources who respect their deadlines. If you work with the press, you have to accept the fact that people will call or e-mail you at inconvenient times with requests for material or interviews. Even if journalists are working on a magazine or broadcast feature that has considerable lead time, there may be production and scheduling factors that require them to gather information quickly. If you want your issue or perspective to be covered, you have to respond expeditiously. If you wait three weeks to return a phone call, you can be sure that your information or point of view will not make it into the story. The journalist will have gathered his facts from someone else, possibly from a doctor. Moreover, faced with the journalistic equivalent of patient noncompliance, most reporters won't call you again and may not respond favorably to an overture you make in the future.

Return the phone call immediately and find out what the journalist wants. You might be able to deal with it quickly. If you are busy, ask the reporter about his or her deadline and try to arrange a more convenient time to talk. If you have a secretary or assistant, ask him or her to arrange a time for a conversation with the reporter. If you are too busy, have your assistant refer the journalist to another nurse who can help.

6. Journalists need sources who will provide them with written documentation.

Nurses must understand that journalists are concerned about making a mistake and wary of going out on a limb without written documentation. Journalists rely on validated information. Although individual accounts are essential to any good story, when a complicated phenomenon arises, data are needed to document the amplitude and effect of the trend. Hoaxes committed by reporters at the *New York Times* and the *New Republic,* as well as public criticism of the use of unattributed sources, have made editors more concerned about checking data and sources.

Do not assume that just because studies are "out there" in the nursing world, journalists know about them. Make it a point to provide journalists with such studies. Be sure to keep internal memos, correspondence, records of meetings, and any other documentation a journalist might need if you plan to go public about an issue.

However, don't e-mail massive amounts of material to a journalist and expect her to take the time to read it, print it out, or download it. As one journalist told us: "I opened my e-mail one day and found fifteen messages on the same subject from someone who wanted me to cover it. Each contained a lengthy document. My heart sank. I e-mailed back and asked them to send me this material through the mail."

If your office has too much documentation to send, you can invite a journalist to your headquarters to look at the data and talk with your experts. The Service Employees International Union (SEIU) gave *San Francisco Chronicle* journalists access to their files for a major investigation on the lack of safe needles in hospitals (see Chapter 9).

Don't ever tell a journalist—particularly one on deadline—to go to a medical library to look up material or to do an online search. Not only does this make the journalist's work impossible, it signals that you are not sophisticated about dealing with the media.

7. Journalists need someone who will interpret complex material from a specialized field so that they can understand and write about it. This means you may have to spend a considerable amount of time explaining what certain data mean or how things work in a certain environment. Journalists need to understand the standard operating procedures in your workplace or field as well as the underlying assumptions that guide your work. In others words, you have to be willing to give journalists a crash course on nursing in general and on your work in particular. You need to be prepared to answer, with grace, what you consider to be elementary or even foolish questions.

8. Journalists need someone to help them frame the story. Sometimes we really want to do a story, but we just can't figure out how to get a handle on it," former public radio editor Madge Kaplan told us. "If a reporter can't figure out how to do the story, the story won't get done."

Journalists rely on trustworthy people who will help them conceptualize an issue and structure their story. Nurses often complain—and correctly so—that most reporters frame health care stories around medicine or money and ignore care and thus nursing. No journalist can take an unusual approach to a story—that is, a nursing-centered approach—without first selling the idea to an editor or producer. The journalist has to feel confident about an unusual "frame" and sources to convince an editor that he has the right "take" on the issue. If you become a trustworthy source, a journalist may well call you and say, "Do you have a minute? I'm thinking about doing a story on *x*, *y*, or *z*. Does this make sense to you?"

9. *Journalists need sources that can summarize issues briefly and quickly and furnish the quotable quote.* The journalist's job is to reach a wide audience. To do this, journalists need sources that can get to the heart of issues in compelling, concise language. Today, the media, particularly TV and radio, depend on tight sound bites.

Reporters working on deadline often call a source, describe the story they are working on, and ask, "Would you comment on this?" Journalists really appreciate someone who will make an immediate, to-the-point comment. This is not the time to tell a journalist that he or she should read all the material you've produced on the subject and then call back with questions.

One of the things that happens when someone becomes a valued source for a journalist is that the reporter feels free to call and say, "I need a quote on this." People who are in the news a lot are there not just because they are experts on their subjects but also because they can provide a good quote at the right time.

One such source is Arthur Caplan, the director of the Center for Bioethics at the University of Pennsylvania and undoubtedly the most quoted bioethicist in the country. A lot of people deal with complex and controversial issues, but what makes Caplan special, at least to the media, is his ability to communicate in ordinary language, his affability, and his availability. Perhaps most important, Caplan isn't afraid to take a strong stand on the most hotly debated issues, and to do so in pithy quotes.

In an MSNBC commentary, prompted by the news that a sixty-six-year-old woman, the oldest ever, had given birth, Caplan noted, among other things, the sexual disparity involved in this issue by asking: "So, how old is too old? Was Larry King of CNN too old when he had a child with his seventh wife at age 70? Was Cheryl Tiegs who had twins at 52 too old? . . . James Doohan (Scotty from the original *Star Trek*) who had children at 80? Donald Trump, 58, now making menacing reproductive noises in the context of his widely publicized third marriage? It is very hard to draw an absolute line and say what age is too old to become a parent, although the idea of Donald Trump mating makes the project a particularly compelling one."

Then, true to form, Caplan took a stand:

"My proposal is that anyone over 65 who is single should not be allowed to use reproductive technology to have a child. If you have a partner, then your total ages should not be more than 130. And if you are a female at or near 55 years of age and hoping to become pregnant, then you should only be allowed to use reproductive technology if you can pass a rigorous physical examination. At age 66, forget it . . .

"In light of the high risks at stake, the medical profession or state legislators should act [to impose limits]. The race to create the world's oldest mom should be declared over."[16]

10. *Journalists need sources who can give them accurate information.* Journalists' stock and trade is the who, what, when, where, why, and how of things. They need accurate and verifiable information. Journalists want to make sure they have the correct spellings of names and institutions, the correct dates and times when events occurred, and the correct words from a quote. This may mean they will call you after you've already spoken to them to check their information.

Journalists usually condense volumes of information into brief reports. This means that your studies and data will be tightly summarized. From what might have been a lengthy discussion of an issue, the journalist might use only a one-sentence or one-paragraph quote. The journalist may paraphrase your words. Or they may not cite you or refer to you at all but use your comments to inform their reporting.

Scrupulous journalists will call or e-mail you to ensure they haven't altered the meaning or added an incorrect nuance when they've simplified, condensed, paraphrased, or translated jargon into ordinary language. Welcome such calls and take the time to help a journalist get the story right. Nurses often complain that journalists always get it wrong. But if you refuse to be available or are impatient, defensive, and irritable and act as though talking to a reporter is a terrible imposition, you're contributing to inaccuracy.

11. *Journalists need sources who will stay in the game.* Even if you establish an excellent working relationship with members of the media, there will still be mishaps and frustrations. At times you may be misunderstood or misquoted. In simplifying complicated issues, journalists will make errors. You might be quoted out of context. In some instances, you, your specialty, and profession may get negative coverage. That's the risk of voice and of being "consequential."

You may spend an hour talking to a journalist and not even get mentioned in the report. The journalist—or his editor or producer—may decide not to do the story. Television documentary or feature producers are notorious for picking a source's brain, implying they will interview them on air, and then going off in a different direction or finding someone else to put on their show. Journalistic demands may prove disruptive to your work and home life. When you try to help and seem to get nothing out of it, this can be infuriating.

But even if your efforts don't produce immediate results, they can have a long-term impact. Most journalists have never talked with a nursing expert. They don't know how to cover nursing, how to think about nursing, or even the first question to ask about nursing. They don't know that nurses can comment intelligently on many health care matters beyond nursing practice. Many don't even know there is anything intelligent to say about nursing practice. When you take the time to talk to a journalist, you're building a foundation for recognition and respect for yourself and your profession.

For example, we recently talked with a television producer who was trying to figure out whether he could do a documentary proving that cutbacks in hospital staff were undermining quality care. The producer knew of an incident that seemed to connect understaffing with serious patient injuries. But was there enough there for a story? he wondered. He didn't have any nursing sources. "I have no idea how to get into nursing," he confessed.

We talked with him repeatedly over the course of a week and gave him the names of several nurses to call. He talked to the nurses and was impressed with their knowledge and accessibility. Two weeks later he told us he wasn't sure he and his colleagues had enough substantiation to go ahead with the project. Whether the project gets on track or not, we know this producer has a more positive view of nursing than he had before. His new knowledge of nursing can lead him to future stories, and he can share his knowledge with the journalists he works with. That, in and of itself, is a positive outcome of a nursing intervention.

Chapter 7

Reaching Out to the News Media

A lot of people believe that if they are doing something newsworthy, the news media, for better or worse, will discover it. Popular culture supports this misperception by depicting reporters as relentless in their pursuit of good stories.

But reporters aren't Lone Ranger–like figures who independently decide what to go out and cover. In general, interested parties draw journalists' attention to significant developments and issues. According to public relations professors Todd Hunt and James E. Grunig, an estimated one-half to two-thirds of news stories are "source-originated."[1]

Often the source is a public relations (PR) professional who works on staff or as a consultant for corporations, government departments and agencies, organizations, or individuals. When investigative stories appear (such as the *San Francisco Chronicle*'s series on needle-stick injuries described in Chapter 9), they've often been inspired by whistle blowers, individual sources, or organizations that have enough factual material to convince reporters, editors, and producers that the potential story was good enough to justify the time and expense of an in-depth probe.

While they are eager for good stories and try to stay on top of newsworthy developments, most journalists aren't looking for scandals. Journalists don't want to be a tool of promoters and marketers, but they also don't want to miss significant stories.

Journalists operate within a network of relationships. One way journalists discover an issue is by seeing a story on it reported by another news outlet. Then they may have to scramble to do their own story on that subject. Another is when they are contacted by those they consider to be credible or on top of things in a given field. These "sources" reach out to them by sending them press releases via e-mail or fax, calling them to underscore the significance of a particular event, inviting them to meetings, press conferences, and organizational or professional conferences, furnishing them with re-ports and studies, arranging discussions with them and their editorial boards, meeting them for lunch or for a drink, and schmoozing with them periodically.

It's impossible to overestimate the value of developing relationships with members of the media. If you provide journalists with a steady stream of usable tips and accurate and pertinent information, and respond in a timely fashion to their needs and questions, at least some of your issues and concerns will be reported on.

Nurses' Outreach Lags

Why aren't nurses in the news as much as they ought to be? Because nursing has not done the media outreach that other groups have.

To find out whether nurses were taking advantage of Internet avenues for outreach, we spent an hour—a lot longer than a journalist might be will-ing to devote—looking for nursing commentary on then then-breaking and continuing story of Terri Schiavo.

The Schiavo case was a nursing natural. It offered commentary oppor-tunities for nurses who had studied withdrawal of hydration and nutrition or who had cared for patients who were in a persistent vegetative state. We looked for nursing commentary by putting keywords into Internet search engines and by looking at the Web sites of nursing organizations.

When we asked Google for information on "Terri Schiavo" on March 26, 2005, there were 2,620,000 references. When we narrowed the search to nursing and Schiavo, we found precious little. At the American Nurses Asso-ciation site, we found a notable exception, a position statement by President Barbara Blakeney saying that Congress and the President, by intervening, "have acted inappropriately in this case." The statement urged people to pre-pare advance directives or living wills.

FOR IMMEDIATE RELEASE
MARCH 23, 2005

CONTACT:
Joan Hurwitz, 301–628–5020
Cindy Price, 301–628–5038
Carol Cooke, 301–628–5027

American Nurses Association Statement on the Terri Schiavo Case. Statement Attributed to Barbara A. Blakeney, MS, RN, President

The Terri Schiavo case raises complex and emotional issues about the end of life. The American Nurses Association (ANA) recognizes the difficulty of the situation, however, ANA has consistently upheld the right of patients, or if the patient is incapacitated, the right of the designated surrogate, to decide whether to submit to or continue medical treatment.

As nurses, we are ethically bound to assist our patients in maintaining control over their lives and to help them preserve their dignity. The ANA believes that it is the responsibility of nurses to facilitate informed decision-making for patients and families who are making choices about end-of-life care. The Code of Ethics for Nurses specifically outlines the nurse's obligation to protect the patient's right to self-determination and the role of a designated surrogate in situations where the patient lacks capacity. In this case, Terri Schiavo's physicians, over many years, have declared her to be in a "persistent vegetative state." Furthermore, there is evidence that Terri Schiavo expressed her wishes not to have her life artificially maintained under such circumstances. ANA believes the Congress and the president have acted inappropriately in this case. It is unfortunate that Terri Schiavo has now become the symbol of so many political agendas.

The positive outcome from this case is that it raises the public's awareness of the importance of discussing end-of-life issues with family members and underscores how an advance directive, a living will and/or durable power of attorney for health care, clarifies and provides evidence of the wishes of an individual regarding end-of-life decisions. ANA encourages everyone to have an advance directive in place. Advance directives are controlled by state law and vary by state. A federal law, The Patient Self Determination Act of 1990, requires that most health care facilities provide patients with information about advance directives and ask patients about the existence of advance directives. Physicians, nurses, social workers and attorneys are often resource persons in the community who can provide information and guidance concerning advance directives.

My thoughts and prayers go out to the family of Terri Schiavo. I recognize that this is an extremely difficult situation. I wish Terri Schiavo the dignity and peace she so deserves and that we would all wish for ourselves and our own loved ones at the end of life.

Sources: Code of Ethics for Nurses with Interpretative Statements, 2001
http://nursingworld.org/ethics/chcode.htm
Ethics and Human Rights Position Statement: Nursing and the Patient Self-Determination Act, 1991
http://www.nursingworld.org/readroom/position/ethics/etsdet.htm

The ANA is the only full-service professional organization representing the nation's 2.7 million registered nurses through its 54 constituent member nurses associations. The ANA advances the nursing profession by fostering high standards of nursing practice, promoting the rights of nurses in the workplace, projecting a positive and realistic view of nursing, and by lobbying the Congress and regulatory agencies on health care issues affecting nurses and the public.

There was not a word about Schiavo at the Web site of the Hospice and Palliative Care Nurses' Association. There was no information for the public on what palliative care or palliative care nursing is and no list of experts that journalists could contact. The Web site, like many organizational Web sites, was devoted to membership issues and services. The American Association of Critical-Care Nurses had nothing on Schiavo on its Web site.

We also checked medical Web sites. The American Medical Association (AMA) had an updated position statement on end-of-life care and numerous ways to access medical experts. The American Academy of Hospice and Palliative Care Medicine didn't post a position on the Schiavo case but did have a definition of palliative care and palliative care medicine. The site was useful in finding medical experts on end-of-life care. A click on its "speakers bureau" listed doctors and the topics they could speak on—for example, hydration and nutrition—and their geographic area and institutional affiliations.

It's a problem for nursing that so little exists on the Internet to lead journalists to nurse experts. Without active outreach by nurses, the default position of most journalists will be: If you need an expert, call a doctor. This was reflected in the coverage of the Schiavo case. The story raised the issue of how people should deal with family conflicts about end-of-life care. In much of the coverage, families were urged to discuss their end-of-life concerns with their doctor and to use him or her as a knowledgeable mediator in family conflicts. Next to doctors, the leading players in these stories were family members, lawyers, and judges. Nurses were largely invisible.

From this coverage, one would never learn that nurses caring for critically or terminally ill patients might have something to say that could enlighten and inform. The visible nurses were two who allegedly cared for Schiavo and who gave what one judge deemed to be "incredible" testimony about her condition.

We also checked letters to the editor and op-eds in several newspapers. Were nurses and nursing organizations utilizing this opportunity to enter the debate about end-of-life care? They were not.

A rare exception to this nurseless view was a letter to the editor in the *Boston Globe*. The writer argued that "To think that the politicians and the courts are better stewards of the healthcare of our most vulnerable members of society flies in the face of everything that I have seen during my two decades in medicine . . . This is an insult to the dedicated physicians, nurse practitioners, physicians assistants, and nurses who have devoted their lives to providing health care." The letter was written by a physician.[2]

The First Step: Deciding Whom You Want to Reach

It is important to define whom you want to communicate with so that you can determine how you will communicate. For example, there are audiences or "publics" that you can reach without the news media. If nurses are trying to explain a new protocol to the clinical personnel in your hospital, they might distribute a memo via e-mail. If patients with a particular illness need to know some specifics about self-care, nurses might prepare a brochure or sheet of instructions that can be taken home or a videotape that patients could watch when they come in for treatment. You might do a mailing to people in your neighborhood or community to advertise new services at your health care facility. You might also purchase newspaper ad space or commercial time on local television. You might send a notice about the program to a variety of electronic Listservs. Of course, you would post the notice on your organizational Web site.

At the same time, you might want to tell the public about some of these things via the news media. This means that you will have to convince intermediaries—journalists and television and radio producers—that your information is newsworthy, so that they will turn it into a story that reaches the public.

Before you pick up the phone or send out a news release, consider what audience you are trying to reach and which media outlets would be most effective.

Perhaps you would like people in your community to know about a nursing program that can serve them. In that case your best vehicle for communication might be weekly community newspapers. You can increase the chances of external media picking up on your program if you provide information on it on your institution's Web site.

Perhaps you will be rallying in front of your state or provincial capitol to support new legislation or regulations. You'll want as much publicity as possible throughout the state so that citizens can tell their political representatives to support your cause. Therefore, you will want to expand your efforts to the media beyond the capital. You'll want to get your advance press releases to newspapers, television, and radio throughout the region. If you're working with a PR professional, he or she should know whom to contact and how to distribute information. You can find out yourself by contacting the capital news bureau and/or pressroom.

Whether you are seeking a national audience or a local one, you will need an up-to-date media list.

Experienced PR specialists who work with nurses have contacts with the press. We discuss the role of public relations practitioners more fully in Chapter 8. But whether you employ a PR person or not, nurses must establish and tend relationships with reporters who can be helpful to them.

Introducing Yourself

You introduce yourself to the media by bringing them something that's newsworthy. A letter, e-mail, press release, or phone call describing a newsworthy event or project can be your introduction. But how do you know if what you are doing is a story? Stand back and look at your work with some objectivity. Have you seen articles or television reports on similar topics? Have you seen a gap in the discussion that you can fill? Does your activity have some of the news values outlined in Chapter 6? Is your issue relevant to the broader audience that a media outlet would reach? Can you present your work in a way that makes its value and relevance obvious? If your work is narrowly focused, ask yourself if it can be generalized. Is it poignant, dramatic, quirky, offbeat (as in man-bites-dog)? Does it fulfill a need? Does it challenge conventional wisdom?

Considering the newsworthiness of all sorts of activities and issues is a constructive activity for nurses inasmuch as the goal is to fully integrate nursing into health care coverage.

Reaching out with a variety of events, activities, or innovations will make a broad range of nursing expertise more visible. It will open the door for nurses to become regular news sources on health matters far beyond those related to hospital working conditions. Professional organizations can broaden the public view of nursing by becoming as vigorous in promoting stories about nursing practice as collective bargaining groups have been in exposing threats to nursing and patient care.

Any research study or program that enhances patient care is a possibility for a nursing angle. When a study reported in the *New England Journal of Medicine*, for example, discusses parental reluctance to stop futile aggressive treatment for children with advanced cancer, nurses have an opportunity to show how they help parents make difficult decisions. Another good patient care story is nurses' involvement in understanding why heart attack patients delay going to emergency rooms and their efforts to teach patients which symptoms call for immediate treatment. A recent story highlighted in *JAMA* had to do with an innovation initially hailed as a solution to medication errors. Author Ross Koppel and his colleagues found, however, that the computerized physician order entry (CPOE) systems created as many errors as they prevented.[3]

This issue has a nursing component that people should know about. Among other things, CPOE systems are supposed to prevent errors that occur when doctors handwrite orders. However, these systems change the process of medication ordering. Isolated with his or her computer, the physician is more likely to enter orders without the input of nurses. The contextual knowledge the nurse has of the patient—such as what drugs they are sensitive to, what has been tried and failed, and what doses of the drug are appropriate—is lost in the electronic ordering process. Although the study didn't cover the nursing component, its publication offered an opportunity for nurses to explain to the public the role nurses play in safe drug ordering and administration.

Opportunities

Be alert to your particular issues surfacing in the media. When the media focus on a dramatic or even sensational event, be prepared to jump in. Periodically an event—a tragedy, a new study, a court decree, a new law—catapults an issue to the top of the news agenda where it receives intense coverage for a while. Nurses must take advantage of these openings even though some may be created by controversial or unpleasant events.

In such cases, the press is looking for credible sources to present various sides of the issue. If you want your side to be represented, you need to be ready with appropriate spokespeople.

In many instances the kind of events that will propel an issue are predictable. If a blue-ribbon panel has been considering a particular problem or policy, most likely the media will cover its findings. Such groups make a point of packaging their reports in a media-friendly way. Journalists will report on a high court's decision in a controversial case. They usually know in advance when the court will hear the case. The agendas of legislative, policymaking, and regulatory bodies can be monitored to predict when news-making

> *"You can leverage awareness campaigns that already exist. February is heart and stroke month. That's an opportunity to show what nurses do in this area. In May, maybe you can get a reporter to follow a nurse during Nurses' Week."*
>
> —Karen McCarthy, director of strategic communication for the Canadian Nurses Association

developments will occur. Journalists often get advance notice of when new research findings will be released. As a profession concerned with health care issues, nurses can stay abreast of these processes and be ready with their stories when the issue is about to crest again.

Focusing the Story

Pretend that you are the reporter trying to tell the story. You'll have to come up with something that can serve as a peg.

Say you are a geriatric nurse practitioner who has initiated a program to release nursing home residents from physical and chemical restraints. Your work could be a timely and relevant story. One peg for a story could be how the health of the residents improved at a particular nursing home where this program was implemented. A research study that shows how this approach prevents suffering and saves money could also be a peg for a story.

For nursing, the point of outreach is to show, in a newsworthy way, how nurses understand patient needs, prevent problems, enhance public health, offer alternative policies, and meet contemporary health needs. It is not to get free publicity for your institution. Reporters will resist that kind of overture.

Unless you are working with a journalist who has demonstrated his or her knowledge about nursing, assume ignorance. The natural tendency of many journalists is to credit physicians with any improvement in health care delivery. That's why you'll have to highlight the nursing component of the story.

Assembling Written Materials

Reporters generally expect to see something written on the story you are trying to pitch. It makes their job easier and more efficient if they have something to read that gives the gist of the story.

Your Turn

Think of a story or two that you could pitch to journalists stemming from your work, institution, practice, research, or expertise.

How does it relate to a timely, important concern or event?

Try spinning the stories in various ways so that the same development can be connected to patient safety, health care financing, or treatment and care for specific groups.

Most of the time this is a brief letter, a news release, or both. Sometimes a news release will be more effective if backed up by research studies or news clippings that have appeared elsewhere. Reporters may pay more attention if they see that other journalists have found the topic newsworthy. However, they will be looking for their own angle.

If you are mounting a campaign like one of those described in Chapter 9, you will want to e-mail materials to journalists or assemble a media kit. A kit is merely a two-sided pocket folder containing pertinent materials. It can be distributed at an event or mailed to journalists. If your organization has sufficient resources, the cover can be specially designed and printed. If you have fewer resources, you can buy folders at a local office supply store and print labels on your computer. The kit might contain some or all of the following:

- A press release or letter that piques the interest of the reader, briefly gives the facts, conveys a sense of immediacy, explains the relevance of the event or issue, and tells how to contact the people involved.
- A simple fact sheet that lists important points or background events or developments.
- A fact sheet or brochure that describes the organization or organizations sponsoring the event or involved in the issue.
- A "backgrounder" or briefing paper that gives in-depth information. If the backgrounder includes statistics or research data, the sources must be listed in a bibliography.
- Biographical sketches of the important players including information on how to contact them.
- Copies of articles that have appeared in the press and brief descriptions of television reports and features that have been done on this or a similar topic. You could include a compact disc (CD) or a digital video disk (DVD) on the subject; however, in general, it is more efficient for a journalist to sift through papers than to view other media.
- Copies of pertinent research articles. You can give a journalist a list of links to these articles so they can download electronic copies.
- A question-and-answer sheet that suggests and anticipates key questions and gives the answers.

News Releases

News releases are the primary tool for making contact with journalists. Journalists often claim they barely look at the scores of handouts that cross their desks or their computer screens. The reason journalists toss or delete the great majority of the news releases they receive is because the form is greatly abused by corporations peddling products and by organizations that indiscriminately crank out statements containing nothing remotely newsworthy. Many releases are poorly written, have no local angle to interest news outlets in a given area, and have no news elements.[4] But when a release is informative and targeted properly, it can be effective in various ways.

A weekly newspaper, for example, might run an excerpt from or even an entire news release on programs of interest to the public or on people in the community. Most of the health service announcements in such publications—a blood drive will be held, flu shots will be administered, a blood pressure screening clinic is operating—originate in news releases. So do many ideas that can be developed into good stories.

Larger newspapers, and radio and television news organizations might use the information for an immediate story. They might cover an event because of a release. A reporter might hold on to a release for use in a future story. She might add the cited expert sources to her address book. Since journalists receive so many news releases through various avenues, they scan them rapidly, usually reading only the headline and the first paragraph.

Neil Rosenberg, the former health editor for the *Milwaukee Journal-Sentinel*, described his modus operandi this way: "I don't know what other reporters do—I'm sure some see Eli Lilly on the envelope and throw it out—but I open every piece of mail. Ninety-nine percent of it is cast aside. I'm like a fisherman; I'm looking for an idea that I can make into a very good story. Some days I get skunk and some days I get muskie."[5]

If journalists don't see a peg for a story right at the beginning, you can be sure they won't spend their time wading around in your verbiage. Like the newspaper reader or the television viewer, they want to know what the story is right away. Then they can decide if they're interested.

Format

Even though many news releases are sent via e-mail and are posted on Web sites with splashy four-color designs, the form remains pretty constant. News releases must be typed on standard letter-sized paper. Use a business typeface, not script or a peculiar font. Put a 1- to 1½-inch margin around the page. Double space the lines or, if you are trying to save paper, at least the first couple of paragraphs. Single-spaced paragraphs should have double spacing between them. It's best to use only one side of the page. Limit the release to one to three pages. One to two pages is preferable.

Note the reprinted news release from the Canadian Association of Schools of Nursing (CASN). The release responded to the announcement that $2 billion in federal money would be allocated to the provinces and territories for health care. In just five paragraphs, the release adroitly linked Canada's "crisis in nursing" to the need for earmarked nursing-education funds.

Federal Budget 2004: Clear Funding for Nursing Education Needed

News Release

Ottawa, ON—March 23, 2004—Despite committing $2 billion for the provinces and territories for healthcare and $665 million to improve Canada's readiness to deal with public health emergencies in today's budget, the federal government still needs to earmark funds specifically for nursing education if the current crisis in nursing is to be resolved.

Last year, the federal budget committed money to increase the number of students in health disciplines, but the number of nurses continues to be a tremendous challenge when it comes to delivering adequate healthcare to Canadians.

By 2008 Ontario alone anticipates a loss of 30,000 nurses due to retirements. This year only about 3,400 nurses will graduate from Ontario registered nursing programs. Nursing programs continue to have large applicant pools of well-qualified men and women—many of which have to be turned away because of a shortage of professors and facilities to support their learning. This means that specific financial support for nursing schools and increasing the number of professors for the many areas of nursing is crucial if we are to end this crisis in the supply of nurses and nurse practitioners.

"Without an adequate, well-educated and well-prepared supply of nurses, and enough teachers to teach the growing numbers of nurses needed to fill the gaps, further investments in the healthcare system will fail to meet the needs of Canadians," says Dr. Carole Orchard, President of CASN.

"Increased financial support for nursing education and research will result in higher levels of university prepared nurses required to care for our citizens in hospitals, in homecare and in communities. But will the schools of nursing actually receive any of the necessary funding?" asks Wendy McBride, Executive Director of CASN.

The Canadian Association of Schools of Nursing (CASN) is the national voice of nursing education, research and scholarship, representing 90 schools across Canada. CASN is also the official accrediting agency for university nursing programs in Canada.

For additional information, please contact:
  Tara Tosh
  Communications Officer, CASN
  Tel: (613) 235–3150 ext. 23
  E-mail: ttosh@casn.ca

Components of a News Release

The news release typically contains the following components:

1. *Letterhead.* Your news release should be printed on letterhead with your name or the name of your organization, mailing address, phone number, e-mail addresses and Web page location. You can create this yourself on a computer if you don't have a printed letterhead.

2. *Contact information* goes at the top of the release. After the word Contact: put the name(s) of the person or persons that a journalist can contact to verify the information in the release and to learn more. Be sure to give their day and nighttime phone numbers and/or pager numbers, and include e-mail addresses.

3. The standard news release identifies itself with the word NEWS or NEWS RELEASE written in large type at the top of the page.

4. Next a *release time* is given. Almost always you just type FOR IMMEDIATE RELEASE, which means the news organization can use the material as soon as it comes in or any other time. Type in the date the release is being issued. Some releases, reports, and studies will have an "embargo" date on them. This sort of release is intended to give journalists time to prepare their stories, but they must wait to publish or broadcast them until the specified time and date.

5. A *headline,* or tag line, goes at the top to catch the interest of the recipient. This is not the headline that the news organization will use. They will write a headline that fits their own format.

Note the headline on the news release that follows from the University of Pennsylvania. Like a news headline, it captures the point of the news release. It uses two present-tense verbs ("find" and "die") to convey not just timeliness but urgency. Try to make your headline dynamic. Employ active verbs when possible. Like the "Finds More Patients Die," in the headline, your release should make as strong an assertion as you accurately can. This is not the time to fudge the issue.

EMBARGOED: Not for release until October 22, 2002, at 4pm EDT

News
Release

Contact: Joy McIntyre Telephone: 215.898.5074; 5673 Fax: 215.573.2114
E-mail: joymc@nursing.upenn.edu
PDFs available at www.nursing.upenn.edu

Penn Research Finds More Patients Die in Hospitals with Lower Nurse Staffing

Philadelphia, PA—In the first study of its kind, University of Pennsylvania researchers have determined that patients who have common surgeries in hospitals with the worst nurse staffing levels have an up to 31% increased chance of dying. More nurses at the bedside could save thousands of patient lives each year, as reported today in *The Journal of the American Medical Association (JAMA).*

The Penn researchers found that every additional patient in an average hospital nurse's workload increased the risk of death in surgical patients by 7%. Patients with life-threatening complications were also less likely to be rescued in hospitals where nurses' patient loads were heavier. The findings impact the national legislative agenda. More than 20 states have enacted or are considering nurse staffing legislation.

For every 100 surgical patients who die in hospitals with 4:1 patient ratios, the number that would die in hospitals with higher ratios would be:

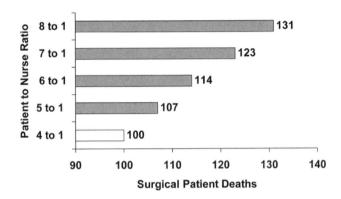

"Nurses report greater job dissatisfaction and emotional exhaustion when they're responsible for more patients than they can safely care for. Failure to retain nurses contributes to avoidable patient deaths," said Linda Aiken, PhD, RN, director of the Center for Health Outcomes and Policy Research at the University of Pennsylvania School of Nursing. "Patients facing planned hospitalization should inquire about nurse-to-patient ratios and choose their hospitals accordingly." Hospital nurse staffing levels vary widely, usually from four patients per nurse on most unit types to up to 10 or more.

Specifically, the Penn nursing researchers found that:

If all hospitals in the nation staffed at 8 patients per nurse rather than four, the risk of hospital deaths would increase by 31 percent, roughly translating to as many as 20,000 avoidable deaths in the U.S. annually. Some 4 million surgeries like the ones studied are performed each year.

Having too few nurses may actually cost more because of the high costs of replacing burnt-out nurses and higher costs of caring for patients with poor outcomes.

Adding two patients to a nurse already caring for four, increases the risk of death by 14 percent; adding four increases the risk by 31 percent.

"It is clear that nurses are saving lives," said Dr. Aiken. "Nurses are the front line of surveillance and early detection of potentially life-threatening problems."

The report, "Hospital Nurse Staffing and Patient Mortality, Nurse Burnout, and Job Dissatisfaction," concluded in the October 23/30 issue of JAMA: "When taken together, the impacts of staffing on patient and nurse outcomes suggest that by investing in registered nurse staffing, hospitals may avert both preventable mortality and . . . problems with low nurse retention in hospital practice."

The study, funded by the National Institute of Nursing Research of the National Institutes of Health, examined data collected from 168 hospitals, 232,342 surgical patients, and 10,184 nurses in Pennsylvania from 1998 to 1999. The researchers examined data on relatively common general surgeries (e.g., gall bladder), orthopedic surgeries (e.g., knee or hip replacement), and vascular surgeries, excluding cardiac surgery such as coronary bypass. Some routine but emergency surgeries were included, such as appendectomies.

The Lead of the News Release

Like a news reporter, never save the best stuff for last. Construct your news release like a news story—inverted pyramid style with the foundation for the story at the top. The first paragraph of a news story or news release is called the *lead*. Like the headline that preceded it, a good lead is a small story all by itself.

A summary lead is the most common type. It usually contains several of the five Ws—who, what, where, when, why (and sometimes how). It does it in one or two sentences. Look at the first sentence of the Penn release: "In the first study of its kind, University of Pennsylvania researchers have determined that patients who have common surgeries in hospitals with the worst nurse staffing levels have an up to 31% increased chance of dying."

- The "what" of the lead is the problem: patients at risk of dying.
- The "why" in this case is the nub of the story: poor nurse staffing levels.
- The "who" refers to researchers at Penn.
- The "where" is hospitals with the worst nurse staffing in the United States. But the location of the researchers is also important.
- The "when" is now.

When writing the lead (and the rest of the news release) don't be melodramatic or flowery. Write the way reporters do—in simple declarative sentences in the active voice.

Body of the News Release

Stick to the facts. Use direct quotations to introduce subjective material, opinions, or allegations. Get in a pithy quote as soon as possible. Quotations are essential to your news release because they allow you to inject "voice," opinion, vigor, and, sometimes, colorful language.

A direct quotation is a good way to make a strong point as experts did in the third paragraph of the Penn release. In the fourth paragraph of the ANA release, Barbara Blakeney makes a personal comment that highlights the poignancy of the issue.

Direct quotations for news releases are anything but spontaneous. The speaker herself might construct one or a public relations person might write it with her or for her. But the quote is carefully tailored to deliver maximum impact and still sound like something the person would say. It should also be conversational and sound as though it was spoken rather than written.

Direct quotations must be attributed to the speaker. Inexperienced writers tend to put the name and the title of the speaker before the quotation. But unless the name is the most important element, advance attribution slows down the eye and lessens the impact of a dramatic or colorful quote. Look at the quotations in this book and at those in newspapers. You will see that the sentence often begins with the quote and finishes with the attribution. Also note the punctuation. In the United States, quotation marks go after the punctuation at the end of a quote.

The *Elements of Style,* by William Strunk Jr. and E. B. White, is an excellent, inexpensive source of information on grammar and style. This slim volume is a classic reference guide used by tens of thousands of students and writers.

A speaker is credible in a news release (or a news story) because he or she has expertise or authority. How is that fact established? By the person's title, position, work, and experience. Nurses often worry that being "just a nurse" is insufficient. For the working nurse, doing the work of nursing is precisely the credential that matters.

Note how Linda Aiken and Blakeney are identified. Aiken has many credentials. She is a PhD, a professor, a researcher, and an RN. Blakeney is an RN with a MS degree. By using the RN credential, both are emphasizing its importance to the subject matter. They are nurses who are authorities.

Be sure to highlight your nursing credentials when you are sending out a news release. In some instances PhDs let their institutions send out news releases with no explicit mention of their connection to nursing. Their name appears as Mary Smith, PhD, or as Dr. Mary Smith. This not only contributes to the invisibility of nursing, it actually risks giving medicine credit for nurses' accomplishments. Although PhD nurses may feel strongly that they have earned their "Dr." title, in this society they will generally be mistaken for physicians unless they make an extra effort to identify themselves as nurses.

When you are writing your news release, plan to spend about half of your time on the headline, the lead, and the first direct quote. These are the most important elements, and it's reasonable to rewrite them until you have reduced them to the essentials. The rest of the release elaborates on the main points. For an inverted-pyramid-style release, you don't need a snappy ending. Just end before you start belaboring the points. Remember the release is designed to be a quick read.

Organizations often end their releases with a boilerplate paragraph that describes the function of the organization, such as in the CASN and ANA releases.

Accuracy

Make sure your news release is accurate. Check and recheck all of the names and other proper nouns for correct spelling. Then have someone else proofread your release. It is astonishing how easily errors can creep in and not get caught. Your credibility could suffer if there are errors in your release. It is a maxim in journalism that if a name is incorrect, then nothing else is believable.

It should go without saying that a release must be honest as well as accurate. You are expected to present information from your point of view. However, you must not mislead, exaggerate, or distort the truth to build your case.

Broadcast Releases

Radio and television stations can use information in a standard news release to create a report, but they cannot broadcast it as is. If they are interested in doing a report based on the release, they will convert its essential information into a short, broadcast-style piece. When you are trying to get media attention for timely events—such as a major nursing demonstration at a state or provincial capital—it might make sense to fax a two hundred–word (one minute long) broadcast release to radio and television stations around the state or province. Small radio stations might use it, although they will probably tighten it further. You would want to include an extra sheet with exact information on where and when the event will take place, and the names of participants on the scene who will be available for interviews.

For broadcast writing, simplify the issues. Write for the ear, not the eye.

Use short sentences. Use colloquial language. Avoid hard-to-pronounce words. Don't use abbreviations. Follow a difficult name with phonetic spelling in parenthesis so that the reader will know how to pronounce it. Spell out numbers. By all means use participants as sources of information, but in most cases, paraphrase instead of quoting directly; for example, "Stella Smith is among the registered nurses who say a safe staffing law will improve the care of patients in area hospitals."

Distribution

There are times when you will want to broadly distribute a news release to news organizations. You might fax or e-mail your release to all the news organizations in the area or, for a fee, get it onto a PR newswire that goes to news organizations. Even with widespread distribution, targeting is important. You will want to make sure that appropriate reporters get their own copy.

In some instances, it's better to contact just a few reporters. If you have a story that you think would be of particular interest to a certain feature writer, columnist, or writer who focuses on health policy issues or would fit the format of a television newsmagazine show, put your efforts into making a good match. Tailor your presentation to that reporter or media outlet.

Write a short letter to accompany your materials explaining who you are and why your project might make a good story. If you are pitching to television, make sure you can provide good visuals, an interesting setting, and people who will appear on air to tell their stories.

If you are seeking attention for new research or for your participation in a health care campaign, don't make the mistake of thinking that a journalist will read your release just because it is on your Web site. Some journalists may check your Web site for news. But nursing organizations and institutions can't assume that journalists regard them, as they do some medical associations, as news producers that require routine monitoring. Even those journalists who pay attention to nursing advise nursing groups not to use materials posted on their Web site as a substitute for assertive outreach to journalists.

Helen Palmer, health correspondent for American Public Media's *Marketplace*, a national daily business radio program that frequently covers health care, explained to us, "I don't have time to check out Web sites on the off chance that there might be news on them, and I certainly can't check out Web sites that I don't know exist. Groups that have something to say need to find out who the journalists are they want to reach and make sure they let us know when they have something that is newsworthy.

"The California Nurses Association and the Massachusetts Nurses Association are very media savvy. They e-mail and fax news releases. The MNA also e-mails and faxes its 'Tuesday Reporter.' It's very interesting. If I were looking for something on a nursing issue I'd be very likely to go to the California Nurses Association or the Massachusetts Nurses Association because they've made themselves known to me. If I wanted to track down a nursing issue or run something by someone on nursing, I believe they would find me a nurse who could talk to me on that particular issue. Diana Mason at the *American Journal of Nursing* is also very proactive. These are people who are very responsive, media friendly and media savvy."

Phone Calls

When you send a news release or a letter containing the elements of a news release, follow up with a phone call. You can't be sure the reporter has read his or her mail, paid attention to the specific piece, or even received it. That phone conversation will allow you to elaborate on the initial communication, or present it if the release hasn't been read or gotten lost. Don't call just to ask if the reporter received it. Use the opportunity to sell the story.

If you've made phone contact with the reporter before sending the release or letter, it is wise to have a written version before you so that you can make your points on the phone without getting flustered.

Getting through to a reporter is not always easy, but keep trying. Many news organizations have voice mail systems that act as fortresses. Try to get the direct extension for the people you want to reach.

Just as patients need advocates in the hospital, nurses need advocates in media institutions, as the following story illustrates.

A freelancer who writes for major media outlets received a press release and a follow-up phone call about a nursing program at a hospital she had written about in the past. Intrigued by the program, she called an editor at the city newspaper, offering to do a story on the program. The editor confessed she had received the same press release, but because she didn't know much about nursing, the release went into the wastebasket. She did, however, respond to the call from a journalist she trusted and assigned her to do the story.

Arranging Meetings with Editorial Boards

One of the best ways of establishing relationships and stimulating interest in nursing stories is to meet with the editorial board of a newspaper. Editorial boards—editorial writers and the editor of the section—frequently meet with experts and community members to discuss current issues. Sometimes the reporters who cover the subject area participate in the meeting.

"For coverage of the news, we depend on our reporters. But in terms of argument on public policy, we depend on advocates to present all sides of an issue," Judy Dugan, deputy editorial page editor of the *Los Angeles Times,* told us. "When we hear the arguments and nuances of the debate, we are more able to form a solid public policy position. The lifeblood of editorial pages consists of frequent meetings with advocates."

Dugan says that those involved in the issues usually call the editorial board. "If advocates have an issue that's on the front-burner—or that should be on the front-burner—we want to talk to them. PR operators all know this and know how to arrange meetings. We try hard to get nonprofits and people who don't realize they can come and talk to us to come forward.

"But don't call to just come in and say, 'Howdy,'" she advises. "Be prepared to discuss your issue in-depth and to respond to hard questions."

If a newspaper has provided good coverage of your issue, by all means compliment them during an editorial board meeting. Poor coverage, or no coverage at all, however, can be the reason for arranging a meeting with the editorial board of a newspaper or with producers at a television or radio station.

One such meeting more than a decade ago helped attract attention to nursing at the *Boston Globe.* Under the aegis of the Nurses of American campaign, four nurses—Claire Fagin, then dean of the University of Pennsylvania school of nursing and president-elect of the National League for Nursing (NLN); Pamela Maraldo, then executive director of the NLN; Joyce Clifford, then nurse-in-chief of Boston's Beth Israel Hospital; and Nancy Valentine, then vice president for nursing of McLean Hospital—arranged a meeting with *Boston Globe* editors and reporters. They were concerned about the *Globe*'s failure to accurately depict the crucial roles nurses play in health care. They talked about what nurses do and suggested avenues for coverage. The journalists challenged the nurses to explain why nursing was newsworthy, and the nurses told them.

As the nurses spoke, one editor recalled that he had been hospitalized when he was a teenager. Like many people, he had had a positive experience being cared for by nurses, but had no broader conceptual framework about nursing. But when he told his story about his nursing care, it was, Fagin recalls, "like a light going on. The tenor of the meeting immediately improved."

That meeting and continuing overtures from the PR professionals at Beth Israel Hospital, the Massachusetts Nurses Association, and others, helped to establish a relationship between nurses and the paper. The *Boston Globe* became more inclusive of nursing in its health care coverage and now covers nursing more seriously than most U.S. newspapers.

"If more nurses reached out to editorial boards," Fagin says, "they'd be surprised at how responsive journalists can be. The only negative that can happen is that journalists might say no. But they also might say yes."

Inviting Reporters to Visit You

Another way you can forge relationships with the press is to invite journalists to your institution to look at a project or an example of innovative practice. You could invite them to seminars or meetings that illuminate current practice. Imagine that a hospital has just opened a palliative care unit in which nursing plays a prominent role. The nursing staff can work through the nursing department or through the hospital's public relation office to inform journalists about this development and show them how it works.

There are many other opportunities to get the media to come to you. When a hospital show like *ER, Gray's Anatomy,* or *House* bursts out of the fevered imagination of a Hollywood writer, it is time to pick up the phone and ask reporters to see the real ERs, as the Emergency Nurses Association did.

You can also ask journalists to come to your group to describe how they work and what they need to adequately cover nursing. After Sigma Theta Tau International released its report on the status of nursing coverage,[6] it scheduled seven regional meetings at which journalists spoke to nurses about how to improve "nursing's voice in the media." According to Nancy Dickinson-Hazard, Sigma's executive officer, journalists explained how they work, the stresses they are under, and what they consider to be news. Nurses told the press "about the uniqueness and diversity of nursing," Dickinson-Hazard said. Journalists and nurses discussed ways to change coverage.

Presentations to Journalists

Nurses can present nursing issues to journalists in settings other than editorial boardrooms. They can ask to appear at chapter meetings of journalistic associations such as the American Medical Writers Association. There are networks of journalists that cover health and aging. Ask journalists you know about these and see if nurses can make a presentation either at a meeting or through an online Listserv.

Journalism school courses on health and science writing welcome guest experts who can tell them what is new in these areas. It's a safe bet that few ever invite nurses, but you can ask to visit. Nurse researchers should definitely alert such classes and conferences to their important work. Nurses can even write articles for publications for journalists telling them what they need to know to cover nursing. This is exactly what Bernice Buresh and Nurse Jeannie Chaisson did in articles for *Nieman Reports,* a quarterly publication for journalists published by the Nieman Foundation at Harvard University.[7,8]

Organizational Meetings as a Form of Outreach

Professional meetings and conventions can be outreach tools by providing a focus for coverage. However, don't expect journalists to pay registration fees. They are there as observers not participants.

One reason journalists will come to your conference is to cover a speech by a prominent person. The simple appearance of a celebrity speaker, however, will not be enough to draw attention. The speaker will have to talk about newsworthy issues.

If a political candidate is using a conference to advocate a policy change, for example, the media may come, particularly if the speaker holds, or is running for, political office. The appearance of entertainers or celebrities known for their social advocacy may also draw coverage if they are speaking about an issue or event that is in the news. Unless your conference is showcasing original research or presenting new information, reporters won't treat your organizational meeting as anything other than a setting for the appearance of celebrity keynoters. They will cover the speech and leave. Only if you link the keynote speech and the experiences or research of your members will a reporter remain to talk with other participants. If that link is made, they may interview people at the conference about their views.

Speakers can help your public outreach if they do more than use your organization to advance their platform or popularity. All too often organizations provide a platform for prominent speakers without asking anything in return. If speakers are well briefed in advance, they can refer to care problems, practice innovations, and policy proposals that will improve patient care or health care delivery. This will help direct coverage to your organization and concerns, not just to the speakers' agenda.

This is, however, a delicate negotiation. Speakers will not respond well if they believe you're trying to write their speeches. On the other hand, speakers like to appear to be knowledgeable about the group they're addressing. So when you're preparing speakers or their representatives, brief them on the critical issues and suggest certain points or research they could highlight that would make the audience more receptive and responsive. Unless the speaker specifically requests such help, it's not a good idea to present speakers with "talking points" or written material that they should insert into their remarks. However, speakers may be grateful if you provide them with background information and the talking points "we give to our members."

If a reporter, producer, or editor, or politician or health policy expert—or any other prominent individual—is speaking at your conference, woo them to your cause. Invite them to a luncheon or reception following their presentation. If they are staying overnight—which is often the case—invite them to dinner. Ask a select group of your members to meet with the speaker. This group might include researchers on health policy or nursing practice, nurses who give direct care, or managers, academics, or administrators who can explain what nurses do and why their work is important.

Prominent keynoters or panelists may decline your invitation. They may be too tired or too busy to attend such a gathering, or they may have other plans. But often they will be delighted to have the opportunity to converse with members of your organization. The point is, give them the opportunity to say yes, and give yourselves the opportunity to take advantage of yet another educational opening.

News Conferences

Because people see news conferences so often on television, they may think that the news conference is the first choice for disseminating information. In reality, it is the last. It is a device that has been so abused by publicity-seeking people or organizations that journalists tend to be wary of them. A full-blown news conference requires labor-intensive organizing and should be used only for carefully defined purposes.

A news conference would be warranted, for example, if several nursing organizations formed a coalition to fight for better patient care to reduce medical errors. They could use a news conference to present the various issues involved from the point of view of nurses and patients. Preconference organizing would include preparing media kits, rehearsing the speakers' presentations, checking audiovisual equipment, and doing extensive outreach to encourage journalists to attend.

A press briefing, on the other hand, can be an efficient way to update journalists. Hospitals often hold news briefings on their premises to keep journalists informed about the condition and treatment of a government official, a movie star, or some other highly visible personage. They use the same forum to update reporters when many people are injured in a massive accident or when an extremely unusual or experimental procedure, such as the separation of conjoined twins, occurs.

Broadening the Story's Impact

The news media are interested in stories that may represent a trend. A *trend*—something that is occurring in more than one place—has currency because it affects a lot of people. Newsmagazines, because they circulate nationally and internationally, seem to specialize in trends, especially those with major economic, cultural, or political impact. National publications and TV news organizations cover trends by having their bureaus contribute information on what is going on in various geographic areas. Correspondents look for dramatic examples that illustrate the phenomenon. The illustrating example requires spokespeople who are willing to talk and, usually, appealing visual elements.

To convince a reporter that you have a good story, you might want to brief her on how the program/event/phenomenon is happening elsewhere and thus is part of a national or international trend. Good nursing trend stories will be unrealized if organizations and institutions promote only what is going on within their walls or among their members. Being unique works in some instances but backfires when a broader appeal is called for.

For example, a nursing department, eager to promote an experiment that allows family members to be present when a loved one is undergoing intense and invasive emergency treatment, may get more attention by telling the media that this program is being tried at another hospital in the area or in other facilities around the country. Similarly, if journalists knew that nurses all over the world—in Ireland, Poland, Canada, and the United States—were striking over similar issues, they might be more attracted to writing about a strike in a local area.

Pitching Your Story

When you're trying to get media attention, be aware that there are many ways of presenting a set of facts, program, activity, or event. When talking about a potential story, an editor will ask a reporter, "What's the angle?" The editor is not seeking just a set of facts. She wants the reporter to explain why the story is appealing enough to displace other competitors for time on the nightly news or space in the morning paper.

To convince his editor, the journalist will have to come up with an attractive angle. Because many stories are multifaceted, you must determine which angles to highlight when you are trying to attract coverage.

Consider the latest nursing shortage. It was just beginning to surface as a story in 1999. The *New York Times* and other newspapers got into the subject by concentrating on the aging-of-the-nursing-workforce angle. Others, such as the Canadian magazine *Elm Street* and the *Boston Globe* focus section, ran pieces suggesting that mistreatment of nurses was a factor in the shortage and was driving nurses toward more militant actions.

In recent years, coverage of the nursing shortage has been driven by studies documenting the links between insufficient nursing care and patient deaths and complications. Other studies have focused on the problems nurses have with overwork, mandatory overtime, and unpredictable schedules. Because one of the remedies proposed by nursing groups is safe staffing legislation, there have been a number of stories debating the wisdom of this solution. These stories have received big play in major newspapers and other media outlets.

However, the media are notorious for having a short attention span. "Many reporters now regard this story as a big yawn," notes Karen McCarthy of the Canadian Nurses Association. "If you want media attention, you have to think about how you can reposition or repackage the issue."

In Canada, McCarthy says, the media and politicians are interested in the length of time people have to wait for health care services and the degree of access to services and procedures. So the challenge, McCarthy says, is to "repackage" the nursing shortage in connection with the issues that are current, and to use "new language to strike a chord with reporters."

The nursing shortage can provide fodder for business coverage. Nurses can point out that a chain of undesirable business and economic consequences are attached to this issue. Some hospitals try to raid nursing staffs elsewhere by throwing monetary incentives at nurses with certain expertise. Temporary, traveling, and immigrant nurses are often used to plug holes in hospital staffs. What are the monetary implications of this? When hospitals increase their demands for mandatory overtime, nursing organizations and unions protest. Stopgap responses to a shortage of nurses lay the groundwork for labor unrest and perhaps nursing strikes. With conditions deteriorating and nurses being poorly treated, more of them will leave the profession, thus exacerbating the problem. This is a realistic scenario that nurses should spell out for journalists.

The nursing shortage also has an educational and policy component that must be brought to the attention of reporters who cover those areas. It is a serious matter when policy makers try to circumvent university education—as they did in Canada, Australia, and the United States—to speed up the production of nurses. Although lip service is constantly paid to the extensive education and training required for contemporary nursing, efforts to produce nurses more quickly and cheaply undercut quality patient care.

Journalists should be encouraged to compare how physician population fluxes are handled. No one would dare implement policies that shave a couple of years off medical training so that more doctors enter the workforce faster. The supply of doctors is manipulated by regulating how many people are accepted and graduated from medical school, not by reducing the time they spend there or by reconfiguring their curriculum.

Keeping a Story Going

In some cases, the goal will be to get one good story on your program or practice. If, however, you are working on an ongoing issue, one good story does not mean it is time to sit back and relax. It means it is time for more action so that the story does not fade from the news.

Stories can either have a long, robust life span or suffer sudden cardiac arrest and die. They can also be banished to the journalistic equivalent of the long-term-care facility where they are pumped up with nutrients from time to time before they peter out. For stories to remain vital, they must be fed with new material and activity.

You need a plan to create new developments and take advantage of those that come along. Start a pipeline to journalists with new studies, surveys, and reports on your issue. Engage in research or analysis yourself and issue reports. Participate in forums organized by allies. Testify at hearings and distribute written copies of your testimony to journalists. Even if you are not called on to testify, you can bring your own documentation to the hearing and distribute it to the press corps. You can use other people's testimony in your reports and analyses as well. Plan media events around the issue.

These are the kinds of things that people involved in reform movements do to keep the story alive. They help to keep issues in the public eye by providing expert testimony at legislative and government hearings, by continuing research into pertinent areas, and by widely disseminating findings to groups that can use them to bring about reforms.

Negative Coverage

Having an active relationship with the news media not only increases the chances of favorable coverage, it is an asset when stories come along that are not kind to nursing.

In recent years, a number of stories have questioned the qualifications of nurses. A dramatic example was an ABC-TV *Day One* program on anesthesiologist fraud broadcast in January 1995.

The program was focused on anesthesiologists "who violate Medicare laws and their own professional rules, who supervise many more operations than they are permitted, are not present at critical moments during surgery, and even fraudulently bill for services they never provide." These renegade anesthesiologists—greedy, incompetent, and negligent as they may be—were not shown to be injuring and killing patients directly. That occurred, the program asserted, when the anesthesiologist was out of the room and the patient was under the care of a nurse anesthetist, also referred to in the program as an "assistant."

The report had a subtext that has often plagued nursing: Although there are individual physicians not worthy of the title, physicians as a class provide safe medical care when they are present. Nurses, on the other hand, are not competent either as individuals or as a profession to deal with patients without close physician supervision.

The program cited four cases in which severe patient injury or death was attributed to the lack of an anesthesiologist in the operating room. The most bizarre involved a nurse anesthetist who, left to her own devices, warmed a bag of blood in a microwave oven. The patient who received the blood died.

Bad press like this understandably terrifies many nurses. They may think if this is what you're going to get by being in the media, it's better to get no coverage at all. There are things you can do, however, to avoid or soften bad coverage and to respond if it does occur.

1. *Anticipate.* When you hear that a story is being developed on an area of nursing that concerns you, contacting the producer or the reporter and offering to provide pertinent information will usually serve your interests better than waiting to see what will happen. In today's world, every profession has to justify its existence. Conflicts and competition among health care professions can be intense and may color news stories. You can anticipate that difficult questions about nursing might be raised. Journalists have a legitimate interest in probing incidents of patient suffering, medical errors, fraud, denial of treatment, and withdrawal of care. Their job is to expose flaws in the system and to question the way things are done.

If it appears that the story will present nursing negatively, try to find out what the issues are and try to help the reporter understand their complexities. Many, if not most, reporters who do serious coverage want to be accurate. They might be influenced in their approach if they are made aware of aspects they didn't know about.

If a producer or reporter insists on forcing the story in a direction that makes you nervous and refuses to listen to you, you don't have to deal with him. But you should weigh this carefully. Opting out of a game you fear you can't control might not get a better result.

The American Association of Nurse Anesthetists (AANA) was confronted with this sort of choice when it learned what *Day One* had in the works. The organization's board decided not to provide on-camera interviews out of concern that cooperating with a report implying widespread anesthesiologist fraud would be detrimental to certified registered nurse anesthetists (CRNAs). As a courtesy, the AANA notified the American Society of Anesthesiologists of its decision.

Later, however, when the AANA thought the program's focus had changed, it sought to put nurse anesthetists on camera as patients' advocates; *Day One* producers resisted the overture.

Day One found nurse anesthetists on its own. It interviewed two in in silhouette to hide their identities. These nurse anesthetists said that to make more money, anesthesiologists regularly violate practice regulations and that nurse anesthetists cover up for them. The program also had no trouble finding a credentialed physician to slam the whole nursing specialty. Dr. Wilson Wilhite—the past president of the American Society of Anesthesiologists, the organization that the AANA treated so courteously—implied on the air that medically directed anesthesiology delivered by nurse anesthetists is dangerous.

Nurses can anticipate that doctor groups under attack are not going to treat them with kid gloves. They may even make nurses the scapegoat. Knowing that you cannot control the content of such a television program relieves you from trying to do the impossible. Then you are free to try to have at least some influence.[9]

2. *Act.* It is impossible to duck scrutiny. If nurses are to have professional credibility and access to the media when they need it, they have to get involved and stay involved.

By doing interviews and taking a tough stance with the *Day One* producers, AANA might have been able to cast nurse anesthetists in a better light. Maybe it would have made no difference. But the overriding urge that nurses sometimes exhibit to protect the welfare and reputation of another profession can limit nurses from acting on their own behalf. Other professions are capable of looking out for their own welfare. When nurses act in their own interest, it does not mean they are being disrespectful of others.

Acknowledging a problem within the profession does not invalidate nursing. Not every nurse is a great nurse; not every nurse gives high-quality care, but of what profession is that not true? Unless you are willing to admit this fact, it is very hard to defend nursing. Indeed, rather than defending nursing or a nursing specialty in the abstract, concretely describe the problems nursing has delivering quality care in the context of the issues being probed. If the subject involves practices that jeopardize patients, this can be an opportunity for nurses to advocate for patients and speak out against practices not under their control.

3. *React and respond.* Don't get tempted into thinking that a strong response will merely fan the flames of criticism. Don't believe for a moment that if you are quiet, it will all blow over. Media reports are powerful because they can leave a lasting impression.

Although AANA limited its ability to shape the story, it did respond assertively. Before *Day One* aired, the AANA sent its members survey forms for recording their responses to the program. They included fact sheets on CRNAs and anesthesia to help nurse anesthetists answer questions from patients or others in their workplace. This groundwork produced a virtuoso response.

Nurse anesthetists were outraged by the show and refused to let it stand. The day after it aired, Mary DePaolis-Lutzo, president of the AANA, sent a letter to the president of ABC, other network executives, principals on *Day One,* and managers of ABC-owned stations stating that the program had misled the public and unfairly attacked nurse anesthetists. Accompanying the letter was a six-page point-by-point rebuttal to nineteen distortions she said occurred in the report. She strongly refuted the assertion that "patients' lives are at risk" if an anesthesiologist isn't in the room by pointing out that CRNAs administer more than 65 percent of the 26 million anesthetics given to patients in the United States each year. She explained that CNRAs are permitted to practice in every state, and that "they work with surgeons independently of an anesthesiologist, or collaboratively with anesthesiologists."

DePaolis-Lutzo put a message on the AANA's president's hotline advising callers where to send protests. Some 2,000 persons called ABC, and 1,500 of those who wrote letters sent copies to the AANA.

Two weeks later, *Day One* acknowledged the "huge response" to the program. For the first time in its history, it quoted on-air letters it had received.

Nurses must respond to serious inaccuracies and misinformation. This means talking to and writing to journalists, editors, and producers. It may mean taking out advertisements.

In the end, even a negative report can help organizations discern what issues they need to address publicly. It can be an opportunity to go forward with new communication activities that will benefit both nursing and the public.

Establishing the Rules of the Game

People inexperienced in dealing with the media may fear they will be at the mercy of reporters. Of course you cannot control everything, but you should expect an honest working relationship with reporters. You should inquire about what information is being sought, why it is being asked for, and how it will be used. You should do all you can to ensure accuracy and clarity. But don't ask for or expect to see an advance copy of the story.

The late Edward L. Bernays, who was a legend in the public relations field, said he always told his clients that there was only one rule in talking with reporters: "If you don't want it printed, don't say it." Always assume that you are speaking on the record to a journalist even if the conversation has an informal tone. Journalists are in the business of conveying information, not in keeping it to themselves. It is in nurses' interest to speak clearly and directly about their work and not shrink from that role.

If, however, there is an instance when you do not want your name or information that you give used, you must make that agreement up front, not after the fact. Here are some ways in which reporters temper information.

- *Not for attribution.* There may be times when you want a journalist to report on something that has happened, but you fear the personal consequences if it is attributed to you. You might be able to work out an agreement with a reporter that the facts can be used but not attributed to you by name. You should discuss with the reporter how general the attribution should be, such as "a clinical nurse specialist in oncology said Tuesday," or "a nurse at the hospital said Tuesday." The more sources a reporter has that can confirm and expand on the information, the more you are off the hook.
- *Off the record.* Contrary to what you see in the movies, these agreements are rare. "Off the record" really means that neither the information nor the source can be used. A person might seek this agreement if he or she was the only person who could have possibly been the leak for something that was explosive or possibly criminal. By making an off-the-record agreement, the journalist is saying that he or she will not use the information unless it can be found from another source without identifying the original source. Journalists don't make these agreements lightly. They know that if a court orders them to reveal a source, they will have to decide whether to comply or perhaps go to jail.

To take advantage of the media opportunities that occur and to craft strategies that will amplify nurses' voices, it makes sense to work with public relations professionals. How they work and how to work with them is the subject of Chapter 8.

Chapter 8

Working with Public Relations Professionals

While effective public communication depends on the participation of large numbers of individual nurses, it is unrealistic to expect nurses to know all the ins and outs of media work. Nurses go to nursing school to learn how to be nurses not public relations (PR) or media specialists. Yet, sometimes nurses who are inexperienced with PR find themselves talking solely with other nurses about how to devise media strategies for their organizations. If nurses don't get expert communication assistance when they need it, they risk spinning their wheels on fruitless activity and growing demoralized when they don't get hoped-for results. This may discourage them from engaging in more productive activities in the future.

Public relations experts have a lot to offer nurses. "One reason to hire a public relations specialist is to get someone who is not inundated in your reality but is sensitive to the issue," says Scott Foster, a communication consultant who has worked with the Hawaii Nurses Association. "A little bit of distance may be needed to shape the information and focus it."

Public relations experts can help nurses develop a media strategy and enlist allies to achieve goals. "I don't operate in a vacuum," Foster explains. "When I work with a group, I bring in other people—say political consultants—who can provide an important perspective and contacts."

"Public opinion is critical in waging a political battle or winning a policy victory," says Joan Hurwitz, director of communications for the American Nurses Association. "Given increasing competition and unprecedented changes in health care—including who makes decisions about how a shrinking economic pie is divided—nursing must be aggressively promoted."

Many of the problems that nursing groups face are more political than they are technical. Therefore, it is essential that nurses find PR consultants or political organizers who are well versed in public outreach and grassroots organizing. "Instead of hiring a traditional adman or PR person, nurses usually will be better off finding a communication specialist who is experienced in community activism and coalition building and who will do it from a nursing perspective," says David Schildmeier, communication director for the Massachusetts Nurses Association (MNA).

"When you are planning a media relations initiative, you need to think strategically," says Karen McCarthy, director of strategic communication for the Canadian Nurses Association. "Is there another group or individuals that can carry your message?"

Not only should a PR person know how to reach the mainstream media, she should be able to connect with patient and consumer advocacy groups, doctors and other health care workers, unions, and organizations with pertinent interests and influence.

A good PR person will help nurses to feel comfortable talking about their work by showing them how to shape information and speak in a way that captures public attention. She should be able to address their real or exaggerated concerns about the media. The job isn't only to convince journalists to talk to nurses; it is to convince nurses to talk to journalists. This may involve a lot of work and patience. The PR professional may have to conduct media-training sessions with leaders and members of the group, and do a lot of handholding to help nurses negotiate this new public arena. An effective PR professional will be acquainted with the mores and culture of the group or individuals he is working with and will know what obstacles come with their territory.

Gaining access to the media is usually easier in a small or medium-sized community than in a major city where there is heavier competition for media attention. Nurses in smaller communities may not find it difficult to place a story on something interesting that they are doing. However, they may feel inhibited about "what people will say" if they are doing something unconventional or if they "step out of character" by assuming a more visible and feisty role. If nurses, for example, decide to wage a campaign over health care and practice issues, they might fear that they will lose whatever public support they may have won through "professional" or caring behaviors. One young nurse expressed this apprehension in the following way: "The public trusts us because we are so caring and compassionate. If we begin to talk about medical and technical things, we risk losing that trust."

A skilled PR professional can and should help nurses weigh such concerns. He might point out that it's hard to imagine that a doctor would fear losing public respect by claiming both technical skill and excellent bedside manners. Doctors understand that by claiming it all, they become even more valued.

Good PR specialists understand the local media market and culture in which they function. Nurses in a big city might be quite persistent and still

> *"Many nurses worry that reporters will misquote them. They will. About 70 percent of the time they won't get it exactly right. But that's close enough to be effective."*
>
> —*David Schildmeier, director of communications for the Massachusetts Nurses Association*

not capture media interest. The challenge in an overheated media market can be determining the right moment to take on a particular issue, the right tactics to use, and the right contacts to make.

An effective PR strategist will need the most recent statistics and research studies in the field. She should make these reader friendly and available to nurses so that they can prepare themselves for discussions with journalists and legislators. She would also disseminate relevant materials to journalists.

When breaking news demands a nursing response, an effective PR operative will craft the necessary press releases and call on nurses who are prepared to talk to the media. He should be able to contact just the right nurse and, if needed, help her construct her argument. He might try to generate a large volume of letters from nurses by sending out an e-mail alert with sample letters. Some issues might require op-eds or letters from nurses with specific expertise. Most PR specialists can help to craft these. When an organization is waging a campaign, the PR person will work with members to produce communication materials such as news releases, slogans, banners, posters, videos, advertisements, and media kits.

Expert PR practitioners not only shape information, they know to whom to take it. They know the phone and fax numbers and e-mail and postal addresses of journalists and have good working relationships with many of them. The PR person cannot guarantee that the story he pitches will be picked up, but he should be at least well enough established with key media outlets to get his phone calls or e-mails answered. A good PR person, Foster says, will have established credibility with journalists who recognize that he is, in turn, bringing them credible clients and information.

Above all, the PR person should not play to the fears or anxieties of nurses who employ him. Nursing groups should also be wary of PR professionals who encourage them to use traditional virtue scripts and images (see Chapter 2) in recruitment, retention, or image campaigns no matter how well intentioned.

Some of the widely distributed ads from the Johnson & Johnson Campaign for Nursing's Future fell into the virtue-script trap. In some of the promotions, nurses were depicted as "unsung heroes" whose work is to make beds and open windows to let in the air, and for whom the "gratitude in a patient's eye" is sufficient reward.[1]

A classic example of the virtue script is the following jingle from the Johnson & Johnson campaign: "You're always there when someone needs you / You work your magic quietly / You're not in it for the glory / The care you give comes naturally / You take my hand / Touch my life / When I need you."[2] We believe this promotion inadvertently undercut the skilled caring that nurses do and the knowledge that nurses have. How does a nurse know what question to ask a patient, what tone of voice to use, or when to hold the patient's hand? We conclude from our observations of nurses that these actions stem from attentiveness, knowledge about the patient and his or her condition, clinical judgment, experience, and well-developed caring skills. But this promotion says that such caring is not knowledgeable work, it's "magic." According to the promotion, caring isn't learned and practiced, it just comes naturally. So, one might ask, why should we support nursing education if nursing comes naturally?

This ad also negates the idea that nursing requires other resources by asserting that you are always going to be there no matter what. Are you always going to be there when someone needs you if you don't get paid, if the nursing agency goes bankrupt, or if you are stretched so thin by a shortage of staff that you can't tend to all of your patients? A literally minded member of the public might wonder, why should I worry about the future of nursing if you're always going to be there "when I need you."

These virtue-script messages are appealing because they reflect the yearning we have for a mother who will care for us when we are sick. They appeal to nurses additionally because they reflect an ideal version of the kind of care some nurses would like to give.

Because nurses and nursing organizations often rely on angelic images to promote nurses, PR and media specialists may think that is the way nurses want to be seen and that these images are realistic. Thus sentimental and simplistic images of nursing continually circulate in a communication loop from nursing to the public and from the public back to nursing.[3]

When you work with PR specialists who know little about nursing, you must be clear about what you want to convey. It is up to you to instruct your communication experts even as they instruct you.

In 1997, the British Columbia Nurses Union (BCNU) produced an ad (see p. 171) that turns the stereotypical view of nurses on its head by showing what is going on behind the pleasant appearance of the nurse.

> *Boston Medical Center*
> *Exceptional Care*
> *Without Exception*
> *A place where nurses walk on*
> *water*
>
> —*headline in* **Hospitals 2004**,
> *advertising supplement to the*
> **Boston Globe**

CAUTION

Your Turn

Here is the original version of a Johnson & Johnson public service advertisement in which a nurse describes his work:

> *Being a nurse is all about holding someone's hand . . . or getting the wrinkles out of the back of a sheet that's causing someone to be uncomfortable . . .*
> *And sometimes just rubbing someone's back is the answer to all their prayers.*

What do you think about this description of nursing? How could it be improved? Suzanne Gordon did this makeover:

> *Being a nurse is about saving patients' lives.*
> *Being a nurse is about making sure a patient doesn't develop a fatal complication after surgery.*
> *It's about paying attention to the small but significant details such as smoothing out the wrinkles on a sheet so a patient doesn't develop an excruciating and costly bedsore.*
> *Sometimes by sitting and talking to someone, I find out the most important things—like whether patients understand how to take their medications, whether they have support at home, and whether they are frightened and anxious.*

Which script do you think more accurately captures the essence of nursing? Which script is more convincing? Which script makes it clear that not just anyone can do the work of nurses?

Now do your own rewrite of the Nurses' Day composition, p. 34.

If your organization does not have in-house expertise, you can get it from PR professionals on a consultancy basis. If your group has little or no budget for PR, you might be able to get help from public relations students at a college or university. There are student groups that take on nonprofit organizations as clients. Some PR and advertising firms do pro bono work. The Public Relations Society of America (www.prsa.com) has professional and student chapters throughout the United States. You could contact your local chapter and invite a representative to speak to your group on what is involved in setting up a PR program.

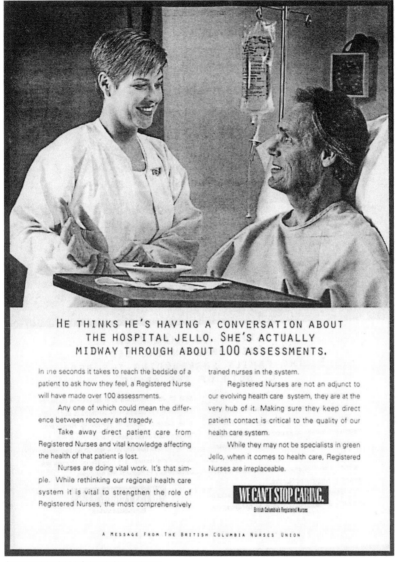

Courtesy of the British Columbia Nurses' Union

"Internal" and "External" Communications

Many nursing organizations, nursing schools, hospitals, and other health care institutions have PR, marketing, or communication specialists working for them. Therefore, it may seem mysterious that nursing still ranks as the least visible health care profession. The mystery can be solved, however, by looking at what many of these PR practitioners are actually assigned to do.

Your Turn

Look at the images that your nursing organization or hospital disseminates to promote your specialty or nursing in general. Do the images reinforce or reverse traditional stereotypes? Do the messages diminish nursing practice or imply that one group of nurses is superior to another? Would you like to see these images or messages reflected by the media? Are there alternative images and messages you might use?

The primary goal of any organization is to serve and retain its members and to recruit more. Most nursing organizations expect their marketing and PR people to do more "internal" than "external" communication. Their mission is to enhance communication and the image of the organization with members and with others in the profession.

In a nursing school, for example, a communication specialist might spend most of her time putting out newsletters and promotional materials for prospective students and alumni. Her duties might also involve promoting the nursing school *within* the university.

In a subspecialty organization, a PR staffer might put out an organizational newsletter, supervise the publishing of clinical journals and books, and help plan and promote conferences and conventions.

While internal communication activities are critical to organizational survival, they do not constitute a viable "external" communication strategy. Internal communication activities do not get nursing into the news, nor do they necessarily raise the public profile of the profession.

This calculus is pertinent to every nursing organization. However, the reality is that the vast majority of nursing organizations, subspecialty groups, and professional associations do very little "external" communication and outreach to

> *"If people don't see nurses playing important roles, then the public and policy makers don't really give nursing what it is due in terms of money and a significant place at the policy table. As a result, nursing research doesn't get funded to the level needed. This affects nursing school budgets and the number of faculty that can be hired, which in turn affects the number of nursing students, which then affects the future availability of nurses."*
>
> —Dan Mezibov, who, for many years, was director of public affairs for the American Association of Colleges of Nursing

journalists. They may produce policy statements or position papers on important issues and may even hire speech writers and media trainers to teach officers how to speak in public, do interviews with journalists, and appear on television and radio. An organization might even invite journalists to a conference to speak about the how-tos of nursing coverage. But these actions are self-limiting if the organization does not engage in consistent outreach to the media on pressing health care issues and help its members to speak out and participate in collective actions that will turn rhetoric into reality for nursing. An unintended consequence of not having an external communication plan is that it reinforces the silence of nurses. When nurses don't see members of their profession in the news, they might conclude that the media aren't interested in their stories and that nothing can be done to change that.

> *"I always tell them to return that call. I think that's the number-one mistake a lot of people make. They hear that the press is on the phone and they freeze thinking it's 60 Minutes doing an investigation. But it's really an opportunity to get attention for their program."*
>
> —Robert Rosseter, director of public affairs for the American Association of Colleges of Nursing (when asked what is the most important thing he tells nursing school administrators and faculty about dealing with the media)

Making the Clinical Workplace Work for You

Many of the health care institutions in which nurses work do not promote nursing and won't unless nurses intervene.

The media officers who work for hospitals and medical centers usually do an excellent job of promoting doctors and medicine. If a journalist needs

Your Turn

Inquire about your organization's or school's public relations mission. What are its stated public relations and marketing goals and priorities? What actions are staff members taking to reach the stated goals? What are the timetables? What resources are needed? List your ideas about the goals you think are important and the actions needed to reach them.

an expert to bring him up to speed on urinary incontinence, for example, he might phone the media relations department at a medical center and ask to do an interview with an expert on staff. Almost invariably—even if the subject is one in which nurses have particular expertise—that authority will be a physician. In pitching stories and responding to requests from journalists, PR people at the institutions where most nurses work are often on automatic pilot. The flight instruction is: Find a Doctor.

A veteran practitioner of medical center media relations suggests that the reasons for this are that most PR and marketing people in health care institutions begin and practice their work in a media culture that devalues nursing, and they develop their careers in institutions whose fortunes are viewed as being synonymous with those of the medical staff. The raison d'être of the PR staff, then, is to promote the medical staff.

Tony Swartz-Lloyd, who was the vice president of communications at Boston's Beth Israel Hospital for twenty-three years, says that many communication staffers view nurses as a quantitative not a qualitative variable in patients' hospital stays. "They understand that hospitals need enough nurses to keep the hospital running," he says. "They say there aren't enough qualified nurses, and that nurses are overworked and underpaid. But their understanding usually doesn't go beyond that. They can't tell you why having an individual, highly qualified nurse is important."

This, Swartz-Lloyd says, is very different from a PR staffer's understanding of physicians' work. "A PR person can easily explain why it's important to have a doctor who is skilled and qualified. They'll explain that if you don't have a good orthopedic surgeon, he could attach your left leg to your right."

But, he says, they don't understand that to patients, nursing is equally important. "They don't understand the consequences of nurses not being able to do their work effectively or not being supported by their institutions. They don't get that you don't just want nurses there to 'answer the bell' but you also want them to do research and teaching and publishing and furthering their own education. This is a good thing, not a ducking-out-of-work kind of thing."

Communication specialists in medical centers also quickly get the message that doctors think anything interesting revolves around them. It's natural for marketing and communication people to absorb the attitudes that some physicians have about nurses. "Because medicine is a 'male' culture," one public relations expert asserts, "doctors don't like nurses who see themselves as being equal to doctors and, worse, who can go about proving it."

Maureen McInaney, senior public information representative at the University of California San Francisco Medical Center agrees. "Most hospital PR staff are not taught that promoting nursing is part of their brief, and too few institutions make it part of their brief. They conceive of hospitals as buildings with patients and doctors in them. Public information professionals are still more likely to seek out physician experts, often forgetting that nurses can respond to many of these inquiries," McInaney explains.

Without institutional support and encouragement, communication specialists at medical centers and hospitals will be wary of promoting nursing even if they would like to. This is why, in the 1980s, the administration of Beth Israel Hospital in Boston gave its PR staff the resources and authority to promote nursing. "It took five years to sell primary nursing, which Beth Israel was developing and implementing, but eventually we did it," says Swartz-Lloyd, who directed the effort. According to Swartz-Lloyd, Mitchell Rabkin, MD, and Joyce Clifford, RN, then the hospital CEO and nurse-in-chief respectively, not only encouraged the communication staff to go in a new direction but shielded the staff from medical sniping. Time and again, through local and national print and television stories, Beth Israel proved that the nursing story is salable.

On the other hand, failure to promote nursing creates a self-reinforcing cycle. Nursing doesn't appear in the media when PR professionals don't send releases or pitch stories about nursing or educate journalists by talking with them about developments in nursing. So when a PR person approaches a journalist, as one Australian information specialist explained, the journalist discounts nursing as too "touchy feely." If a PR staffer doesn't know how to counter that view of nursing, she may simply give up trying to pitch nursing stories. With no one initiating or pursuing the conversation, PR people don't get inquiries from journalists about nursing and thus conclude that nursing is not salable, and thus might discourage nurses who approach them with good stories.

Nurse executives and deans of nursing can provide the impetus to break that cycle. At the University of California San Francisco (UCSF), Nursing School Dean Kathleen Dracup and Medical Center Vice President of Nursing Anne Wittenberg have urged the public information staff to learn about and promote nursing. "Nursing leaders in the hospital have helped PR people understand that nursing practice, research and innovations are salable," says McInaney, the public information specialist there.

But such interventions by top nurses apparently are not the norm, as evidenced by a short survey of nurse executives in the southern United States who attended a "Silence to Voice" presentation in 2002. All but five of the sixty respondents said that their institutions were experiencing a nursing shortage.

But only ten said they meet with their institution's PR staff to educate them about nursing. Ten said their hospitals had sent out press releases pitching nursing stories, and eighteen said that they have given PR staff the

names of nurses doing interesting work in their hospitals, but few had engaged in follow-up.

In a remarkable statistic, only two of the sixty said that they and/or their
staffs had ever met with reporters. Thirty-three—more than half of the respondents—had done no work at all with their PR departments. Indeed

Southern Health: A Notable Example from Australia

Kim Sykes, who in 2003 was director of nursing of Southern Health (the
largest hospital system in Melbourne, Australia), worked with the system's
public relations department, leadership team, and nurse managers to launch
a systemwide project to encourage nurses at all levels to speak about their
work to the public. A key participant in this effort was Andrew Williamson, the
executive director of public affairs and a former producer for the Australian
Broadcasting Company.

"Andrew has expertise that can really help us get the message out," says
Sykes, who later became interim chief nurse of the state of Victoria. "But
what Andrew knows about nurses is only as good as the knowledge we share
with him and the information we make available to him."

"When I came to work at Southern Health," says Williamson, "I quickly
realized that the directors of nursing and senior managers in our hospitals
were highly educated and well respected. I used them as spokespeople for
Southern Health on key issues." But, Williamson says, he didn't know how
skilled and knowledgeable the nurses were. "Too often nurses miss out on
valuable opportunities to explain the knowledge, skills, and innovative
thinking that goes on in their work. They also miss opportunities to take
credit for their contribution to medical achievements, and this colors the
views of public relations professionals who often present a narrow view of
nurses as nurturing and caring but little else."

Southern Health's communication project began with a series of
breakfast seminars for nurse managers and senior clinicians that featured
speakers on topics ranging from the history of nursing culture to
contemporary nursing stories that might be of interest to the media. A
daylong "Silence to Voice" workshop was conducted as part of the project.

Williamson says that these seminars and interaction between PR staff
and nursing have generated a number of nursing story ideas. Southern Health
has also set up a Web site so nurses can communicate with each other and
alert the PR department to interesting stories. "We don't know what the
stories are if nurses don't tell us," he says. "We can't educate the media if
nurses don't educate us."

most of the nurse executives reported that their PR departments did not send out releases that included nurses and that the media did not include nurses in whatever reporting was done on their institutions.

As those PR staffers who promote nursing tell us, relationships are as critical to getting the PR staff to work for you as they are to quality patient care. Get to know the PR people so that you can bring them up to date on what is going on in nursing. Suggest potential stories based on nursing activities and events that contain some of the news values outlined in Chapter 6.

Think about inviting a PR staff member to follow an RN for a day. Suggest that she invite journalists to do the same. Compile a list of nurses who are doing interesting work in the institution and ask the PR staff to pitch stories about them. Write a brief description of the relevance of their work to the public. Ask the PR staff to refer reporters to nursing sources for expert comment. Give the PR department a list of nurses with expertise in various areas and include information on how to contact them.

If the PR staff insists that journalists want to talk only to doctors, persist. You can explain that you're not in competition with doctors or trying to displace them, but by giving visibility to nurses, the hospital raises its public profile. To buttress your case, collect news stories about nurses from elsewhere.

If the PR people remain cool, nurses have other avenues for getting their stories out. Let's say that the critical care nurses at a certain hospital develop a new protocol for working with cardiac patients, but the hospital doesn't pick up the ball by putting out news releases or talking with health care reporters about it. There is no need to let the story die. The nurses' professional organization or union can pitch it to the news media. The nurses involved can then speak to journalists as representatives of their professional organization or union.

Roles of Unions

Unions, because they so often interact with the media, have numerous opportunities to promote the professional work of nurses. In large part because of unions, nursing is in the media much more than it was when we first began tracking nursing coverage in 1989. But the major way that nursing is visible now is in connection with workplace and contract issues—nursing shortages, staffing ratios, pay demands, and overtime policies. It is legitimate for unions to focus on the problems that nurses have doing their work, and it is important that the public know about these problems. But the public also needs to hear "practice narratives" that show what nurses actually do (p. 204).[1]

Picking a Public Relations Consultant

There are many books that can tell you how to pick a good PR staffer or consultant. We summarize guidelines of our own:

- Be wary of someone who unknowingly reflects societal stereotypes of nursing.
- Pick someone who respects the core of nursing and is not trying to turn nurses into something they consider more "professional," respectable, or legitimate.
- Seek candidates who can showcase the complexity of nursing by communicating its caring, medical, technical, and body-care facets.
- Hire someone who will respectfully make demands on nurses to be more assertive, more willing to speak, and more able to take on controversial issues.
- Hire a person who understands that promoting positive images of nursing and taking assertive stands on health care issues is as much political work as it is communication technique.
- Don't have unrealistic expectations of what a PR expert can do for you. He or she can talk with you but not for you and can make contacts that will facilitate your work but not be a substitute for it.

"The PR professionals who work for nursing unions or collective bargaining associations are generally very experienced and active in external communications," says Rand Wilson, a veteran union organizer formerly with the Service Employees International Union. "They could expand their outreach beyond workplace conflicts by making the practice of their members visible and utilizing academic research so that the public would understand why a nurse who's just worked a ten-hour shift cannot safely care for patients if she's forced to work another ten-hour shift. These are issues of concern to patients and the public. Increasingly, contract issues aren't settled at the bargaining table, they're settled in the court of public opinion. That's why an effective communication strategy is essential."

Chapter 9

Constructing Campaigns That Work

In 1999 California, despite heavy opposition from the health care industry, became the first U.S. state to pass legislation mandating safe nurse-
patient staffing ratios. A year later, the state of Victoria in Australia became
the first place to actually implement staffing ratios and no-lift policies to
protect nurses and patients.

These watershed commitments to nursing and patient care didn't just
happen. They were the hard-won victories of thousands of nurses who engaged in strategic planning, collective advocacy, and extensive public communication to reverse the erosion of nursing care brought about by relentless budget cutting. Their determined activism on behalf of their profession
and patients was far from novel. They were acting in the finest tradition of
nursing, which, throughout its history, has waged campaigns to win practice and patient-care advances.

Although many don't think of Florence Nightingale as a whistleblower
or lobbyist, she was both.

It was the press that first drew Nightingale's attention to the poor treatment of British soldiers in the Crimean War. William Howard Russell, the
first British war correspondent to file dispatches from the front, reported in
The Times that cholera and other enteric diseases—not artillery fire—were responsible for hospitalizing 20 percent of the expeditionary force. Because of
abominable hospital conditions, these soldiers were more likely to die than
survive. Moreover, while France provided nurses to care for its sick and
wounded soldiers, Great Britain did not.

When Nightingale learned of this, she contacted her friend Lord Sidney
Herbert, the Secretary at War and the person in charge of finances and supplies. In November 1854, after extensive negotiations, Nightingale em-
barked for the Crimea with thirty-eight nurses. During her stay in the
Crimea, Nightingale used the popularity she gained through newspaper ac-

counts of her activities to lobby for money to finance her efforts. When she encountered military, medical, and bureaucratic recalcitrance, she got much of what she wanted in part by threatening to inform the press of opposition to her cause.

After she returned to England, Nightingale used every means to improve military and civilian hospitals, to provide home care to the sick poor, and to give respectable women paid work outside of the confines of the Victorian household. One of the first health care statisticians, she used research findings to bolster her arguments. Nightingale also collaborated with a notable female political writer, Harriet Martineau, who was then a columnist for the *Daily News*.

As Lois Monteiro writes: "Nightingale contacted Martineau when her attempts to pressure reform in the Army in 1857–58 were going too slowly; she turned to public opinion as the pressure source." In 1858, Nightingale sent Martineau a "private reading" copy of a report she had produced on army reform. Over the years, Nightingale continued to feed Martineau information that later appeared in the journalist's columns. Martineau's book, *England and Her Soldiers*, grew out of the two women's working association.[1]

Nursing's major advances have come about through nurses' individual and collective advocacy. Their earliest struggle "was the effort to distinguish trained nurses from everyone else who purported to care for the sick," says nursing historian Joan Lynaugh. "It involved the insistence that nursing work required education and standards." This campaign took place from roughly 1860 to 1915. But, finally, according to Lynaugh, the idea that "there is a distinct thing called nursing" requiring a distinct education achieved worldwide acknowledgment.

"Efforts to bring about significant change require coalitions that have a purpose, leaders who won't give up, and public activity," Lynaugh asserts. "They grow out of the awareness that the only way you can achieve anything is to connect your own little world to other worlds in which people share your views, at least about one particular issue."

There have been a number of important nursing achievements in recent years. Nurses who specialize—nurse midwives, nurse practitioners, and critical care nurses among others—have won acknowledgment for their distinct work and nurse practitioners have obtained reimbursement and prescriptive authority. Nursing schools have started PhD programs, the National Institute of Nursing Research in the United States has launched cutting-edge research, baccalaureate education has become the standard for entry into practice in the majority of Canadian provinces, and nursing has been added as a clinical category to the Canada Health Act. These achievements came about by mobilizing coalitions from within and beyond the nursing profession.

The nuts and bolts of advocacy campaigns are described in the following five case studies. Campaigns are created to deal with a pressing issue or problem. They are grounded in a convincing analysis connecting the issue to larger public concerns. They are aimed at winning sufficient backing to bring about the desired solution to the problem. A campaign is not a one-shot event. It continues over time until the issue is decided. A campaign for a specified remedy, however, is almost always part of a larger, long-term program.

The campaigns described in the following case studies are characterized by the creativity, persistence, and assertiveness of nurses.

Case Studies

1. The Fight for Safe Hospital Staffing Legislation in California

As nurses debate solutions to an ongoing nursing shortage, a number of countries and U.S. states are exploring mandatory nurse-to-patient ratios to ensure adequate levels of nurse staffing to patients and reduce intolerable workloads for nurses. In the United States, California is a bellwether state. It was the first state to dramatically reduce the number of nurses in hospitals during the cost-cutting rampage of the 1990s. Then it was the first to try to reverse the damage by legislating staffing ratios. Staffing ratios were mandated in California because nurses campaigned for them for several years. Even though the legislation was finally signed into law in 1999, the campaign continued because of attempts by the California Hospital Association and the state governor to derail full implementation of the ratios.

The staffing bill was a response to the hospital restructuring that began in the early 1990s. To save money, hospitals were laying off registered nurses (RNs) and replacing them with unlicensed assistive personnel who lacked the training or experience necessary for proper patient care. Nurses complained that the restructuring resulted in expanded RN workloads, understaffing, and assembly-line treatment of patients who were forced out of hospitals by length-of-stay reductions imposed by health maintenance organizations (HMOs). In 1994, the California Nurses Association proposed its first staffing bill. With a Republican majority in the assembly, it never got out of committee. But the Association was mobilizing for the long haul. One of its most innovative tactics was to advertise to find patients who had suffered from short staffing.

"It's 3 A.M. Who will come when you need help?" asked ads that ran in California newspapers and the *New York Times*. The ads asserted that "hospitals and HMOs are cutting care to make record profits. Patients are paying the price." They explained that nursing staffs were being reduced and that "unlicensed staff, often with no clinical background or experience, are being forced to make decisions about your health."

The ads asked people to write to the Association's "Patient Watch," program, "If your care or the care of your loved ones has suffered because of short staffing or inadequate care."

The Association received many responses. Some told tragic stories. "Our family has suffered from the death of our daughter because of short staff and/or inadequate care in a local hospital," one parent wrote. At about 3 A.M., Tuesday, June 7, she vomited and aspirated the vomit, causing cardiac arrest and then seizures. She then went into a coma and was in the coma until she died."

For the most part, the patients and family members who wrote in did not blame individual nurses for the terrible neglect they had experienced. They saw it as a system problem. "Nurses do a terrific job, but more nurses are needed to nurse the patients in the hospitals, not just to hook up patients and take the vitals," said a San Francisco respondent.

In 1994, activists were pursuing every avenue to halt the decimation of nursing care, including national legislation. But the news media were treating managed care largely as a business story. Reporters had trouble finding working nurses who would talk to them about the human costs. Gag orders, threats, and employer retaliation against nurses made it difficult for RNs to come forward. Some did, but only if reporters cloaked the nurses' identities. One nurse interviewed by NBC News was shown only in silhouette behind a screen.

In this atmosphere, the "Patient Watch" stories were an invaluable tool even when the names of patients and hospitals were withheld to avoid lawsuits. To encourage coverage, the Association faxed a new patient horror story to journalists each night (when the phone rates were the lowest).

With support from unions and other organizations working for health care reform, Democrats regained control of the California assembly in 1996. A new, safe-staffing bill finally made it through the legislature in 1998 only to be vetoed by Governor Pete Wilson. That fall, Californians elected a Democrat, Gray Davis, as governor. Davis had told the California Nurses Association he would be favorable to the legislation.

The union knew that even with a friendlier governor and Democratic majority in the legislature, a staffing bill would face intense industry opposition. Only thousands of nurses—working with other health care and patient groups—could overcome this opposition.

To mobilize nurses, the Association built a statewide campaign network. Articles in its publication, *California Nurse*, explained why hospitals were so short staffed and why legislation was necessary to ensure better patient care.

Activists distributed leaflets on the issue in both unionized and nonunion hospitals. In their workplaces, RNs sent signed petitions to unit managers and administrators and asked them to support the bill. Although Association members recognized that few of these administrators would actually support the bill, for some nurses, the action of signing a petition was the first step toward greater involvement in the campaign.

The Association distributed educational material to all California nursing schools. It used its own as well as other nursing Web sites and Listservs to distribute a continuous stream of information.

Association members and other supporters were asked to write letters to state senators and assemblymen. Model letters were made available, but nurses were encouraged to tell their own stories in their own words. Nurses spoke at hearings on the bill, before church and consumer groups, and on television and radio shows. Patients and the families of patients who had suffered were encouraged to join the lobbying effort. They also testified at hearings, wrote letters to the editor, and contacted legislators.

Nurses organized press conferences and used research available on staffing to buttress their case. They met with the editorial boards of all the major newspapers in California and won a number of supportive editorials. Individual nurses also wrote letters to the editor and op-eds.

After the California assembly passed the staffing bill in the summer of 1999, the California Nurses Association organized large rallies to encourage the more reluctant senate to follow suit. When the senators were set to vote on the question, 2,400 RNs gathered at the state capitol in Sacramento. Hundreds more from fifty different hospitals—union and nonunion alike—rallied in Los Angeles. The outpouring of grassroots support pushed a sufficient number of fence-sitters to cast pivotal votes for the bill.

But the governor's signature was still needed to turn the bill into a law. Although Gray Davis had signed other propatient measures, he complained that the legislature was sending him too many bills on health care. He refused to sign a major nursing home reform measure that he worried would place too great a burden on the state budget. He hesitated to sign the staffing bill.

Eleventh-hour lobbying by hospitals and HMOs was intense. Nurses feared that Davis would be swayed by the industry's argument that the bill was too rigid. Campaigners turned up the heat with more letters, faxes, and phone calls, trying to make it politically unacceptable for Davis to refuse to sign. To get the governor's signature, Assemblywoman Sheila James Kuehl, the sponsor of the bill, agreed to offer a follow-up bill the next year postponing implementation of staff ratios from 2001 to 2002 to give the state time to work out the correct ratios.

In 2000, after confronting intense lobbying on the part of the California

Hospital Association, which wanted much higher caseloads for nurses, the CNA was able to win a phased-in set of ratios that approached what nurses had hoped for. Although the ratios varied considerably depending on the patient unit, in 2004, medical-surgical nurses were not permitted to care for more than six patients at a time. This ratio was slated to go down to five patients on January 1, 2005. Some hospitals, like Kaiser Permanente's, had already begun staffing in accordance with the newer ratios.[2]

For a number of reasons (none of which had to do with the staffing legislation), voters became extremely dissatisfied with Davis's performance and voted him out of office in a special recall election. Actor Arnold Schwarzenegger defeated other replacement candidates and became governor of California in 2004. In November, the day after President George W. Bush's election to a second term, Schwarzenegger issued an emergency order suspending continued implementation of the ratios until 2008. Schwarzenegger's order allowed emergency departments to override four-to-one patient-to-nurse ratios during any "unexpected and unpredictable influx of patients."[3] Since it is in the nature of ERs to experience unexpected and unpredictable influxes, this meant that staffing ratios would be almost permanently on hold.

The governor contended that ratios were an added expense that California's hospitals could not afford. He blamed the closures of about a dozen hospitals, and emergency room diversions and closures, on the difficulty of implementing the ratios. He insisted that there were not enough nurses in California or the rest of the country to fulfill the new staffing requirements, and that they placed an inordinate burden on hospital managers and administrators.

The governor's action kick-started a whole new campaign against both him and his action. The California Nurses Association, joined by the Service Employees International Union and consumer and patient advocacy groups like the Consumer Federation of California, insisted that the ratios worked and were not the cause of hospital closures. California nurses quickly mobilized to create public and political pressure on the governor to rescind his executive order. The central argument of their campaign was that the governor was not acting in the interest of California patients, but was doing the bidding of the hospital industry and other special interests as evidenced by the $26 million he had received in campaign contributions from such industries.

Nurses picketed the governor at almost every event he attended. Then in December, Schwarzenegger made a critical error when a handful of nurses interrupted his remarks before approximately ten thousand people at a women's conference in Long Beach. The governor stopped his speech and said: "Pay no attention to those voices over there. They are special interests. Special interests don't like me in Sacramento because I kick their butt."[4]

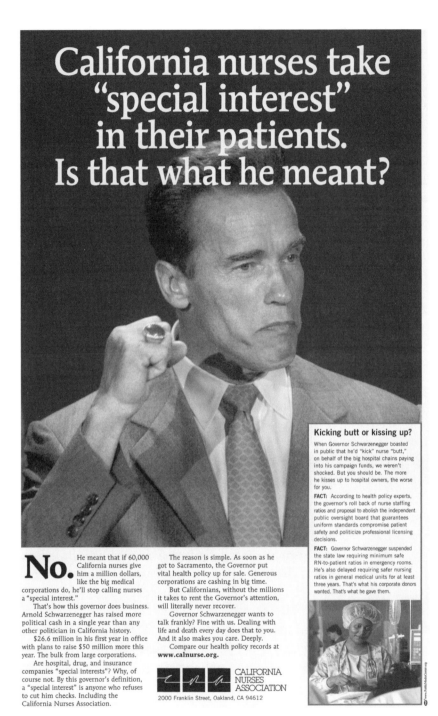

California nurses take "special interest" in their patients. Is that what he meant?

Kicking butt or kissing up?

When Governor Schwarzenegger boasted in public that he'd "kick" nurse "butt," on behalf of the big hospital chains paying into his campaign funds, we weren't shocked. But you should be. The more he kisses up to hospital owners, the worse for you.

FACT: According to health policy experts, the governor's roll back of nurse staffing ratios and proposal to abolish the independent public oversight board that guarantees uniform standards compromise patient safety and politicize professional licensing decisions.

FACT: Governor Schwarzenegger suspended the state law requiring minimum safe RN-to-patient ratios in emergency rooms. He's also delayed requiring safer nursing ratios in general medical units for at least three years. That's what his corporate donors wanted. That's what he gave them.

No. He meant that if 60,000 California nurses give him a million dollars, like the big medical corporations do, he'll stop calling nurses a "special interest."

That's how this governor does business. Arnold Schwarzenegger has raised more political cash in a single year than any other politician in California history.

$26.6 million in his first year in office with plans to raise $50 million more this year. The bulk from large corporations.

Are hospital, drug, and insurance companies "special interests"? Why, of course not. By this governor's definition, a "special interest" is anyone who refuses to cut him checks. Including the California Nurses Association.

The reason is simple. As soon as he got to Sacramento, the Governor put vital health policy up for sale. Generous corporations are cashing in big time.

But Californians, without the millions it takes to rent the Governor's attention, will literally never recover.

Governor Schwarzenegger wants to talk frankly? Fine with us. Dealing with life and death every day does that to you. And it also makes you care. Deeply.

Compare our health policy records at **www.calnurse.org.**

CALIFORNIA
NURSES
ASSOCIATION

2000 Franklin Street, Oakland, CA 94612

© 2005 California Nurses Association and Public Media Center.

Many people were appalled by his comments and recalled accusations that he had groped women and made demeaning comments about them. The California Nurses Association took advantage of the fact that people like nurses, trust them, and don't appreciate vulgar attacks against them. Schwarzenegger also provided fodder for campaigns by labeling nurses "special interests," and then, in his January State of the State speech, extending the category to include teachers, police officers, and firefighters. The Nurses Association, and other groups, stepped up their demonstrations and publicized Schwarzenegger's outbursts as much as possible through TV and print ads. One of these that ran in the West Coast edition of the *New York Times* showed the governor apparently shaking a fist, with the caption, "California nurses take 'special interest,' in their patients. Is that what he meant?"

According to Charles Idelson, communication director for the California Nurses Association, more than six thousand nurses protested at two enormous rallies at the state capitol in Sacramento. Nurses protested at Schwarzenegger's "normally discreet" fundraising dinners in private homes and hotels. A light plane also flew over Schwarzenegger events, towing a banner reading, "California is not for sale."[4]

In February 2005, after protesters blocked the red carpet for a film premiere that Schwarzenegger was attending in Sacramento, Nurse Kelly Di Giacomo, who had a ticket to the event, was detained and questioned by a plainclothes security officer (and later by a bodyguard for the governor) about whether she intended to harm the governor. Di Giacomo asked why she would be considered a threat to Schwarzenegger. "Well, you were wearing a nurse's uniform," was the reply. The press, of course, reported this incident.[5]

On March 4, the sixty thousand–member Nurses Association won the lawsuit it had filed challenging the authority of the governor to overrule the legislature. It had argued that patient safety, not hospital finances, should govern mandatory staffing. California Superior Court Judge Judy Holzer Hersher ordered the immediate implementation of the five-patient limit.

Nurses savored the moment. They carried signs outside the courthouse reading, "Nurses 2, Arnold 0" (referring to the governor's earlier reversal of his decision to abolish the state nursing board), and sang, "Arnold fought the law, and the law won."[2]

In 2000, a world precedent was set when the Australian Nurses Federation (ANF) won a legislative framework for staffing ratios in all public hospitals in the state of Victoria. As in California, the ratios themselves were developed through an administrative rule-making process, in this case conducted by Victoria's Industrial Relations Commission. Organizers drew on U.S. studies connecting inadequate nurse staffing with patient mortality. Rather than going for a strict one-to-four ratio of nurses to patients, however, the ANF formula required five nurses for every twenty patients on medical-surgical wards, and various ratios for other patient populations. (In Victoria, unlike other states in Australia, no patient care assistants are used in acute care public-sector hospitals.)

ANF leaders believe they have a flexible formula that takes into account nurses' levels of experience and training. "Somebody senior might have five patients, while a more junior nurse might have only three," explains Belinda Morieson, past secretary of the ANF in Victoria. "A nurse with very sick patients might care for only three. It's up to the charge nurse to allocate the patients, but there will be five bedside nurses for twenty patients."

In Victoria, "no lift" rules assure nurses that there is sufficient safe-lifting equipment available to handle heavy and immobile patients. Safe-lift rules were passed by the California legislature in 2004, but opposed by the hospital industry. They were vetoed by Governor Schwarzenegger.

With its new ratios as the main incentive, Victoria launched a recruitment campaign to encourage nonpracticing RNs to return to the workforce. The ANF negotiated a government-paid, thirteen-week reentry training program for those who'd let their nursing certificates lapse. In addition, nurses receive guaranteed educational leave time. A part-time nurse receives three paid days off annually to attend seminars and conferences, while a full-time nurse gets five days for this purpose. As news of the ratios and related reforms spread, four thousand nurses returned to the workforce, resulting in few remaining nursing vacancies in Victoria's public hospitals.

In 2003, the Labor government announced that it wanted to replace the ratios with the kind of computerized nurse staffing allocation systems that are common in the United States. The ANF and Victorian nurses immediately launched a campaign dubbed "5-4-20" (signifying five nurses for every twenty patients) to maintain ratios.

The ANF committed $150,000 to advertising, media activities, and plastering the "5-4-20" symbol on everything from taxis to nurses' badges.[6] After trying to bargain with the government for five months, in early 2004 nurses announced that they would take industrial action to protect ratios. "Victoria is the only state in Australia that does not have a severe nurse shortage because the state government was the only one able to advertise

(continued)

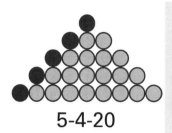

5-4-20

5-4-20 nurse-patient ratios, Australian Nursing Federation (Victoria Branch).

nurse–patient ratios," Lisa FitzPatrick, secretary of the ANF's Victoria branch, told us. "We are taking this action to ensure patients have a mandated minimum, not maximum, number of nurses on each shift to provide a safe and proper level of care."

Because of the nurses' actions, the staffing ratios remained in place and the ANF continued to work to improve their provisions.[7] Many nurse managers in Victoria said that they favored ratios because they protected nursing budgets.

2. Massachusetts Whistleblower Legislation

On November 16, 1998, an unusual column appeared in *Newsweek*. It was written by Massachusetts Nurse Barry Adams, who recounted his efforts to alert administrators to unsafe patient conditions in his Cambridge, Massachusetts, rehabilitation hospital. The article begged members of the public to support a national Patients Bill of Rights that would include whistleblower protection for health care workers.[8] Adams's action was part of a widespread campaign to protect health care workers who were "blowing the whistle" on unsafe conditions in their workplaces.

Reports from nurses and other caregivers about institutional failures eventually prompted the press to turn a critical eye on the growth of managed care in the United States. Whistleblowers risked their jobs to protect the public from hidden health care risks. But one whistleblower, Nurse Adams, became a symbol for the need for legislation that would protect caregivers from retaliation wherever they worked.

The Massachusetts Nurses Association (MNA) had lobbied for whistleblower protection in 1996. MNA leaders understood that passage of such a bill would require public support. But few members of the public were then aware of what was happening to patient care in hospitals and other institutions. Nor did they understand the risks of retaliatory dismissal of those caregivers that revealed unsafe conditions to the public or to governmental agencies.

Members of the MNA had tried to raise public consciousness about this problem. When Adams was fired and the story hit the press, the public was given a vivid illustration of the restraints on caregivers who try to protect their patients.

Four years previously, Nurse Adams had gone to work at the Youville

Health Care Center, a rehabilitation hospital in Cambridge. As the facility experienced mounting pressure to cut costs, Adams witnessed a dangerous erosion in patient-care standards. He documented cases of poor wound management and mistakes that occurred because newly graduated nurses were not adequately supervised.

Adams tried to address these problems in-house. He talked with his immediate supervisor and two other managers who were also alarmed by the eroding quality of care. But when Adams tried to discuss his concerns with Youville's director of nursing, she refused to meet with him. So he sent a memo to the director of nursing and to the chief hospital administrator, who was also a nurse. Both dismissed his reports. As the risks to patients mounted, Adams persisted. The director of nursing threatened to fire him for documenting his concerns. Suddenly his supervisors claimed he was having "time management" problems.

On October 15, 1996, Adams went to the Massachusetts Board of Registration in Nursing (BORN) and filed a complaint of "unprofessional conduct," "unethical conduct," and "patient neglect" against the director of nursing and the administrator of the Youville Center. He asked for clarification of nurses' responsibilities under the state Nurse Practice Act, specifically, whether nurses who were in charge of institutional finances were responsible for the safety of care given under their administration.

Three days later, the hospital dismissed Adams. Two other nurses who had protested were forced to work rotating shifts and resigned soon after.[9]

Although Youville was not unionized and Adams was not an MNA member, he contacted the association. "I'd never been involved in any political or union activity," he said. "But I knew they were the professional organization for nursing in the state, so I called them and said, 'I just got set up and fired.' They talked to me, told me they would help, and said that the first thing I needed was an attorney."

The MNA put Adams in touch with Marie Snyder, an attorney who had been a nurse. She filed a wrongful dismissal suit in state court. She contended that it was a violation of the public trust to fire a nurse for speaking out on behalf of patient care.

Adams and the two other nurses filed a complaint of unfair labor practices against Youville with the National Labor Relations Board (NLRB), the enforcer of federal labor law in the United States.

While these cases were pending, Adams went to work for the Visiting Nurse Association of Boston, whose members were represented by the collective bargaining arm of the MNA. The MNA asked Adams if he'd be willing to talk publicly about his experience. "You bet your boots I would," he responded.

After Adams completed his six-month probationary period at his new job, MNA's director of communications, David Schildmeier approached the

Boston Globe with an offer of an exclusive on the Adams story. Coincidentally, *Globe* reporters had been digging through Massachusetts department of public health records and discovered that a Youville patient had died from an accidental drug overdose. They learned that the health department had cited Youville for eight deficiencies in patient care. Two were specifically for "patient-care neglect" and two were for "lack of professional and technical services" in the department of nursing.

The *Globe*'s story incorporated this information into the saga of Adams as a health care whistleblower. The story generated widespread media coverage.[10] Adams became a symbol for all of the health care whistleblowers who had been penalized. The MNA recognized that Adams was a focal point for the issue and helped him hone his media skills.

Soon after the *Globe* story appeared, the American Nurses Association (ANA) unveiled its Patient Safety Act, a proposed federal bill to provide whistleblower protection throughout the country. Adams was a featured speaker at an ANA press conference on the legislation held at the National Press Club in Washington, DC.

In May 1997, the NLRB held a two-day hearing on the complaint of Adams and his two colleagues. Six months later federal administrative law judge Arthur Amchan ruled that his firing was an "illegal attempt to silence [Adams] and retaliate against him." Amchan found that Youville's disciplinary actions against the three nurses were discriminatory, punitive, and carried out with "animus." He dismissed testimony by the hospital nursing director and ordered the RNs reinstated with back pay. The judge also ordered the hospital to post a notice reassuring employees that they would not be harassed, fired, or disciplined for joining together for mutual aid or protection.[9]

While Adams won this case, he lost his wrongful dismissal suit in state court. Adams and the MNA saw the state court verdict as a demonstration of the need for statutory protection. One reason Adams fared well with the NLRB was that he could show that he had acted in concert with two other nurses. Under U.S. labor law, workers—even nonunion ones—cannot be legally fired or disciplined if they engage in "group" activities related to wages, hours, and working conditions. They have protection if they can act as a group. Many nurses, however, are unaware of this and act alone, sometimes because their colleagues are afraid of what will happen if they speak out with them. While NLRB rules do not discriminate between union and nonunion workplaces in this regard, state courts usually offer no protection to "employees at will" in nonunion workplaces, unless there is a specific statutory ban against recriminations.

In March 1998, a measure to provide such a statutory ban was again introduced into the Massachusetts legislature. Adams appeared on radio and television as a spokesperson for the bill. To keep the whistleblower story alive and draw national attention to legislative activity in the state, Schildmeier later that year contacted a reporter at *NBC Nightly News*. After extensive discussion, NBC carried a piece on the Adams case.

Joan Hurwitz, the ANA's communications director, then suggested that Adams submit an article to *Newsweek*'s "My Turn," a premier forum for personal experiences that have national implications. With the ANA's help, Adams wrote the article and submitted it. *Newsweek* published it on November 16, 1998.

The *Newsweek* column provoked national reaction. Thanks to Adams, and all the nurses who had spoken out, whistleblower legislation was passed in Massachusetts in 1999 and signed by Republican governor Paul Cellucci.

"Being a public speaker and a spokesperson for an issue has been very intimidating to me," Adams says. "But I can cope with this kind of scrutiny because no matter what kind of legal wizardry or spin is placed on what I say, it's still the truth. Getting the support of other nurses and learning that I can deal with even the toughest questions has been very rewarding to me because it has helped nurses improve their working lives. If I had to do it all again, I would."

Over the next several years, a number of states passed some form of whistleblower legislation to protect health care workers against retaliatory action from their employers, but some of the laws provide incomplete protection.

3. *SARS in Ontario*

Over the past decade and a half, it has become a truism that when health care systems start restructuring in order to cuts costs, nursing is likely to take the biggest hit. This was certainly the case in Canada. As Monique Bégin, a former national health minister, told members of the Canadian Nurses Association in 1998: "The restructuring of the health care system in our provinces was done—and is still done—on the backs of nurses. In the last few years, it is mainly, almost only, nurses who have lost full-time employment and income and, worse, in my opinion, who are witnessing the deprofessionalization of their occupation."[11]

In Ontario, the provincial home of Canada's largest city, Toronto, budget cuts led to massive layoffs of full-time nurses. In 1998, half of Ontario's RNs were without full-time jobs. By 2003, there was slight improvement, but more than 43 percent of nurses were still working on a part-time, agency, or "casual" (ad hoc) basis, according to the Registered Nurses Association of Ontario (RNAO), a professional association affiliated with the Canadian Nurses Association.[12]

The restructuring theory was that health care institutions could hold down costs by creating a "flexible 'accordion-like casual work force' that [would] expand and contract on demand," RNAO executive director Doris Grinspun explained. But, "as cost-cutting policies collided with reality, we got a nursing shortage of epic proportions."[13]

Nursing leaders warned that decreased nursing capacity was making it difficult to ensure safe patient care under normal conditions, much less meet the demands of any health emergency. In 2003, even as nurses were expressing these concerns, the epidemic that became known as SARS (severe acute respiratory syndrome) was silently making its way from China's Guangdong province to Toronto, where in little more than four months, it would infect some 375 persons, many of them health care workers, and kill forty-four persons, among them two nurses.[14]

The story of how SARS quickly spread from China to the other parts of the world reads almost like a script for one of television's hospital dramas. An infected physician, since immortalized in the medical literature as Patient A, traveled from Guangdong province to Hong Kong to visit family. He checked into the Metropole Hotel where in the course of his stay, he infected twelve other hotel guests. Those travelers took the illness to Hong Kong, Vietnam, Singapore, Ireland, Germany, and Canada.

The first Canadian casualty, Kwan Sui Chu, a 78-year-old Toronto homemaker, and her husband had been in Hong Kong in February to visit relatives and stayed on the same floor of the Metropole as Patient A. She returned to Toronto on February 23, where she suffered respiratory problems and died at home on March 5. A coroner ruled that she died of a heart attack. No autopsy was done.[15,16]

A week later her 43-year-old son died. His case and that of four other family members who became sick in Toronto was dismissed as tuberculosis, despite a hunch by a Chinese-speaking nurse at Scarborough Grace Hospital that it was an emerging virus she had read about emanating from southeast China and Hong Kong. According to a retrospective analysis by the *Toronto Star*, even after SARS was identified, in many cases infection control was lax and the observations and recommendations of nurses were ignored.[17]

With the onset of the disease in March, the twenty thousand–member RNAO and the Ontario Nurses Association (ONA) union, which represents 51,000 RNs and allied health professionals, immediately began to hear complaints about workplace problems. But even more troubling was what happened during a lull in May when the World Health Organization took Toronto off the list of places with local transmission and politicians turned to luring tourists back. Nurses at North York General Hospital tried to alert doctors about patients with SARS-like symptoms and were told that the cases were not SARS. In fact, seventeen of the forty-four SARS deaths were produced by a second outbreak, a toll that nurses said could have been avoided.[18,14]

During the emergency, the RNAO helped to set up a SARS Nursing Advisory Committee that brought together representatives from all the nursing organizations and involved health care facilities in the province. It created a specific online chat room where nurses could share information and support each other. The ONA posted a dedicated Web site to keep members updated about the latest developments in the epidemic. Nurses were informed about their right to refuse unsafe work, problems they might have if they were pregnant, or what they should do if they were exposed to SARS and were quarantined and thus couldn't work.

Among other things, the SARS epidemic revealed just how ill conceived the manipulation of the nursing workforce had been. The cut in full-time jobs meant that thousands of nurses were working on a part-time or "casual" basis, the latter with neither the benefits nor workplace protections of full-time workers. Many who needed full-time employment cobbled together several jobs, often traveling from one institution to another in the same day or on alternate days, an obvious problem for containing SARS. During the epidemic, the movement of casual nurses was prohibited, thus depleting the workforce more and causing economic hardship for individuals.

Cost-cutting created other containment problems, reported Barb Wahl, then ONA president. Hospitals were skimping on protective gear and failing to educate nurses about the need to wear gowns, gloves, and masks when they were in contact with patients suspected of having SARS. Both the ONA and the RNAO complained that hospitals did not give nurses good protective gear. When they had appropriate gear nurses often didn't have enough time to put on the cumbersome face shields and apparel that might protect them from the respiratory droplets that are the main route of SARS transmission. "We urge you in the strongest terms," Wahl wrote to Ontario Premier Ernie Eves, "not to stand back and knowingly aid and abet those employers who continue to put our members' lives at risk."[19]

The nurses who took care of SARS patients worked long hours and endured tremendous stress. They risked contracting the illness themselves or being carriers of the virus. At least 5,200 health care workers were placed on "working quarantine," meaning they were allowed to go to work in hospitals and other facilities but at home had to remove themselves from any contact with their families, friends, or roommates. Some of the nurses were shunned. "The neighbors were not going outside if I was in my backyard," one nurse reported on the RNAO chatline. "They were afraid of me."

"I can remember worrying about whether I should have left my socks at the hospital as I drove home, recalled Nurse Yvonne Warner. She said that when she arrived at home, "the first stop was my laundry room; then it was into a hot, hot shower where I scrubbed until my skin was almost raw." Warner said that for an entire month, she never once hugged her children or husband for fear of contaminating them. Evenings were spent sitting on the other side of the room from them.[20]

The media and politicians did acknowledge the extraordinary work of nurses during the epidemic. When Nurse Nelia Laroza became the first health care worker to die from SARS, the premier and cabinet ministers attended her funeral along with hundreds of nurses, some of whom stood at attention and saluted her casket as part of a formal honor guard.[21]

But this was far from sufficient to address the workforce policies that had put nurses and patients in peril. In June, the RNAO demanded a full investigation into the handling of the SARS crisis. The organization insisted that the investigation be in accordance with Canada's Public Inquiries Act so that a judge or commission would have subpoena powers and those who testified would have whistleblower protection.

To get maximum media and public attention to pressure the reluctant Eves government, nursing organizations mobilized nurses to speak about their experiences and the issues that needed to be addressed and provided them with factual material and talking points. Nurses conducted informational pickets. Nurses showed up at one press conference in the provincial parliament wearing white facial masks with the words "muzzled," "silenced," or "ignored" emblazoned on them.[22]

The RNAO named three key issues that needed to be investigated: the ability of the health care system to respond to SARS and to protect the health and safety of health care workers and the public, the impact of "excessive reliance on casual, part-time and agency nurses" on the "quality and availability of nursing services during the SARS outbreak," and the circumstances of the second outbreak of SARS and the reasons nurses' early warnings were ignored.

The nurses also wanted the government to declare what measures it was prepared to take to "ensure the preparedness of the Ontario health-care system for health emergencies."[23]

Citing issues of patient confidentiality, Premier Eves rejected the call for an investigation under the Public Inquiries Act and instead named Ontario Superior Court Justice Archie Campbell as an independent commissioner "to investigate how the SARS virus came to the province, how the virus spread, and how it was dealt with." Significantly, the commission did provide whistleblower protection to those who supplied information.[24]

In July, ONA President Wahl met with Campbell and reported to members on the ONA Web site, "He wants to hear specific examples of what happened and when it happened from individual nurses and allied members who actually had the experiences, wherever possible." Wahl reported that Campbell wanted to know the impact of pay inequities from reliance on part-time, casual, and agency nurses and wanted to hear from nurses "who were pushed to work on SARS units, from nurses who had to work without masks or with masks that did not fit. She said that the commissioner wanted "copies of e-mails sent by employers indicating (infection control) restrictions could be tailored to specific hospitals." The ONA told its members it would work with them to help prepare testimony.

In August 2003, the RNAO conducted fifteen focus groups and fifty-one personal interviews for its own inquiry. In its report the organization called for whistleblower legislation "to ensure nurses and other health care workers can express concerns without fear of reprisals from employers," and implementation of what it calls "the 70 percent solution," an increase to 70 percent full-time employment for RNs along with staffing levels high enough to cover contingencies.

RNAO President Joan Lesmond said that the SARS outbreak was an "experience our profession will never forget and to many nurses, it was the worst of times. Their voices are at the heart of our report."[25]

Since 2003 some progress has been made. The federal government provided new funding to the provinces to improve their health systems and set up a cabinet-level health agency to work on health promotion and emergency preparedness. A new provincial government was elected. In fall of 2005, 59 percent of Ontario's nurses were working full time.

At that time, SARS seemed to be gone in the world, but it is not forgotten. It is widely regarded as a wake-up call to health systems that may have to deal with new fast-moving epidemics. SARS had infected some 8,100 people in 29 countries and killed 774.[16] Many of those who came in contact with it suffered ongoing physical, psychological, and emotional effects.

In August 2005, a judge ruled that at least three lawsuits involving Toronto nurses infected with SARS could legally proceed. One of the suits was a $600 million class action; another brought by the family of Nurse Laroza sought $12 million in damages; and the third, launched by the ONA on behalf of 53 nurses, including Nurse Tecla Lin who died from SARS, sought $17 million in damages. The suits alleged that the Ontario government had put the economic health of the province's tourism industry ahead of that of its nurses.[26]

Commissioner Campbell made two interim reports outlining changes in authority and procedures to improve health emergency response, and calling for whistle-blower protection for health care workers. His final report was scheduled for 2006.

"It might inspire a whole new campaign to get the recommendations implemented by the government," Sine MacKinnon, director of communication for the RNAO, told us. She pointed out that provincial elections scheduled for fall 2007 are a time for nurses to influence politicians who hope to get their votes.

"We first started talking about the 70-percent solution in 1999," Mac-Kinnon said. "We're just now seeing some of our recommendations being put into effect. It takes years to get legislation and funding, so you have to be absolutely persistent."

4. The Service Employees International Union (SEIU) Campaign to Prevent Needlestick Injuries

On Monday, April 13, 1998, readers of the *San Francisco Chronicle* opened their newspapers to find the first installment of a three-day series of articles on "Deadly Needles."[27] *Chronicle* reporters Reynolds Holding and William Carlsen reported that some one million nurses, physicians, nurses aides, hospital housekeepers, lab techs, home care nurses, and other health care workers in the United States each year experienced accidental needlesticks that exposed them to the human immunodeficiency virus (HIV), hepatitis B and C, and other diseases; thousands of health care workers became infected from needlesticks; and hundreds eventually died from their illnesses. Most of this, the reporters asserted, was the result of corporate greed, hospital penny pinching, and regulatory agency indifference that had prevented the widespread use of safer syringe needles.

In a total of twelve articles, Holding and Carlsen laid out the "chilling pattern of indifference and neglect within the nation's medical industry" that they had uncovered during six months of investigation.

The reporters found that the hazards posed by conventional needles were widely known by the early 1980s and had stimulated a variety of approaches toward making needles safer. Indeed, the reporters learned that executives at Becton, Dickinson, and Company, a medical device corporation that has largely controlled the global market in syringes, knew by the 1960s that hepatitis B could be transmitted both by the reuse of contaminated needles and through accidental needlesticks. Ironically, although patients were protected from contamination by the use of disposable needles, health care workers were not.

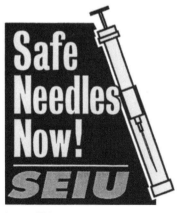

Couresty SEIU.

Safer needle options have existed for almost two decades. But Becton Dickinson, whose revenues reached

$2.8 billion in 1997, refused to jeopardize its existing market share by introducing safer needles. Hospitals, in turn, declined to spend extra money to purchase safer needles from other suppliers. For their part, the U.S. Occupational Safety and Health Administration (OSHA) and Federal Drug Administration (FDA) dawdled and delayed actions that would have protected workers. In 1985, the Centers for Disease Control (CDC), knowing there was a needlestick problem, recommended that health workers wear gowns, gloves, and masks to protect against infection and receive the hepatitis B vaccine as a precaution. But the CDC did not recommend the use of safer needles. By then, the reporters pointed out, needlesticks were already spreading a mysterious new disease—AIDS—that was killing with brutal efficiency. In 1988, the *New England Journal of Medicine* published a landmark study that blamed needlesticks on syringe design rather than on the carelessness of health care workers and asserted that needlestick injuries could be reduced by 85 to 90 percent by using safer needles.[28]

Reynolds and Carlsen cataloged the tragic consequences of corporate, institutional, and governmental disregard. They profiled health care workers who suffered terribly, like Ellen Dayton, a nurse practitioner at the San Francisco General hospital and a University of California drug clinic, who in 1996 was accidentally pierced with an HIV- and hepatitis C infected needle. She contracted hepatitis C, for which there is no vaccine or cure, and she became ill with AIDS even though she took the prophylactic medications that sometimes stop or slow the development of the disease after exposure to HIV. Dayton, a member of SEIU local 790, sued Becton Dickinson, contending that the company made and marketed an unreasonably dangerous product.

The *Chronicle* series was a pivotal event for the hundreds of thousands of nurses, physicians, and other health care workers who had been working for years through the SEIU and other unions and health care groups to get safer needles. The series appeared just as SEIU was launching its biggest effort yet—a campaign for safe needle legislation in California and other states.

For almost fifteen years, the SEIU had engaged in aggressive and sustained public communication in its pursuit of educational, legal, regulatory, and contractual remedies to the needlestick problem. Early on, for example, it published educational materials and conducted workshops to teach members how to avoid needlesticks.

Between 1992 and 1994, the union negotiated safe needle requirements in some of its hospital contracts. It filed complaints with California's workplace safety agency, CalOSHA, against the Kaiser Health Plan. This action led to a CalOSHA citation against Kaiser that required the HMO to evaluate and purchase safer needles throughout its California facilities. This was a step forward, but there were still questions about which needles were the safest. Implementation was uneven, and health care workers in other facilities were still unprotected. Without strong state laws, there would be no industrywide implementation to protect all workers.

SEIU and its allies began lobbying hard for such legislation. One of the most active groups in unveiling this hidden menace was the SEIU Nurse Alliance, which represents the union's nurses.

Communication was especially critical for gaining public support. It was central to organizing a grassroots force powerful enough to be heard by legislators.

In January 1998, SEIU's campaign communication department devised a list of "crowd events" and "non-crowd events" that union locals could use to attract media attention.

The categories of crowd events as outlined in an internal memo were:

- *Rally*—requires a large crowd and could include state legislators and community leaders as speakers in addition to nurses.
- *Speak-out*—workers standing on capitol steps taking turns talking about their fears or actual experience of contracting a deadly disease from needlesticks.
- *Candlelight vigil*—"even a few dozen people carrying candles at dusk can make a powerful statement."
- *Lobby day*—health care workers (in purple scrubs) showing legislators and others how safe needles work by injecting oranges.

Recommended non-crowd events to illuminate the problem included hearings at which health care workers and outside expert witnesses could testify to the dangers of needlesticks; news conferences; donations of a day's worth of safer needles to a hospital; setting up information booths in hospitals and at other health care facilities; informational pickets to distribute leaflets in front of hospitals and regulatory agencies; and "fax-ins" to generate large numbers of messages directly to the governor or to a central location from which they can be forwarded.

In 1998, the year of the most intense effort in California, the SEIU readied an arsenal of communication materials to inform and mobilize its members, allies, and the general public and to encourage reporters to pursue the needlestick story. These included workplace posters, leaflets, model laws, instructions on how to file complaints with OSHA, and a media "tool kit" for union locals.

This tool kit, and another one developed at a later stage of the campaign, was designed to help activists persuasively tell the story of the needlestick epidemic and featured a list of talking points.

There was a question-and-answer sheet that responded to arguments that might be raised, such as the suggestion that safer needles would be prohibitively expensive.

"They range in cost from 17 cents to 45 cents per unit for safety needles versus 8 cents per conventional needle," the SEIU response sheet stated. "However, these costs are based on demand, which at this time is virtually non-existent because most hospitals are not purchasing them. If manufacturers were to make these devices in large quantities, the unit costs would go down dramatically. And any analysis of cost ought to include liability costs or the cost of sending a health care worker home to their families with hepatitis B or C or HIV."

The tool kits contained prototype op-ed articles that a nurse or a union official could adapt and submit to a newspaper. They contained a draft of a letter that a group could send to a newspaper editorial board to arrange a meeting on the issue. There was a draft pitch to television outlets that suggested interviewees (nurses who had been stuck by needles) and a story peg (pending legislation) that could be used for a TV feature or talk show. It was accompanied by a videotape aptly named "Killer Needles: Our Fight to Stop a Health Care Epidemic."

The SEIU's press work helped pave the way for the *San Francisco Chronicle* series, which was the most influential media report on the subject. The series was spurred by other developments as well. One was a report by the CDC (renamed as the Centers for Disease Control and Prevention) in 1997 that using safer needles could reduce needlestick injuries by 76 percent. Around that time, Retractable Technologies—an upstart firm trying to manufacture and market safe needles—contacted the *Chronicle* because its reporters had been covering AIDS and worker safety. During the same period, Nurse Ellen Dayton, a member of SEIU, went public about the consequences of her needlestick accident. The situation had the components of a great exposé. The *Chronicle* assigned Holding and Carlsen to investigate. They spent several days in Washington, DC, combing through relevant documents at the SEIU headquarters and speaking to union experts.

"The *Chronicle* series illustrates how newspaper coverage can act as a catalyst on an issue," says Jamie Cohen, an occupational safety and health expert who is the coordinator of the SEIU Nurse Alliance. "Information on the dangers of needlestick injuries had been around for more than a decade before this series came out. But this series brought it all together."

It had an immediate impact. California Assemblywoman Carole Migden, a Democrat from San Francisco, worked with the SEIU to draft a bill setting a timetable for study and implementation of safe devices. Union members, particularly the SEIU Nurse Alliance, mobilized to support the bill. The union sent out a full set of campaign materials to activists including sample news releases and other tip sheets and checklists. To lobby legislators personally, nurses went to the state capitol in Sacramento armed with safer needles and oranges.

On September 1, 1998, the California legislature became the first in the nation to pass a bill requiring the state OSHA to enforce the use of needles with retractable sheaths and other protections that would reduce accidental needlesticks. But a huge obstacle remained. Earlier that year, Republican governor Pete Wilson vetoed the California Nurses Association nurse staffing bill. He was likely to do the same to the needlestick legislation.

To sway the governor, SEIU members faxed him 1,200 messages. Activists organized candlelight vigils in Los Angeles and San Francisco. Kaiser Permanente, the largest health care insurer in California, and the California Health Care Association (an industry group that had initially opposed the legislation) urged Wilson to sign the bill. He did so on September 30, 1998.

As we write this, twenty-four states have safer needle laws on the books. In 2002, the federal Needlestick Safety and Prevention Act was passed. Still, "aggressive monitoring" suggests that the incidence of needlestick injuries ranges from 14 to 839 per 1,000 healthcare workers per year.[29] The SEIU Nurse Alliance is continuing its campaign to ensure that the laws are adequate and enforced, to provide information about the best devices, and to get unsafe sharps removed from the market.

5. *The Center for Nursing Advocacy*

Nurses frequently complain about the misuse of their image and inaccurate representation of the profession by marketers, television writers, and journalists. From time to time there have been nursing protests against distorted media depictions of nurses, but there has never been an established vehicle to consistently track and respond to media and commercial depictions of nurses and their work. In 2002 that changed when the Center for Nursing Advocacy launched its excellent and provocative Web site, www.nursingadvocacy.org.

The Center was prompted by seven graduate students at the Johns Hopkins University School of Nursing who met to talk about the nursing shortage and concluded that resources for staffing, education, and research were negatively affected by inaccurate images of nursing. One of those students, Sandy Summers, now executive director of the Center, drew upon her colleagues, family, and friends to make the Web site a reality. She recruited prominent nursing figures and communication experts to form a nonprofit

The Center for Nursing Advocacy Mission Statement

The Center for Nursing Advocacy seeks to increase public understanding of the central, frontline role nurses play in modern health care. The focus of the Center is to promote more accurate, balanced, and frequent media portrayals of nurses and increase the media's use of nurses as expert sources. The Center's ultimate goal is to foster growth in the size and diversity of the nursing profession at a time of critical shortage, strengthen nursing practice, teaching, and research, and improve the health care system.

corporation and to serve as directors and advisers.* The Center's budget comes from modest membership donations, individual and organizational contributions, and grants. "What Sandy is doing is incredible," says pioneering media researcher Beatrice Kalisch, who is chairman of the Center's board of directors. "We all need to support this vital service."

The Web site serves three major functions: (1) It tracks depictions of nurses in the news, entertainment, and advertising media. (2) It serves as an early warning system to alert nurses to problematic images and to mobilize them to respond so that purveyors of such images will either withdraw or amend them. (3) It maintains an accessible archive of these materials and reports on significant studies and developments in nursing.

Of these, the Center's most important function, we believe, is its mobilization of nurses to protest problematic media images of nurses and to seek accurate and respectful ones. Its director and board understand that powerful media groups will not respond to a single protesting letter or phone call. Like the organizations mentioned earlier that use the power of thousands as citizens to vote for or against particular politicians, the Center uses the power of nurses as consumers. It also provides encouragement and censure by giving awards to the best and the worst images of nursing.

In just a few years, the Center for Nursing Advocacy has waged a number of successful campaigns against major advertisers who used vulgar and semi-pornographic images of nurses to peddle their products.

For example, in August 2003, nurses who had signed up to receive the Center's e-mails, were informed that the Skechers shoe company was planning to launch a global "Naughty and Nice" ad campaign featuring the pop star Christina Aguilera in three different ads: as a police officer confronting

*Disclosure: Bernice Buresh is a member of the Center for Nursing Advocacy's board of directors, and Suzanne Gordon serves on its advisory panel.

a woman bending over a car, as a schoolteacher confronting a student sitting at her desk, and as a nurse confronting a patient sitting on a hospital bed.

"In each photo," the Center noted, "Aguilera plays both figures, and there is a strong element of sado-masochism, with the authority figures as the dominants. All figures are dressed and posed in sexually suggestive ways, often with exposed bras and/or short shorts. In each case the dominant wields a symbol of her physical authority in a threatening, if goofy, way: the teacher holds a ruler, the cop some handcuffs, and the nurse is about to inject a patient with something that looks like a huge 100 cc metal syringe connected to an 8 gauge needle."[30]

The Center reported that it had learned from the business and advertising trade press that the three print ads, with all the figures wearing Skechers shoes, were to run in pop culture and teen magazines, and that the images would be placed in retail stores around the world.

The Center urged nurses to send a letter posted on its Web site (or their own version) to executives of the company urging them to pull the ads and refrain from using nurses in future ads. More than 3,000 nurses and nursing supporters did just that. Within two weeks, Skechers released a statement from its director of corporate communications announcing that it pulled all U.S. distribution of the advertisement and was discontinuing international media placements.[30] The Center followed up by urging nurses to send a thank you letter to Skechers for pulling the ads.

This is just one of several campaigns the Center has waged. It got Procter & Gamble to pull its commercial for Clairol's Herbal Essence Shampoo featuring a nurse that abandoned her patient so that she could wash her hair in the patient's bathroom and experience an orgasm over the results. After nurses and nursing organizations, including the American Nurses Association, wrote to the company, and after an influential nurse spoke directly to a high-ranking executive of the company, Procter & Gamble stopped the ad and sent a letter of apology to the ANA.[31]

The Center has also focused on the popular television show *ER*. Communication researchers have measured *ER*'s effect on perceptions of the U.S. health care system and health issues. A 1997 study sponsored by the Kaiser Family Foundation documented the impact of just one episode of *ER* that introduced the topic of emergency contraception following date rape. "The entire 'date rape' vignette is no more than a couple of minutes long, and the mention of using birth control pills for emergency (postcoital) contraception is less than a minute." Yet, a week later, "the number of *ER* viewers who knew that a woman has options for preventing pregnancy even after unprotected sex increased by seventeen percentage points."

In 2002, another study by the foundation found that "entertainment media are also likely to play a role in shaping viewer's broader conceptions of the health care system." Viewers of hospital dramas believe they're being "taken behind the scenes to see the hidden forces affecting whether there's a happy ending or a sad one. There are good guys and bad guys, heroes and villains and innocent bystanders."[32]

In that light, in 2001, the newly launched Center held a one-hour conference call with *ER* producers and the show's medical advisers to relay its concerns and urge it to depict nurses more accurately.

"The reach of *ER* is broader than any other health care show ever," says Center executive director Sandy Summers. "It is seen by millions across the globe. It wants to give the impression that it accurately depicts what clinicians do in hospitals. While other television shows ignore nurses, *ER* has some nurses doing something—collecting vital signs, throwing IV bags back and forth—so that viewers think this must be what nurses really do. But nursing is consistently under-portrayed and the show has doctors doing the work of nurses."

Summers says the nurses' main function on *ER* is to date doctors and that the show follows the love-lives of the main nurse characters more than those of the doctors. Case in point: When *ER* character Abby Locklear was a nurse, the writers dwelled on her love life. "But then they decided she was 'too smart' to be a nurse anymore and to take that grief from physicians, so she became a physician. Now they don't portray her love life at all," Summers says.

The Center tried to conduct a dialogue with the show's producers, but when that didn't prove fruitful, it alerted members and others to write to *ER* to protest its view of nursing. Then it fired off news releases on its concerns about *ER*, which resulted in worldwide press attention.

"*ER* is the most influential purveyor of the handmaid image," Summers told us. "Getting that to change takes massive effort by nurses. Perhaps there has been slight improvement, but they have light years to go, and we need to keep up the pressure."

In all of these campaigns, nurses weren't just trying to polish their image and upgrade their status, they were, and are, campaigning to secure resources to defend a profession central to health care and to protect the health care delivery system itself. In the process, they not only showed the public the power of nursing but helped nurses understand the potential of collective action.

Chapter 10

In Your Own Voice: Letters to the Editor, Op-Eds, and Blogs

Letters and opinion sections in newspapers and magazines or on the Web, and the more recent blog sites, can be powerful forums for nurses.

Many news publications and radio and television news outlets provide a page or a Web site for the publication of readers' and listeners' views. Here readers may complain about or praise coverage, give their slant on an issue, set the record straight, or highlight their own or their group's activities in connection with a current issue. The key is to do it briefly.

News organizations welcome timely, well-written letters, even though they often receive many more submissions than they can publish. A number of the letters are simply unpublishable because they are diatribes, libelous, or nonsensical. Small and medium-sized newspapers might publish a high percentage of the acceptable letters they receive. There is much more competition at big-city newspapers and national magazines. Nevertheless, a letter to such a publication may influence coverage even if it is not published.

Today the Internet makes it possible for letters to broadcast and cable outlets to be "published" as well, and published in large volume. Before the development of Web sites, there was little opportunity for the public to know how viewers and listeners were responding to television and radio broadcasts even though their letters might well have had an impact. Few programs emulate National Public Radio and CBS's *60 Minutes,* which both schedule on-air time to read letters from the public.

However, the major television networks and many other television and radio news organizations have a feedback section on their Web sites that resemble the letters-to-the-editor page in the print media. Newspapers and magazines also have Web sites, and letters from their readers may be posted on them whether or not they appeared in the print version. Because Web sites archive material, it's often possible to see letters that have been sent over a period of time. So your "published" letter may be available to others for a significant amount of time.

Many news publications and some consumer magazines also provide a place for guest opinion columns. Most newspapers reserve part of a page or a full page for opinion columns. In journalism jargon this is the "op-ed" page because it is usually situated opposite the editorial page. The opinion pieces found on these pages are also referred to as op-eds.

The Web log, or blog, is the newest and fastest-growing vehicle for expressing and distributing personal opinions. Some blogs look like letters to the editor or op-ed pieces, but most are freewheeling, quirky, anonymous, and so overwritten that they are probably more satisfying to the writer than to the reader. Still, for all its unreliability, the blog is a form that is rapidly evolving and here to stay.

Writing Letters to the Editor

The letters page or section is the bridge between the readers and the publication. "It is the one vehicle for regularly publishing citizen comment," says the Boston media writer Mark Jurkowitz. "It facilitates lively community debate not possible on the news pages. And, it is often the only recourse for those who feel offended or damaged by something they read here."[1]

For nurses, writing a letter to the editor is one of the simplest and most effective ways to do the following:

- Correct an error
- Increase nursing visibility
- Express an opposing point of view
- Affirm and encourage positive news coverage
- Educate journalists and the public about a particular issue
- Try to change the way a topic is perceived or covered

Letters to the media can provide editors, producers, and reporters with feedback on their coverage, as does the following letter.

A Portrait of Class in America

MAY 19, 2005

To the Editor:

"Life at the Top in America Isn't Just Better, It's Longer" ("Class Matters" series, front page, May 16) reveals the true inequities in our "top notch" health care system with the comparative experiences of a heart attack for three different social classes of citizens.

Letter
to the
Editor

We spend more per capita than any other country for our health services, get less in outcome than any other country, and still extol the virtues of our system. It is our own caste system, and this kind of gold standard no one should emulate.

Our system is innovative in diagnosing and designing, but it is also costly, unfair and unstable. We can do better.

Carole Ferguson
Lexington, Mass., May 16, 2005
The writer is a pediatric nurse practitioner.

If you see coverage that is erroneous and must be corrected, or coverage that deserves praise, respond quickly with an e-mail *and* a phone call. When Mark Jurkowitz was ombudsman for the *Boston Globe*, he asked nine editors how readers who want "to connect with a newsroom decision maker and force the paper to rethink its coverage" could do so. The editors suggested that readers should first call the reporter and bring the problem to his or her attention. If there is no resolution, or the reporter can't be reached, the caller should try to get through to the editor of the section.[2]

A direct but courteous approach works better than a harangue. Maintain an even, reasonable tone in all contacts with the media, oral or written. "No matter how angry you are, avoid conspiracy theories and vicious personal attacks," Jurkowitz advises. In a letter to the editor or in personal contact or correspondence, never accuse a journalist of maliciously fabricating information if you are concerned about a factual error. A good way to build the bridge is to say you appreciate the reporter's effort and then calmly state your criticism. Give specific examples of what was underplayed, overplayed, or misreported, and suggest what should be handled differently.

Newspaper editorials that deal with health care or with the nursing profession provide a great opportunity for nurses to publicly highlight their expertise through responding letters to the editor. Above all, nurses must write in to correct stereotypes and misconceptions about nurses and nursing.

Today, the cost of nursing education is a topic that frequently arises. In Australia, the baccalaureate degree is now required for entry into nursing. Periodically, politicians and policy makers question whether this level of education is necessary for nurses, the implication being that such educational resources are too costly. The Melbourne newspaper *Sunday Age* ran an editorial opining that university degrees were not as important as nurses' "people skills." A nursing historian immediately responded citing nursing outcomes research to show that the editorial's quaint idea of what it takes to be a nurse is out of synch with the reality.

August 22, 2004 (*Sunday Age*)

To the Editor:

It is disappointing that Victorian nurses are once more confronted with the hoary old chestnut that their education belongs in the realm of "people skills and life experience." This time, the purveyor of the myth is none other than the *Sunday Age*.

How is it that accountants, lawyers and architects are not told that their "applied" knowledge and skills disqualify them from admission to university? Nor do our colleagues in physiotherapy or occupational therapy suffer the same devaluating of their knowledge and skills.

Research shows that every patient in excess of four that a nurse has to care for has a seven per cent increase in risk of dying. Is this because of nurses' interpersonal skills? It is also official that medical error is the fourth-largest cause of death overall in the US.

So can one seriously argue that nursing is simply the work of good, kind women, "clever with their hands?"

Sioban Nelson (Professor) School of Nursing,
University of Melbourne

Pointers on Submitting Letters to the Media

If you have something to say, write a letter and say it. Most letters pages have information on where to send your letter. More information is usually available on the publication's Web page. The following guidelines from the *Milwaukee Journal Sentinel* are fairly typical. Note the suggested two hundred–word limit. Editors are ready to condense letters submitted to them, but only up to a point. If you submit a letter that goes on and on, you are making it a better candidate for the delete button than for the letters page.

1. Generally, we limit letters to two hundred words.
2. Name, street address, and daytime phone are required.
3. We cannot acknowledge receipt of submissions.
4. We don't publish poetry, anonymous, or open letters.
5. Each writer is limited to one published letter every two months.

The *Journal Sentinel*'s Web site has a form on which a letter can be typed and submitted electronically. The site also gives the postal address, but it's better to e-mail the letter because the window of opportunity is tight. If an article that you want to respond to appears on December 2, it's best to write and send your letter that day. Indeed, you may see responses in the next day's newspaper. The more days that pass, the lower your chances of getting published.

Note that all publications will want your name, address, telephone and fax numbers, and e-mail address. News publications do not run anonymous letters, and some call to verify that you are the writer. Under rare circumstances, the publication might withhold your name if you ask. But one of the reasons for writing letters to the editor is to make nurses more visible.

Here are some other guidelines:

- A letter that contains news values (see Chapter 6) will be more publishable than one that doesn't.
- If you are responding to a particular article or articles, include the name of the article and the date that it appeared.
- Include your credentials in both your signature (e.g., "RN") and the body of your letter ("As a nurse . . ."). The reason for doubling up is that some newspapers (the *New York Times* is one) print MD after doctors' names but do not list nursing degrees (possibly because the general public would not be familiar with any other than RN). The only way that readers will learn that you are a nurse is if you say so in the letter and also after your name so that editors can't miss it. If you are a PhD and use only that as a credential, the nursing connection is likely to be lost. Note that Carole Ferguson's academic credentials did not follow her name, but the *Times* identified her as a pediatric nurse practitioner from information that she provided.
- Make sure your facts are accurate. News publications discard letters with obvious factual errors or exaggerations. Some publications even fact-check letters before publishing them.
- A publication may ask you to condense your letter or, more likely, will do it for you. An editor may ask you for additional information. Most of the time you won't see the editing changes until the letter is published.
- Send copies of the letter to the reporter who wrote the story, to the editor of the section in which it appeared, and perhaps to the ombudsman (a staffer who represents the interests of readers and investigates their complaints) if there is one. You can find the names on the publication's Web site or by calling. If you're writing about a disputed issue, you might also want to send copies to the editor and managing editor whose names are on the publication masthead.

You don't have to be a specialist or a nursing professor to respond to coverage. You are an expert on your experience as a nurse, and your observations can educate the public about nursing and health care, as did the following letter from two Canadian nurses.

Broken Legs or Broken Condoms, the ER Staff Cares

January 13, 2000 (*Vancouver Sun*), Letter of the Day

Letter
to the
Editor

To the Editor:

Crisis in the emergency department! This is news? It exists, but it is far from new.

As nurses working at St. Paul's emergency department, we have, for many years, had to battle overcrowding, struggling to care for patients expediently while attempting to assuage our guilt about making patients wait. However, there are many reasons to be proud of working at Vancouver's inner-city hospital. We would like to express a more positive view than has been recently portrayed in the media.

We have a highly educated nursing and medical team who are supportive, caring and collaborative in their approach to treating a diverse community of patients. Despite it being a challenging environment, staff who have left often choose to return to our unique department.

Patients can expect to be treated in a nonjudgmental way whether they seek treatment for a broken leg, a broken heart, a broken condom or a broken needle in their arm. We provide a safe, albeit noisy, environment with humour and warmth.

Certainly from the trenches the solutions seem evident:

1. Build more extended care facilities for convalescent and geriatric patients.
2. Increase home-care services.
3. Open a temporary unit in each hospital for overflow emergency patients.
4. Increase the admission capacity of nursing schools.
5. Make nursing a more attractive career choice through public education, increased compensation for shift work and more opportunities for growth and development within the profession such as advanced nursing practice.

Lisa Moralejo and Michelle Gilbertson, Vancouver

Timing Is Everything

In letters to more than one newspaper, Claire Hale, the professor of clinical nursing at the University of Leeds, weighed in on one of the most vexing "solutions" to the global nursing shortage—using foreign nurses from less-developed countries to increase the number of nurses in industrialized nations like Great Britain. Her letters were prompted by an article in the *Times Higher Education Supplement*, a weekly newspaper for universities and colleges, on the proposed elimination of scholarships to foreign, non–European Union nursing students.

Letter to the Editor

To the Editor:

One of the main reasons the UK has a shortage of qualified nurses was the Conservative government–induced reduction in the number of nurse training places in the early 1990s. To redress the shortage this created, many NHS [National Health System] trusts are now having to recruit qualified nurses from overseas.

It is against this background that Labour is set to abolish the system of offering bursaries and tuition support to prospective nursing students resident outside the European Union. The reason for this change in policy, as stated in your report, is the concern that taxpayers' money might be spent on overseas students who are not planning to work in the UK.

We do not know how many of these overseas students stay in the UK to work as qualified nurses. Even if all or most do return to their own country on completion of their training, that should not be a reason for abolishing their eligibility for a bursary. If Labour is prepared to condone the depletion of the qualified nursing resource of less developed countries, then it has an obligation to help to replenish that resource. To do otherwise is morally reprehensible.

What price an ethical foreign policy now?

Claire Hale, Professor of Clinical Nursing, University of Leeds

Hale told us that many hospitals were recruiting aggressively overseas in response to the nursing shortage in the United Kingdom, which she asserted was "largely of government's own making." She said that at the time she wrote her letter, all students accepted for the nursing diploma program were eligible for a government scholarship that would cover fees and provide approximately 5,000 British pounds. "This was quite attractive to some students," Hale said, "particularly those from countries with old colonial links to the United Kingdom such as Zambia and Zimbabwe. Some schools take quite a lot of overseas students."

However, the government was about to drop the scholarships for non–European Union students and require them to pay overseas student fees. "This might not be an unreasonable thing to do if we had plenty of nurses and potential students in the UK," Hale said, "but as long as we have hospitals touring the world looking for staff, then it is quite insensitive."

Hale said that after she wrote her initial letter, "I was so pleased with it that I decided to send it 'cold'" to two major British newspapers, the *Independent* and the *Guardian*. The *Guardian* apparently had covered the issue and thus ran her letter. The following week the topic was debated at the Royal College of Nursing, and the *Independent* reported on it. Hale speculated that had she waited a week before writing to the *Independent*, she might have been published there as well.

A year and a half later, Hale saw an article in the *Independent* on the recruitment of overseas nurses, and she e-mailed her opinions to the writer and sent a revised version of her original letter to the letters page. The *Independent* published it. "It just shows that timing is everything, and you can get a lot of mileage from one letter," she said.

Blogs

Instead of or in addition to writing letters to newspapers and magazines, many people are dashing off their opinions and posting them on blog sites, on electronic bulletin boards, and in chat rooms.

Blog readership grew significantly in 2004, driven, according to a study by the Pew Internet and American Life Project, by events that people urgently wanted to discuss, such as the tsunami disaster. Twenty-seven percent of online adults in the United States said in November 2004 that they read blogs, compared with 17 percent in a February survey. Even so, only 38 percent of Internet users knew what a blog was.[3]

Bloggers have been credited with unearthing damaging and significant facts about politicians, celebrities, and news operations. "Blogging is a huge part of the public conversation now," Jurkowitz told us. "As an entity the blogosphere is certainly growing in clout." He explained that journalists now routinely monitor certain blog sites or the work of particular bloggers for news leads and to get a sense of what people are talking about. "Some blogging is reporting, it's fact-based information," Jurkowitz said. "The flip side is that a good deal of it is unvarnished opinion, unverified fact, and rampant speculation. It's not always easy to tell whether bloggers are adding information or just standing on a corner soapbox."

The biggest problem with blogs (and with reader and viewer postings to the electronic bulletin boards of news organizations) is that most are anonymous, and thus the writers are unaccountable for what they say.

Some blog sites do have operating rules and provide a platform for nurses who want to engage in serious discussion. One such site is *www.nurseblog.org* operated by the Service Employees Industrial

> *"The difference between letters to the editor and blogs is that letters are vetted, they are edited, and if they have obscenities they don't appear."*
>
> —O. Ricardo Pimentel, *editorial page editor*, **Milwaukee Journal Sentinel**

Union (SEIU) Nurse Alliance of Florida, which posted this introductory course on blogging for the uninitiated:

What is a blog?
Blog is short for web log. It's an interactive online journal. The blog is also a spirited forum for discussion.

What's the point?
The blog also allows you to join in discussions with other people interested in the same topics.

What sort of things get posted on the blog?
Entries about what nurses are discussing, union activities, topics of interest.

Why are some words on the blog in bold purple letters?
These words are links to others pages. Clicking the bold words will take you to the page.

What does it mean to link?
We provide links to relevant stories, articles, or Web sites. However, NurseBlog.org does not endorse and is not responsible for the content of external sites linked to from the blog.

Can anyone visit the blog?
Yes, NurseBlog.org is free, though a free registration is required to make comments and blog entries.

How do I join the online discussion and community?
Just enter the asked-for information on the sign-up page, then follow the instructions in the e-mail sent to you.

What's the difference between a blog and a comment?
Comments appear in the threads and can be posted by anyone.

Can I post a comment?
It's easy. After signing up, at the end of each blog entry, is a link that says "comment" ... and links that let you "reply to" other comments. ... Clicking on "reply to" or entering a comment in either of these places will allow you to make a comment.

Can I write anything I want?
We encourage you to stay on topic, but we do not edit comments with which we disagree. We reserve the right to delete comments that are rude, derogatory, discriminatory, libelous, or offensive. Remember: civility is the foundation of our democracy.

Can I change my comment once I've posted it?
No. Your comment is saved permanently in the archives and can be read by anybody.

Does anyone actually post comments?

Yes, especially as the site grows in traffic.

Does anyone actually read them?

Yes, people like you will read them, the SEIU organizers will read them, and others that are visiting the blog as well.

When can I post a comment?

You can join a discussion anytime of the day or night. Typically the most lively discussion happens on the most recent thread (on top).

What is a lurker?

Someone who reads the comments threads but doesn't post his or her own comments. (That's not a bad thing, but feel free to join the discussion!)

What is a troll?

A troll is someone who deliberately disrupts the discussion in the comments thread. (It comes from the fishing term—a troller drops his lure hoping someone will bite.)

What do I do if I think I see a troll?

Please remain seated. Do not panic. If trolls are making posts that violate the comment policy, the best thing to do is to give them a low ranking. Responding to a troll simply prolongs the disruption of the discussion.

How do I find an old entry or thread?

All entries are saved in the archives, which can be found on the right-hand column.

What else?

NurseBlog.org is fun, thought provoking, and addictive. Sign up here, and have fun!

A blog site can be a useful forum for nurses analyzing political developments and health care policies, as this blog on Medicaid by Betsy Marville, and the commentary following it, demonstrates.

Medicaid   Blog

POSTED BY BETSY MARVILLE, RN

January 17, 2005

If you don't hear the word MEDICAID every day for the next six months then you aren't listening enough. Medicaid is under attack in Florida and many other states at the state and federal level. President Bush is calling for deep cuts to the states in Medicaid funds from the federal government, and his brother wants to privatize and limit Medicaid services in Florida. As more people lose their benefit-providing jobs and therefore their healthcare insurance, as premiums become prohibitive, the demand for Medicaid has increased each year.

President Bush and his brother seem to forget that these dollars that fund Medicaid come from our taxes and are really our money, not theirs. Taxpayers fortunate enough to have insurance understand that the need for healthcare will not just go away if it isn't funded. Instead more people, taxpayers themselves, will be denied access to preventative care resulting in loss of quality of and life itself. The sad reality is that more money will be spent in the long run by denying relatively cheap prevention.

Medicaid isn't the answer to the healthcare crisis, but until all have coverage it is helping a large amount of people in need. How do we justify cutting them off from something many of us take for granted? Why do we cut the safety net to those of us with the least in resources? Where are we naive enough to think they will go?

Remember what Scrooge said when told that people would rather die than go to the workhouses? He said to let them die and be rid of the surplus population. He changed his attitude when he learned that he was referring to Tiny Tim in that group. Let us not turn into Scrooge and remember that there for the Grace of God go all of us. As healthcare workers particularly we need to look out for all of our patients and find ways to prevent the proposed cuts.

It is time to contact our state and federal legislators and demand that our tax dollars support Medicaid and not privatize it for corporate profit or cut it.

Blog

Surprising Facts about Medicaid

POSTED BY NURSE ALLIANCE STAFF

JANUARY 17, 2005

MYTH: The private health insurance sector is more efficient than the public Medicaid program.

FACT: Private insurance costs nationally increased by just under 14 percent while Florida's per capita Medicaid cost increase was just under 5 percent. (Winter Park Health Foundation Policy Brief July 2004)

MYTH: All Medicaid costs are out of control.

FACT: Growth in Medicaid as percent in state budget actually declined from 14.1 percent in fiscal year 1994–1995 to 11.5 percent in fiscal year 2000–2001. (AHCA Presentation to Senate Health Care Appropriations 1/13/05)

FACT: The primary causes for Medicaid cost increases are increased enrollment due to the lagging economy and the rising price of prescription drugs. (Winter Park Health Foundation Policy Brief July 2004)

MYTH: All Medicaid recipients are unemployed or the children of unemployed parents.

FACT: Low wage employers are using Medicaid as subsidy. Over 50,000 Florida employers have employees receiving Medicaid benefits. (Tallahassee Democrat 12/19/04)

Op-Eds

Despite the popularity of blog sites, the op-ed sections of newspapers and newsmagazines remain powerful forums. If you have enough material for a 750-word essay, by all means write an op-ed. There's also no reason why a letter to the editor or a blog couldn't be shaped into an op-ed.

The op-ed page is now a fixture of newspapers, but it only dates back to the early 1970s when the news media were being pressured to grant greater access to "non-establishment" points of view. The political movements of the 1960s and 1970s for expanded civil rights, an end to the war in Vietnam, and women's liberation challenged the status quo of many institutions including the news media. Some complaints came from journalists themselves who, in a rash of new journalism reviews, accused the mainstream media of being the mouthpieces of those in power rather than forums for diverse, and even unpopular, views. Various advocacy groups demanded greater public access to news and editorial sections. The op-ed page was one of the most notable results.

Although the first op-ed page seems to have appeared in the *New York World* in the 1920s, it was limited to pieces by professional columnists. The *New York Times* can thus claim credit for creating the open-access op-ed page.

In 1990, in a commemoration of the twentieth anniversary of the *Times* op-ed page, Robert B. Semple Jr., who edited the page for many years, wrote that editors initially had no idea how many submissions the page would get. An early trickle quickly turned into a flood of manuscripts—some sixty a day. In twenty years, Semple wrote, more than 350,000 manuscripts had been submitted to the *New York Times* op-ed page. Some 21,000 were published.

Semple described the process of selection: "Each incoming manuscript is read by several editors; even the articles solicited by the editors are not guaranteed publication. And those chosen for publication nearly always undergo editing.

"Long odds—but not, obviously, a significant deterrent to anyone with something to say."[4]

The popularity of the op-ed quickly spread to other newspapers and to magazines. They varied greatly then, and still do, as to the types of pieces they prefer and what they pay to contributors ($0 to roughly $450; with higher fees for longer Sunday "think" pieces). Today this essay form is found in weekly newspapers as well as dailies, and some newspapers even provide additional slots for op-eds in their business, health, or other sections. *Newsweek*'s long-lived "My Turn" column and *Maclean's* biweekly "Over to You" are notable newsmagazine examples.

What Are Op-Eds About?

- An op-ed can propose a solution to a pressing problem.
- An op-ed can present an unaddressed aspect of an issue or give an unusual twist to the discussion.
- An op-ed can expand on news coverage.
- An op-ed can present a personal experience that relates to a public issue.

Op-ed pages usually contain a mixture of pieces by regular columnists (on staff or syndicated) and submissions from outside contributors. A contributor may be involved in a newsworthy issue or have a particular expertise to offer. Professional journalists write the majority of op-eds. Op-ed editors sometimes solicit a piece when they think that certain points of view haven't been represented.

Submissions that are accepted most likely will also be published online, which means that more readers and those beyond the print distribution area may see it.

Some women's and consumer magazines run essays from outside contributors. These range from opinion pieces to slice-of-life features. Business magazines provide another market for the op-ed contributor as do many magazines that serve specific "communities" such as college alumni or members of religious denominations. Although the *Times*, like many big-city newspapers, regards its op-ed page as a magnet for policy analysis, from the conception of the page, Semple wrote, "there was a conscious effort to leaven the relentless discussion of geopolitics with offbeat and sometimes whimsical essays."[4] Some publications reserve slots for longer unsolicited analytical pieces. Sunday week-in-review and analysis sections of newspapers may accept pieces up to 1,500 words. Public policy magazines may also accept longer submissions. This kind of piece covers more facets of an issue than the typical op-ed. A potential contributor usually talks over a proposed piece with the editor to see if there is any interest and to determine what angle would be most appealing.

Even with stiff competition for access, the op-ed remains a forum of choice. For nurses, time dedicated to learning how to compose op-eds will be well invested. Expect to rewrite your essay many times. It takes skill to deliver a snappy op-ed. That skill develops from practice. Don't be discouraged when your submission is rejected. Submit it somewhere else. Above all, try, and try again.

An op-ed should address a timely issue, one that has been in the news

The Nuts and Bolts of Op-ed Writing

An op-ed is only 750–800 words long, 2½ to 3 double-spaced, typewritten pages. The standard form consists of four parts: (1) lead, (2) focus, (3) elaboration, and (4) kicker.

1. The opening paragraph, or lead, sets the scene and tone for the reader. It may state the main point or direct the reader toward the point. The lead could be in the form of: (a) an anecdote or scene-setter; (b) a summary of what has happened before; or (c) A direct statement calling for a specific action.

2. The second paragraph usually contains the focus of the piece (if it isn't already in the lead). The focal paragraph is known in journalistic jargon as the "nut graf" (meaning the core paragraph or "graf" for short) or "billboard" (meaning the paragraph that "advertises" to the reader what the article is about). Every op-ed, indeed every type of article, must have a nut graf. If you start submitting articles for publication, sooner or later an editor will ask you about your "nut graf" maybe in just those words.

3. The rest of the article elaborates on the focus and moves from point to point in an interesting manner using some or all of the following: (a) factual statements; (b) statistics; (c) examples; (d) quotations; (e) anecdotes; or (f) explanations.

4. The kicker, or the last paragraph, wraps up the op-ed and ties it with a bow. The kicker could be: (a) a different, dynamic, or snappy restatement of the point; (b) a direct call to action; (c) a quotation; (d) an anecdote; or (e) a warning.

but has not yet been talked to death. It must confidently express an opinion. Unlike a news article, an op-ed is not designed to present only the "facts" or to take a "on-the-one-hand, on-the-other-hand" tone. An op-ed demands an assertively articulated point of view.

The op-ed must be concise. Most op-eds run no longer than 750 or 800 words, and some may be only 400 to 600 words. Submissions that vastly exceed the standard length run the risk of rejection on that basis alone.

The first and second paragraphs of an op-ed must offer an engaging or novel point of view. An editor sifting through submissions may not read much beyond the first two paragraphs before consigning a manuscript to either the "further consideration" or "reject" pile.

Some editors may be so intrigued by a strong point of view that they will go beyond the normal editing and offer to help cut or reshape the piece. This

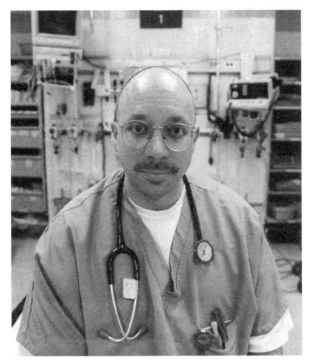

Paul Duke, RN. Photograph by George Waldman, www.DetroitPhotoJournalism.com.

is rare though. Longer commentaries—those between 1000 and 1500 words—should be directed to sections that accept that length.

An op-ed—even a humorous one—must address something that people do or should care about. Health care certainly offers enough facets to keep op-ed writers busy for years. Precisely because of the broad nature of health care, however, the op-ed writer must resist the temptation to address several points in one essay. While an op-ed can be about any number of things, the successful op-ed is about only one. The secret to op-ed writing is to organize the article around one point and stick to that point.

The best time to get published is when the news media are paying attention to an issue—not before it has been raised or after it has crested. But an op-ed can give a new perspective to an issue as did Paul Duke's first-person anecdotal consideration of the causes and results of the nursing shortage that was published in *Newsweek*'s "My Turn" column:

Op-Ed   **If ER Nurses Crash, Will Patients Follow?**

BY PAUL DUKE

February 2, 2004 (*Newsweek*)

I was sprinting down the hall when a patient waiting to be seen by a doctor asked me for a blanket. She was in her mid-70s, cold, scared, and without any family or friends nearby. Did I have time to get her that blanket, or even stop to say a few words to let her know she wasn't alone? No, I didn't.

As an emergency-room nurse, I'm constantly forced to shuffle the needs of the sick and injured. At that particular moment, half of my twelve patients were screaming for pain medication, most of the others needed to be rushed off to tests, and one was desperately trying not to die on me.

Was that blanket important in the grand scheme of things? Not really. She wasn't going to die without it. So it got tossed on the back burner, along with my compassion.

I often find myself hopping from task to task just to keep everyone alive. By the end of the shift I often wonder, did I kill anyone today? I go home tired and beaten down, praying like mad that I didn't make any mistakes that hurt anyone.

For five years I have worked in one of the busiest emergency rooms in southeastern Michigan. For the last two I have picked up overtime by working in four other hospitals, including the busiest emergency room in inner-city Detroit. No matter where I am, I experience the same problem—too many patients, not enough staff.

> *"I'm so overworked that I go home at night praying I haven't made a mistake that might hurt someone."*

When I started emergency-room nursing five years ago, I would typically have four or five patients. I could spend a few minutes chatting with them and answering their questions. Let's face it, when you are in a drafty emergency room in just a flimsy paper gown and your underwear, it is nice to have someone actually talk to you. It's a scary experience to get poked and prodded in various parts of your anatomy.

But now on an average day I have ten to twelve patients. Once I even had twenty-two. On that night I was feeling swamped, so I went to the charge nurse for help. She was as busy as I was, so she told me to take the five sickest patients and keep them alive, and get to the rest when I could. Now, here's a question: do you want to be one of the five sickest who get attention right away, or one of the others who have to wait maybe seven, eight, or even ten hours before someone gets to you?

That night I staggered home grateful that nobody had died. But I wondered, do I really want to do this job? I love the emergency room, but I was so damn frustrated. Was it just me?

I did an informal survey of the emergency rooms where I work. Every nurse I spoke to said the patient load had at least doubled in the last three years. None of them expected the situation to get better soon.

Troubling, but hardly scientific, so I did a little digging for some real statistics. According to the Centers for Disease Control and Prevention, from 1997 through 2000 the annual number of emergency-room visits went from 95 million to 108 million, while the number of ERs decreased. So who picked up the slack? The staff at emergency rooms, like mine, that are still standing.

The journal *Nursing 2003* reports that approximately three out of ten RNs believe their hospital has enough nurses to provide excellent care. Not exactly what you want to hear from the people responsible for your loved ones' health.

The future doesn't look any brighter. Studies show that by 2010, 40 percent of all registered nurses will be over fifty. That's when most of us are getting ready to cut back our hours or switch from direct patient care to chart review. By 2020 there will be an estimated shortfall of 808,400 nurses, partly because many will have retired or become so dissatisfied that they've quit, but also because fewer people are entering the profession. Yet the number of Americans older than sixty-five is expected to double from 35 million to 70 million over the next two decades. As someone who knows just how often the elderly visit ERs due to heart attacks, strokes, and falls, I see trouble ahead.

Don't get me wrong—my colleagues are some of the hardest-working and most professional nurses you will find. But when you're given twenty patients when you should have six, well, you're only so good.

After all this you must wonder why I don't quit. The truth is, I love nursing. It's what I am good at. I love the challenge of not knowing what will come crashing through the doors. Emergency-room nurses rise to the occasion. But we are being steamrolled, stretched thin and beaten down, and the best of us are frustrated.

At the end of my eighteen-hour shift I got that little old lady her blanket and spent a few minutes talking to her. She took my hand, smiled, and said thank you.

I'm frustrated, but I'll be back.

Duke lives in Southgate, Michigan

Conveying Real-Life Experiences and Describing What Nurses Do

Snapshots of physician practice are a staple of op-ed pages. Many physicians contribute stories about their moral dilemmas, relationships with patients, and successful, and unsuccessful, interventions. These narratives position physicians as the primary actors in weighing and resolving the ethical dilemmas that confront our advanced technological societies.

If nurses are to convince the public that they too are storehouses of human insight and health care expertise, they must dramatize this fact with compelling narratives. This is what nurse Jeannie Chaisson did in her op-ed–style article for *Technology Review*, a magazine published by the Massachusetts Institute of Technology (see "Asking the Right Questions" in chapter 2). It ran as a sidebar to a longer piece on contemporary nursing.[5,6]

Chaisson showed that doctors aren't the only ones who diagnose patients' problems. Without condemning physicians, she allowed salient facts to emerge from the narrative. Chaisson cleverly introduced another person, the patient's son, to pay tribute to nursing. "Nobody has ever asked her about these things before," he says. "Nobody has cared what it is like for her."

In her kicker, Chaisson spoke from her own agency to assert that a health care system that ignores the human experience of illness can produce neither health nor care. Without being boastful, she underlines her contribution to this woman's care and, by extension, teaches the reader what nurses have to offer.

Placing Your Op-Ed

Compose your op-ed with specific publications in mind. For each one:

1. Find out the name and contact information for the op-ed editor. If it is not given in the publication, call the op-ed department.

2. When you have written the op-ed, mail, e-mail, or fax it directly to that editor, preferably with a note briefly citing your credentials or experience with this issue. If you are e-mailing, paste the text of the op-ed into the body of the e-mail rather than sending it as an attachment.

3. Give the editor a few days to read it and follow up with a phone call. If you are successful in reaching the editor, be prepared to answer any questions, address any reservations, and enthusiastically "sell" the idea and its importance.

4. When you do reach the editor or leave a message, encourage the editor to use it, but then get an answer as to whether it will or won't be used. If your article is rejected and it's still timely, send it to another publication. Large papers get so many submissions that they usually send a form rejection letter. It's unlikely they will take the time to discuss your piece with you or tell you how you might improve it. Smaller papers might give you useful feedback.

5. If you are trying to get a response to an idea for an op-ed, explain who you are, why the issue is important, and why your point of view will add to the debate. In many cases, an e-mail query will work better than a phone call. Sometimes editors won't respond to either. In that event, send in your written essay.

6. If you have personal contacts that can be useful at a publication—a reporter in another section, a staffer you met at a social event, or a neighbor who knows an editor at the paper—don't be shy about using them.

7. All op-eds are "on spec," which means that editors do not guarantee publication. Don't be discouraged by the lack of a firm commitment.

8. You can submit your op-ed on spec to any number of publications. However, you should say that you're doing multiple submissions. Unfair as it may seem, some large publications expect exclusive consideration.

9. Acceptance is not the end of the process. Editing comes next. Editors may make suggestions for revisions and most of these will strengthen your piece. Be prepared to accept good suggestions, but argue against those that seriously alter your meaning or tone.

Revising a Nursing Journal Article

An op-ed can be a piece from a nursing journal that is revised or shortened for a general audience.

The cardiac critical-care nurse and Yale professor Marjorie Funk wrote a poignant account of her father's death in a critical-care unit for *Image: Journal of Nursing Scholarship* (below). It was an ideal candidate for an op-ed for a general audience as well because it linked her experience to those of other sons and daughters concerned about the quality of their parents lives and deaths

Funk's article is very well executed. Her repeated use of the phrase ". . . and said no," draws the reader's empathy to her deliberation, decision making, and sadness.

Op-Ed

Caring

BY MARJORIE FUNK

Summer 1992 (*IMAGE: Journal of Nursing Scholarship*)

On Saturday, April 27, 1991, my father had chest pain. He was evaluated in the Emergency Room of Bristol Hospital, where they determined that he was having an acute MI. They discussed giving him thrombolytic therapy to dissolve whatever clots might be occluding his coronary arteries. His history of GI bleeding and TIAs were relative contraindications to this type of therapy—but the decision was mine. I thought about it carefully . . . and said no.

Because there were no ICU beds available in Bristol Hospital, he was taken by ambulance to Yale–New Haven and admitted to the Coronary Care Unit. He arrived about 10 P.M. The issue of thrombolytic therapy was again raised. Again, I deliberated . . . and said no.

He was attached to a monitor, had his vital signs taken frequently, and received continuous infusions of IV nitroglycerin and heparin—all usual care for patients with acute MIs. He continued to have intermittent chest pain. They gave him a little morphine. He seemed to be having a little trouble breathing and his oxygen saturation dropped. Maybe he was going into congestive heart failure. A pulmonary artery catheter would provide the necessary data to guide further therapy. They suggested taking him into the Procedure Room and inserting this device. I considered it . . . and said no.

A little later we discussed whether he should be resuscitated if he arrested. I carefully considered this . . . and said no.

I stayed at his bedside all night. He slept some. Although his breathing seemed a bit labored at times, he did not appear uncomfortable. About 7 A.M., his blood pressure dropped and he suddenly became unresponsive. For a brief moment, I shifted gears—I had worked as a nurse in that unit for years. I knew exactly what to do. Lower the head of the bed, call for the code cart, get the arrest board under his back, begin CPR, prepare to administer . . . They asked me if I wanted them to do anything. I took a deep breath . . . and said no.

I continued to hold his hand. A number of people gathered quietly in the room—nurses, physicians, and even some of my students—my friends. He died about five minutes later.

I was alone. My favorite person in the whole world had just died. Where was the rest of my family? Mom was back in the convalescent home where she shared a room with Pop—they both had Alzheimer's disease. She would never know that he died. My brother was home sleeping—he was planning to come in a little later to be with Pop so I could go home to sleep.

No, I wasn't alone—my friends were there. They hugged me; some cried. I felt caring and support.

They seemed to support my decisions to forgo all the technology. How ironic—my professional life had been centered on the highly technical critical care environment. In my practice, I had worked to master the technology. I had tried to teach my students the technical skills necessary for the delivery of proficient care—maintaining that being technically competent was one of the most visible ways a nurse can exhibit caring. My own research concerns the safe and appropriate use of technology.

Over the last 12 hours, I had deemed just about all the available technology inappropriate for my father. Will I ever be totally at peace with these decisions, made alone, but deliberately and contemplatively . . . ?

Two sorts of revisions made Funk's essay more marketable for a general audience: (1) converting initials (e.g., MI, GI, ICU), nurse-speak ("relative contraindications," "thrombolytic therapy"), and the names of drugs (nitroglycerin, heparin) into everyday language for a lay audience and (2) clearly explaining why she deemed the available technology inappropriate for her father. She further connected her experience to that of others by showing empathy for laypeople who must go through this trial, and by pointing out the obstacles posed by managed care.

When she submitted the revised piece to the *Boston Globe*, it was accepted.

Op-Ed   **Doctors, Nurses, Don't Forget the Human Touch**

BY MARJORIE FUNK

May 30, 1994 (*Boston Globe*)

Late on a Saturday afternoon my 88-year-old father, who had Alzheimer's disease and had been in a nursing home for three months, developed chest pains. He was rushed to the emergency room of our local hospital, where physicians determined that he was having a heart attack. They discussed giving him medicine to dissolve the blood clots that were presumably blocking his coronary arteries and causing the heart attack. His history of small strokes increased the danger of this type of therapy—but as his daughter, with power of attorney, the decision was mine. I thought about it carefully and said no.

Because there were no intensive care beds available in the local hospital, he was taken to a nearby urban teaching hospital and admitted to the coronary care unit, where I worked part-time as a staff nurse and taught students as a professor of nursing. The issue of administering the clot-dissolving medication was again raised. Again, I deliberated and said no.

He was attached to a monitor, had his vital signs taken frequently and received intravenous nitroglycerin and heparin—usual care for patients with heart attacks. He continued to have intermittent chest pain. His nurse gave him a little morphine. He seemed to be having a little trouble breathing, and the oxygen level in his blood dropped. The doctors and nurses worried that he might be going into congestive heart failure. A pulmonary artery catheter would provide the necessary data to guide further therapy. They suggested inserting this device. I considered it, and said no.

A little later we discussed whether he should be resuscitated if he had a cardiac arrest. I carefully considered this, and said no.

I stayed at his bedside all night. He slept some. Although his breathing seemed a bit labored at times, he did not appear uncomfortable. About 7 A.M., his blood pressure dropped and he lost consciousness. For a moment, I shifted gears. I had worked as a nurse in that unit for many years. I knew exactly what to do. Lower the head of the bed, call for the resuscitation cart, get the arrest boards under his back, begin CPR. The staff asked me if I wanted them to do anything. I took a deep breath, and said no.

I continued to hold his hand. A number of people gathered quietly in the room—nurses, physicians, some of my students—my friends. My father died about five minutes later.

For years, my professional life has focused on the highly technical critical-care environment. In my nursing practice I have worked hard to master the technology. I have tried to teach these technical skills to my students. I have long maintained that being technically competent was one of the most visible ways a nurse could exhibit caring. Even the research I have been conducting concerns the safe and appropriate use of technology.

Yet over 12 hours, I had deemed just about all the available technology inappropriate for my beloved father. As an experienced health care professional, I had a realistic sense of the odds. I knew that after a massive heart attack there would be little chance of full recovery. I knew that dependence on medical technology, such as a ventilator to assist his breathing, would have increased the confusion of his Alzheimer's. I was aware of myriad possible complications. Even knowing all this, I agonized. I needed all the support I received from the nurses and physicians, who also happened to be my professional colleagues and friends.

As I reflect on my own experience, I am struck by how difficult it must be for the average person, with no medical background, to make these decisions. We health care providers hide behind our legalistic strategies of living wills, advance directives and health care proxies and assail patients' families with statistical data on the probability of recovery. We assume that people who are facing the most frightening decisions a human being can confront and who have entered an alien medical culture can somehow engage in a complex series of rational deliberations.

My decisions were made a bit easier not just by my familiarity with the highly technical hospital environment but also by the support I felt from the hospital staff. Somehow, we as health care professionals have to extend that level of understanding and attention to all patients and their loved ones. We need to encourage dialogue about options, and we need to create systems that enable this to happen.

It is alarming to realize that the managed care that has become so pervasive may be doing just the opposite. We seem to be racing patients through the system and denying providers time to work with and support them, as my colleagues worked with and supported me. As we design and debate health care reform, human exchanges aimed at understanding must be valued as much as heroic interventions aimed at cure.

Try and Try Again

In writing letters, op-eds, and longer articles, remember that you can't succeed without trying. There are many publications—major newspapers, regional newspapers, small town dailies or weeklies, newsmagazines, women's magazines, and business publications—that are looking for intelligent, fresh points of view. This is what Jean Logan, a nursing professor at Grand View College in Des Moines found when she started writing opinion pieces and tried to place them.

"I got started writing for the *Business Record* because I could not get the *Des Moines Register* to publish anything other than letters to the editor," she told us. "The *Business Record* is owned by a woman (I like to think that helped), and once I got my foot in the door they published everything I submitted. I used your tips about describing exactly what nurses do in lay language. I got tremendous response from my non-nurse friends like stock brokers, etc., male and female. Recently I wrote an op-ed about being a nurse and being a trustee of a public hospital, something I think is vitally important for nurses to do. Again, the *Business Record* published it."

Op-Ed   **Nurses Struggle with Overtime Rule, Safety Issue**

BY JEAN LOGAN

Sunday, September 5, 2004 (*Des Moines Business Record*)

Quality of health care and access to care are major issues in the presidential election campaign this year, as they are in most elections. This time, in the midst of a heated campaign, Congress passed a bill that might limit overtime pay for some nurses.

The American Nurses Association believes the federal regulations that took effect August 23 will allow employers to increase forced overtime for nurses. This is because salaried employees are not required to be compensated at time-and-a-half. The result? Many nurses will be hit by a double whammy as they're called upon to work more hours but not be rewarded for their extra effort the same way other workers are.

Most news accounts have said that hospitals and long-term-care agencies will continue to pay overtime to nurses because there is a shortage of personnel, a shortage that will continue to spiral upward until 2020 when there will be a 20 percent vacancy rate in the profession. Access to and quality of health care will both be affected by the severe deficit of professional staff.

Even today, in order to provide patients access to nursing care, employers are asking nurses to work more and more overtime. Some employers mandate overtime, while others encourage the practice and reward volunteers with lucrative hourly earnings. Nurses can boost their income significantly by working overtime.

But do we really want nurses working those added hours?

A recent study of 393 registered nurses led by researcher Anne Rogers at the University of Pennsylvania found that the number of mistakes nurses made multiplied as they worked beyond a 12-hour shift. Nurses who worked an average of between eight- and 12-hour shifts committed errors in 12 of 771 shifts or 1.6 percent of the time. Nurses who worked an average of 12.5 hours committed errors in 103 of 2,057 shifts or 5 percent of the time.

That finding does not surprise exhausted nurses. "Joe" works in an intensive care unit in the Des Moines area. He could work extra shifts almost every day should he volunteer. He is in his twenties, physically fit, and has no children. He is far younger than the 48-year-old average working RN in this country, yet he tells me he's weary.

Given the skills required to monitor acutely ill patients—everything from the ability to recognize subtle changes in a patient's color to adeptness in changing intravenous medication dosage when blood pressure plummets—patients' lives literally are in nurses' hands. Federal regulations limit how many hours airline pilots can be in the air. Truck drivers are also very closely monitored for hours logged on the road. Falling asleep in the cockpit or at the wheel is not good. Neither is giving the patient the wrong dose of medication or missing an erratic heartbeat because one's attention span wanes.

So the problem becomes less about paying nurses for overtime, which I believe most institutions must continue to do, and more about patient safety.

Health care policy decisions at the state and federal levels need to include further discussions about limiting the number of hours nurses work per week. This dialogue will be difficult given the 24-hour staffing that is needed in hospitals and long-term-care centers. Staff nurses need to be included and asked for input into possible solutions.

Would you want an exhausted nurse bending over you or your loved one's bedside? I wouldn't.

Jean Logan is a registered nurse and a professor in the division of nursing at Grand View College

Nurses who are frequently published in letters pages or op-ed sections rarely have all or even most of their work accepted. "I've had many letters to the editor published in major newspapers like the *New York Times* or *Philadelphia Inquirer*," says Claire Fagin, dean emerita of the University of Pennsylvania School of Nursing. "I've succeeded because I've written so many. When I see something I like, I write to compliment the reporter. When I see something that concerns me, I go to the computer and express my views. Because people see me in print, they think that my scorecard is better than it is. For all the pieces I've had published, I've had many more rejected. In fact, I could publish a volume called The Unpublished Letters and Articles of Claire Fagin. My advice is just keep writing."

Our advice is, if you come across something that concerns you in the papers, on the radio or TV, in the movies, or in any of the mass media, do something about it. Write a letter, make a phone call, send an e-mail, start a blog. If you don't like what you hear or see, don't keep it to yourself. If you like it, praise it (the media needs as many pats on the head for the good things it does as slaps on the wrist for the bad). If you're an oncology nurse, and you see something erroneous written about pediatric nursing, don't wait for the pediatric nurse to write a letter to the editor, do it yourself. If you see something disturbing written about health policy, don't hesitate to respond because you're "just a nurse," not a PhD in health policy. You have more real experience with health than most of the highly paid consultants who tell administrators—or even national health systems in many countries—how to organize their services. Speak up, speak out, make a difference.

Chapter 11

Appearing on Television and Radio

One fall morning, Cindy Dalton, a nurse who works in a Montreal community health center, was about to make her television debut. As she waited in the greenroom near the set of the program *Montreal Today*, she reflected on the fact that the sum total of her media experience consisted of being interviewed for five minutes on the radio. Now she was about to appear on a major television show to talk about the nursing crisis in Quebec. Her fellow guest was Suzanne Gordon. Dalton told Gordon that she was nervous. Gordon suggested that she rehearse. Gordon pointed out that the segment on nursing would be only six minutes. "Deducting the time spent on questions from the host, we'll each have about two and a half minutes," she said. She suggested that Dalton prepare an anecdote so that she could use that time to convey the importance of what nurses do.

Dalton thought for a moment. "I work as a community health nurse in the area of family health," she began. "I begin working with families during pregnancy and continue until the kids are six years of age. The other day a pregnant Chinese woman had trouble getting her needs across when she visited the obstetrician. Doctors don't have much time these days, so it's important to ask them the right questions. I worked with her to prioritize her questions and make a list."

Since it was close to airtime, Gordon interrupted. "The problem with this anecdote is that it doesn't focus on you, the nurse," she said. "It focuses on the physician, on the busy man or woman who has no time. You want to highlight the importance of nursing. Is there another anecdote you could use?"

Dalton considered the question. Then she described her home care work with a multiple sclerosis patient who could no longer walk on his own. The man spent his days sitting on the sofa while his wife cared for their two children, a two-and-a-half-year-old and an infant. Although he was unsteady using a walker, the patient refused to use a wheelchair or modify his home to accommodate his condition. He was depressed because the only thing he could manage was to go to the bathroom. He was so afraid he would drop his infant that he wouldn't even hold the baby. As she began explaining how she helped this patient, Dalton suddenly stopped.

Gordon asked her why.

Dalton looked frozen. "I can't use that anecdote. It's private," she said. "The patient might listen to the show. Telling his story would be a breach of patient confidentiality."

"Just change the details," Gordon said. "Make him a woman, change the ages of the children."

"But if I do that, I'm lying," Dalton protested. "Then I'm going to have trouble being truthful while I'm on the air." Dalton said she was also concerned that if she pared her story to a few sentences, people would not "hear the nursing."

Gordon assured her that she would feel more comfortable with a little practice and that if she talked about her nursing work, listeners would not miss the point.

As the two approached the set, Gordon coached Dalton to "take advantage of whatever opening the host gives you to bring up your anecdote."

When the cameras rolled, host Leslie Roberts immediately said to Dalton: "Tell me a bit about your work if you can. You've been a nurse for twelve years. Is it getting worse? Do you see the crisis, or is it being blown up by the media?"

"Definitely, nurses are more challenged in the present health care system," Dalton said. "Every time there's a challenge you have to adjust to it, and today the challenges are coming more quickly, and the period of adjustment is shortened."

The host had been asking for a general description of nurses' problems. But Dalton astutely took advantage of the opening he gave her to bring the audience into the world of daily nursing practice.

"I can give you an example of the kind of work I do," she continued. "At the moment I'm working at a CLSC [community health center] with families with young children. But I also work with people who have chronic illnesses. When I went to visit one family in their home recently, I found they had a newborn baby and the wife had multiple sclerosis. It was a challenge for me to work with her because she was very depressed. The husband was taking on more and more work with the newborn baby. For the first time in her life, the wife couldn't walk but was reluctant to use a wheelchair. I knew she could fall, and if she fell, it would cost more health care dollars because she would need more services." Dalton then explained that she helped to rearrange the house so the wife could navigate in her wheelchair, taught the

Nurses at the Microphone

Nurses, as well as doctors, can become health care experts and hosts on TV or radio. Local cable television shows offer an excellent way to enter the television market.

Diana Mason, the editor-in-chief of the *American Journal of Nursing*, has co-hosted the radio program *Healthstyles* on WBAI in New York City since 1985. The award-winning weekly program was one of the first in New York to talk about the politics of AIDS and the resurgence of tuberculosis. "This is because we talked with public health nurses in the field who described their experiences," Mason explains.

"Nurses," Mason advises, "shouldn't underestimate the skills they have communicating with the public. Nurses know how to interview people. They know how to analyze a situation. And they have an understanding of issues grounded in clinical practice."

wife how to safely hold her baby, and helped the family alleviate her depression.

After this anecdote, Roberts interviewed Gordon about the problems nurses face in the United States. Turning to Dalton, Roberts asked if Canadians should solve their health care crisis by becoming more like the United States.

Although Dalton is not a health policy expert, she did not hesitate to voice her opinion. "No," Dalton answered. "The solution is to strengthen the present health care system. My own personal opinion is that under privatization there would be people who need services and couldn't afford them or would not get good services."

Roberts argued that Canada already has a two-tiered health care system with some people getting better care than others. Dalton agreed that while "there are some services you can pay for and get quicker, we still have universal health care and we should maintain it. It's very important."

Then she bridged to more discussion of nursing.

"Nursing is also very important," she explained. "When you go to the emergency room, the first person you see is a nurse. When you're going to have an operation, the person who prepares you before surgery is a nurse. What's the first thing that happens when you open your eyes? Who are you going to see at your bedside? Who will make sure that you recover with no complications? A nurse. When you're going to ring your call bell at night for help because you're in pain, or you're worried about being sent home the

Basic Rules for Appearing on Radio and Television

- Prepare, prepare, prepare
- Create three "bumper stickers"
- Be credible
- Be enthusiastic
- Speak with conviction

next day, who's going to come to your room and make sure you know how to take your medications safely at home? A nurse."

After the show Dalton was exhilarated. "As I started to talk about nursing, I became more and more energized," she said. "At first I was preoccupied by the set, the lights, the people walking around making strange signals to one another. Because the host kept nodding his head, I was worried that I was taking too much time and that he wasn't interested in what I had to say. I was too focused on his agenda. I was letting the setting paralyze me.

"Then I remembered why I was here. I was here for a purpose—for nursing. I realized I had to focus on my agenda. Once I got comfortable, the ideas started coming to me. At the end, I felt I could do this again. If I did, I would be much better."

With preparation, a sense of purpose, and the conviction that nurses have a right to speak for themselves and their profession, most nurses will find that it isn't all that hard to speak on television or radio, in front of a live audience, or to a journalist who is interviewing them for a story.

How to Feel in Control

As with patient care, the best way to feel you're in charge is to get as much information as possible in advance.

If a reporter or producer calls you to arrange an appearance on a radio or TV program, ask the name of the show and of the host who will be interviewing you. Producers rather than the on-air reporters or talk-show hosts usually make the initial contact.

Find out if the show is on health care or public policy. Is it an entertainment show? Is it a show that encourages conversational dueling? This will tell you what kind of audience it attracts and how to prepare.

Ask how much time you will be allowed to talk. We've been on radio and television news programs where we've had less than two minutes to present our case.

There are different kinds of television and radio programs. Some are fast-paced entertainment shows that rely on glib retorts. Some try to generate controversy for controversy's sake. Others are more interested in drawing out solid information on a particular problem. You can find out about these shows by asking the host, a friend, an organizational PR person, or by tuning in yourself. It's a good idea to observe the format of the show, particularly if you don't have a great deal of on-air experience.

You'll need to know if a show is live or taped and if it is done in a studio or if, in the case of radio, the interviewer will call you at home or work. Most radio interviews are done outside the studio. Some shows are taped in advance and aired later. You will want to know if the show has call-ins. Callers' comments limit your on-air time. In addition, you'll have to respond to differing perspectives and to a wide and unpredictable variety of questions.

Ask the producer or interviewer if there is a particular slant to his or her thinking on the subject that will be addressed. Ask if you will be the only guest or one of several. Ask how many and who they are. Get a sense of their expertise or point of view. If you know you will be debating someone with an opposing point of view, consider what they are likely to say. Find out how long you will be on the air. You need to know whether you will have two minutes or half an hour in which to make your points.

Many shows do a preinterview to screen potential guests. This is useful to both you and the show's producers and reporters. Your responses to questions and your stage manner will help them decide if they want you on the program. This preinterview will give you an idea of the slant so that you can prepare your comments for the show.

Your attractiveness as a guest will depend on your ability to get your points across vividly and succinctly. The syndicated newspaper columnist Ellen Goodman once told us that when she is unenthusiastic about being on a show, she tells the preinterviewer that the subject has many facets and then she proceeds to elaborate on all of them. Interviewers quickly terminate the call.

It's important to know how a show plans to use nurses—for their clinical or health care expertise or for entertainment value. When a television show ostensibly focuses on the "health care team," producers tend to position the show around a physician or physicians and use nurses as props for the physician-centered narrative.

Several years ago, for example, Sally Jesse Raphael planned a show on the care of her son who had been in an automobile accident and was hospitalized for a month. A group of nurses was invited to the program. To thank the doctors and nurses who had cared for her son, Raphael presented video clips of his hospital stay and asked the experts to talk about his treatment.

The "experts" were all MDs. Dressed in suits and ties, they sat with Raphael on the show's main set. The young man's nurses, on the other hand, had been invited en masse. Dressed uniformly in scrubs, they sat in the audience where they dutifully applauded or laughed on cue. None was asked to speak about either the medical or nursing issues that were involved in the complex case.

The same dynamic was at work in a four-part documentary, "ICU," that aired in August 2003. Set in the pediatric cardiac surgery department at Arkansas Children's Hospital, the series was promoted as an in-depth look at a *health care team's* work with young "children whose hearts have failed them" and the "doctors and nurses who save them." For sixteen months, the hospital worked extensively with the ABC producers and crew. When the series was broadcast, however, it did not focus on the ICU health care team but on the OR where the work of one pediatric cardiac surgeon, Dr. Jonathan Drummond-Webb, took precedence. Operating room nurses and neonatal intensive care nurses were shown on camera but in professionally problematic ways. To personalize them, the doctors and nurses were shown both in their working and home lives. They discussed their family dilemmas, relationships, divorces, and attempts to adopt a child. In this regard, the nurses and doctors got more or less equal airtime.

But, in the professional setting, the nurses were relegated to stereotypical traditional roles as nurturers, physician handmaids, or cheerleaders for the surgeon. In one introductory bit designed to perk viewer interest, a nurse was featured saying of Drummond-Webb, "You can do anything. You're our hero."

Although the cardiovascular OR nurse manager Jean Ann Philips was spotlighted, she was never shown making a clinical decision but rather talking mostly about her personal life and her respect for Drummond-Webb. Other nurses on the neonatal ICU made cameo appearances, but the producers focused exclusively on the comfort they provided to and concern they showed for their young patients. The program did not illuminate the clinically demanding medical and technical work they do to ensure their patients survive Drummond-Webb's operations.

The public affairs officer who helped arrange the show and the hospital's vice president for nursing said that they thought the program conveyed the knowledge and skill of nurses. But we wondered if they were confusing visibility on the screen with real illumination of the work that nurses actually do in critical-care units.

It's important to be aware that producers may impose a television template that shows nursing only as emotional work. Resist the temptation to

> ## Your Turn
>
> Imagine that your hospital PR department informs you that a TV crew will be in your hospital filming a documentary on your emergency department. You're a nurse manager in the ED. How will you prepare yourself and the nurses in the department to talk to the journalists? What do you want the nurses to highlight? How will you help them to avoid traditional stereotypes? How will you alert them to possible pitfalls? What will you do if you see a doctor-centered nurse-as-cheerleader narrative emerging?

go with the flow in order to gain visibility. The tendency will be to portray caring not as a complexly skilled activity but as sentimental and heart-warming niceness. Care giving activities must also be amplified with depictions of the medical, technical, and body-care activities that are a routine part of nurses' work.

When working with the media, nurses' public relations specialists and nursing administrators need to hash out in advance what is significant about nursing work and what needs to be shown. Nurses must use their leverage to avoid reinforcing images that aren't going to help them or the public. The media needs you and your cooperation as much as you need media attention. It's a two-way street.

In response to Sally Jesse Raphael's request, the hospital public relations and nursing departments should have insisted that at least one nurse be on the panel to talk about nursing care. That should have been a condition for nursing's participation. If Raphael refused, the nurses could have refused to appear. Even more hardball, nurses had the power to embarrass a daytime woman's-show host whose son was saved by nursing yet wouldn't allow his nurses to appear on a panel of experts. This would have been a good story to leak to the news media. Similarly, the nurses who appeared in the "ICU" series needed to have their own agenda and arrive at an understanding with the PR department about what their roles would be and what activities would be highlighted in this documentary. The PR department had the power to argue with producers if the show was getting it wrong.

Using nursing's leverage in this way may sound risky. Nurses may be concerned that they will alienate the media—or their institutions—if they do so. Hospitals that want free publicity may pressure nurses to cooperate with media requests that demean nurses. But why should nurses agree to reinforce inaccurate stereotypes? The very process of negotiating these matters might teach reporters and PR staff to show more respect toward individual nurses and their profession. For decades, doctors have negotiated the rules of engagement with television. What is being sought is not propaganda for nurses but an accurate and complete picture of what nurses do.

Being Interviewed at Work or at Home

Some shows will ask you to come to their studio. Others will interview you at your workplace or home. Communication satellites make it possible for radio or television programs originating across the country or the globe to set up a telephone conversation or live appearance that sound and look as though everyone is in the same room.

In the case of radio, if an interviewer calls for a comment and you are in the middle of something or just feel unprepared, ask them to call back in a few moments so that you can pull your thoughts together. Sometimes interviewers will be on deadline and will want you immediately. Buy a little time to think by asking a few questions about the show.

If you don't feel ready, you don't have to agree to the interview. But remember, you're the health care expert. The program is seeking your expertise. Try to compose yourself and speak from your heart about what you know. Most of the time people sound and look much better on radio and television than they think they do.

If you have advance notice of an interview that will take place at your home or workplace, give yourself a little breathing space. If you've just seen ten patients or had your management skills tested to the limit, and you are stressed and harried, don't go directly to the phone. Try to take a fifteen-minute or even a five-minute breather. Take some deep, relaxing yoga breaths and collect your thoughts.

Do the same if you will be receiving a call at home. If it's an early morning show (you'd be surprised by how many are) set your alarm to wake you at least a half-hour before you're supposed to be called. Have a cup of coffee or tea. Put on your clothes. It's amazing how talking on the radio in your bathrobe at six in the morning can undermine your professionalism even though no one can see you. Some people like to stand up to give radio interviews because it makes them feel more dynamic and authoritative.

It is not unusual for television programs to bring their cameras to you, in which case you will want to be prepared to receive them. If you are going to a radio or TV station for an appearance, give yourself plenty of time to get there. It's better to arrive fifteen minutes early than exactly on time but frazzled. Air times are locked in stone. If you're five or ten minutes late, you may miss the opportunity to be on at all.

Appearance

How you appear and behave on radio and television affects the way the audience receives your message. Whether you're a staff nurse or a researcher, you want to appear knowledgeable and credible. Your dress and body language will help or hinder this effort.

Look professional. Women should never appear in mid-thigh skirts that hike even higher when they sit or low-slung pants and skimpy tops that bare their midriff and even more. Wear neat, tailored clothes. Don't be bland, but don't be jarring. You should have some color in your attire, but bright reds and oranges go neon on the screen. Whites tend to fade out. Keep away from checks, herringbone tweeds, small stripes, and other small patterns that tend to wiggle on TV. Avoid flowered, sweet, or cute clothing. Men should wear suits, or sports jackets, and ties.

Since television's bright lights tend to wash out even the rosiest complexion, it helps to wear some makeup. Foundation, rouge, and powder will do. Men may also want to apply some powder and perhaps foundation too. Some national shows have staffpersons who will apply your makeup. Assume, however, that you won't be made up there and apply your own cosmetics before you go to the studio. If you are going to appear on television a lot, you might want to invest in a lesson from a makeup artist.

Avoid excessive jewelry, particularly the clanking variety. You don't want necklaces or bracelets to jangle against sensitive microphones or strike desks or chairs. Dangling earrings are a distraction. So are long, Barbra Streisand–type nails. The grunge look or an elaborately teased hairdo also compromises a credible presentation.

When you are seated, try to look alert but relaxed and comfortable. Don't slump. Sit up straight and lean forward slightly. This is an attentive posture. If you are asked to stand for the interview—a format at some stations—stand up straight, try to look relaxed, and let your hands hang easily at your sides. Make eye contact with the host.

Don't worry about the camera. It will follow you; you don't have to follow it. Try not to be distracted by camera people and producers who are signaling one another or the show's host. These people are not signaling because you've made a mistake. They are communicating with the host or each other about timing and production details. If the host looks at people in the studio while you are talking, or reviews his notes, or seems to be listening to what someone is saying in his earpiece, he knows the camera is on you and he is counting on you to continue talking.

Always assume that your microphone is on and recording even if the show goes to commercial breaks or seems to be over. Don't say anything during these breaks and only begin talking normally when your mike has been removed.

With today's automated sets, you might find yourself in a booth or in a newsroom with a remotely operated camera aimed at you. This will be the arrangement if you go to a studio to be interviewed for a program based in another city. Your "face-to-face" with the host will be via his image on a monitor or his voice in your earpiece. This can be unnerving. Keep in mind that on television it will look like you are actually having a conversation with the interviewer. Your job is to regard the robotic camera (which may advance and back away eerily) as though it were a human being and talk directly to it. You will get an indication of when the show has gone to a commercial and you can relax for a moment. But when the discussion is going on, don't assume that you are not on camera because someone else is talking. A camera may be taking reaction shots of you. This is such an artificial environment, you may feel as though they have put you in isolation and forgotten about you. But you are very much part of the program. If you have something to say, and no one has given you a chance, politely, but assertively, interject.

When you are asked a question, don't look toward the ceiling as if waiting for the angels to send you an answer. Keep your eyes on the host (or robot camera). Some people blink rapidly when they are working their way through an answer. If you have this tendency, consciously override it so that you have a steady look. If you're responding to another guest on the show, look at him or her (or at the robot camera as though it were he or she). Make hand gestures, but don't let them get out of control. You want viewers to listen to what you say, not get caught up with your mannerisms.

When someone else is talking, look interested. Don't scratch your head, scowl, roll your eyes, or snicker if you think what the person said is absurd. The camera might pan toward you at any time and catch your reaction. When someone is asking you a question or making a statement, resist grunting or uttering affirmative "uh-huh" sounds. Similarly, don't automatically nod your head. Affirmative nods and sounds are intended to show the other person that you are taking in what he or she is saying, but they can be a distraction and may give the impression that you agree with what the person is saying even if it is outrageous or contradicts your argument. Just looking attentive is sufficient. This is also the correct demeanor for participating in a panel discussion or engaging in questions and answers from a lecture podium.

State Your Qualifications and Set Ground Rules

Before you go on air, establish how you will be identified and how the host and other guests will address you. This is essential. Tell the producer exactly how you want to be identified.

Give the correct spelling of your name and title for the identifier that will flash on the screen when you are talking. Make sure "RN" or "nurse" is included in the identification. If you have another title, like professor, your nursing identification may disappear unless you insist on it being present. Identifications in radio and TV land (and even in most mainstream publications) are short, so get in the essentials, and accept that no one is interested in the fact that you are the Florence Nightingale/Lavinia Dock/Lillian Wald professor of physiological and anatomical nursing at the University of such and such school of nursing. What they need to know is that you are an expert on a certain subject and a professor at the University of such and such School of Nursing.

Make sure you establish ground rules for oral introductions. Ask to be introduced with your specialty and perhaps the number of years you have been a nurse, as in: "Joanne Clarke is with us today. She's been a psychiatric nurse for twenty years and works with adolescents." If you are a staff nurse, provide additional details too. For example, you might want to be introduced as "Tom Smith, who has been a medical-surgical nurse at General Hospital for ten years. Nurse Smith works extensively with elderly patients."

If you're a PhD nurse, beware of being called "Doctor" over and over again. The audience will probably think you are a physician. If you use your "Dr." title, be sure to preface statements with, "As a nurse . . ."

If you are not a PhD and you are going to be on air with MDs or PhDs, insist on being addressed as Mrs., Miss, Ms., or Mr. (last name) or Nurse (last name). Unless you intervene, hosts will call doctors "Dr.," professors "Professor," and you Joan or Jim. Even if you have to intervene while on the air, do not allow yourself to be called by your first name while others are being addressed with titles that convey expertise.

Tone of Voice and Interview Etiquette

Tone of voice is important, especially so on radio. Maintain an even, measured tone of voice even if you are provoked. Don't get riled by what a caller, another guest, or the host has said. Maintain your composure just as you would with a difficult patient. Combat their comments with a powerful argument, not by raising your voice, making personal attacks, mocking, or being sarcastic.

To be polite and still make your point, you can say, "That was interesting, but let's think about this aspect of the issue," and move on to your message.

Regard negative and insulting comments as opportunities to make your points. For example, if a host says, "It's surprising to me that nurses know so much about diseases and medications," pick up on the host's language and respond, "You know, what's surprising is that you're surprised." Then describe what nurses know. For example, "I've been an oncology nurse for ten years. I am very familiar with toxic chemotherapy drugs and how to administer them so that patients don't develop fatal complications."

If you're talking about the consequences of a shortage of nurses or understaffing on hospital floors, a host might concur in a way that subtly demeans nurses. "So what we're missing in health care," he might offer, "is the TLC nurses bring."

To this, you can reply: "Nurses definitely bring a great deal of caring and compassion to their patients and to their patients' families. But the real problem with a shortage of nurses is that there won't be anyone in hospitals to rescue patients from complications that could lead to death. That's what nursing is, a matter of life and death."

If you're on a show where the host or her guests are constantly interrupting and shrieking at one another, your challenge will be to resist retreating into frustrated silence or joining in the shouting match. Try an amused tone to interject: "Well, if I could just get a word in edgewise," or "If one of you would just let someone finish a sentence." When someone interrupts, you can say firmly, "I've given you the courtesy of letting you respond. I'd appreciate the same courtesy."

The most important thing is to be interested, enthusiastic, and cooperative rather than withholding and monosyllabic. When Dick Cavett had a conversation show years ago, we watched him interview the famous Russian ballet dancer Rudolf Nureyev, who appeared wearing a snakeskin suit and matching platform boots. Cavett asked the dancer an intelligent question, to which he responded "yes." Then Cavett asked another excellent question, to which the dancer responded "no." Another perceptive comment received a terse, "yes," followed by "yes," "yes," and "no." After the first few minutes, it must have been agonizingly clear to Cavett that he was living the interviewer's worst nightmare: He had to fill up air-time with a talk-show guest who refused to talk.

If you're nervous or suspicious, don't pull a Nureyev. The way to deal with this is to be prepared, and then talk your way out of your anxiety.

Be Prepared

You must know in advance which points you want to make. Years ago Christopher Lydon (the former host of "The Connection" on National Public Radio) told Bernice Buresh before interviewing her on television that she should think of her points as "bumper stickers." This is a useful image. Bumper stickers represent the essence of your message and are easy to remember. You can embed your bumper sticker into an anecdote, example, or rejoinder. But the main point must be short and clear. Realistically, you may not have time to make more than three points and may only get a chance to make one, but you can make it count.

Earlier we talked about preparing three anecdotes on nursing. For television and radio, these anecdotes must be reduced to a few sentences that can be delivered quickly in a conversational style to make a point. Write down your points, and the statistics or facts that will bolster them, and take them with you to the studio. Review the points before you go on air.

Remember to translate jargon into ordinary language. It's critical-care unit, not CCU; cancer, not CA; heart attack, not MI or myocardial infarction.

Bridging

Bridging is a technique for getting to your bumper stickers. It means using a question or comment as a bridge to make your point.

That's what Cindy Dalton did on *Montreal Today*. She briefly answered the host's question then seized the opportunity to describe the challenges nurses face in their daily practice. Later, when the discussion turned to health care policy, she directed the conversation to the nursing component.

A bridge is merely a transitional statement, such as the following:

- "You know that's an interesting issue, but so is this . . ."
- "Let me tell you about . . ."
- "While we're talking about what's important to patients, consider this . . ."
- "The real issue is . . ."
- "Here's another factor that hasn't been mentioned . . ."

Questions from interviewers come in various forms, some of which may surprise you. Here are a few common types and possible ways to respond.

Hang In There!

The advice to be prepared with bumper stickers has come in handy on more than one occasion but no more so than on an early-morning television news show in Milwaukee that Bernice Buresh appeared on in 2003. In preparation, she talked with the producer the day before and asked how much time she would be given. The producer said three minutes.

Buresh started out the next morning at 5:30 A.M. and drove through blowing snow to get to the station in advance of the 6:20 A.M. segment. At the station entrance, she rang the buzzer repeatedly until someone from security came and let her in. A newsroom assistant greeted her and briskly led her into the newsroom, sat her on a stool, stuck an earpiece in her ear, clipped a small microphone onto her sweater, and disappeared.

After a while, Buresh motioned over a news writer she spotted across the room and asked when she would be on and how much time she would have. The news writer relayed the question to the hosts who were visible on a monitor but situated in a studio elsewhere in the building. Buresh heard the voice of one of them in her earpiece. "Oh, Bernice," she said. "We're so sorry. We're only going to have about a minute and a half because we need to talk more about the snowstorm." Buresh politely protested that she had been offered three minutes and made the trip downtown on that basis. "Well, maybe we can stretch it to two," the host said.

Buresh, seated on the stool in front of a robot camera, looked at the piece of paper on which she had written five bumper stickers, and crossed out two. She quickly rehearsed in her mind how she would present the remaining three.

The two women hosts, who had a format in which they chatted with each other, spent a lot of time discussing a new survey about whether cats or dogs are more popular as family pets. Then abruptly one of the hosts segued to a thirty-second intro on the nursing shortage, which cited Milwaukee hospital vacancy stats, introduced Buresh as a journalist, former Milwaukeean, and co-author of a public communication book for nurses, and then noted, while footage of hospital nurses at work appeared on the screen, that applicants were being turned away from nursing schools because there weren't enough slots available.

In a thirty-second answer directed to the camera in front of her, Buresh documented the extent of the nursing shortage, worked in the name of the university that had set up her appearance ("as I told students yesterday during my lecture at the University of Wisconsin–Whitewater"), and emphasized the serious consequences of the nursing shortage (the closing of ICUs, emergency room diversions).

(continued)

One of the hosts asked a twelve-second question on what could be done about the nursing shortage.

Buresh replied that money wasted in the U.S. health care system needed to be shifted into resources for nursing because of the critical importance of nursing. She said that nurses were leaving clinical settings because of poor working conditions and that the nursing shortage would not be remedied unless nurses could have long-term satisfying careers so that working nurses would want to stay on the job and the best and brightest candidates would want to enter the profession and stay for the long term. Her answer took fifty seconds, the latter part of which was overlaid with more footage of nurses at a Milwaukee hospital.

The instant Buresh was finished, her camera shut off. One host turned excitedly to the other and said she was dying to hear the answer to the important question posed earlier—were dogs or cats more popular?

After learning that it's cats, and after getting a pro forma thank you for her appearance, Buresh morosely made her way out of the station into the dark early morning thinking the whole thing had been a waste of time.

It wasn't. A lot of people saw the segment and remembered it even though it ran only two minutes and two seconds in its entirety. When she reviewed the tape later, Buresh saw that the segment was informative about nursing and had used positive images of nurses doing their work. The program had gotten her name and identification right, and, amazingly, she looked relaxed and cheerful on camera, in contrast to how she had felt.

1. *The Flattering or Gift Question*

An interviewer might say: "Oh, nurses are wonderful people. They do such important work." Or, "It's just terrible what's happening to nursing."

These "non-questions" can derail you because it's hard to know how to respond. Treat them as an invitation to take the conversation in the direc-

---

Your Turn

Think of three bumper stickers you'd use to describe your work or make your point. For example:

Nursing is a matter of life and death not TLC.

Nurses are the ones who see patients first in the emergency department; nurses decide how sick they are, how urgently they need to be treated, and who needs to treat them.

tion you'd like to go. "Thank you," "Yes, that's true," or "I'm glad you feel that way" are reasonable prefaces to a follow-up such as "Nurses hope the public will transform private gratitude into public support for nursing. Those listeners who share your views about nursing may want to call their political representative to support increased funding for nursing education, staffing, or research. In fact, there's now a bill in the state [or provincial] legislature that would allocate more money to nursing. We need public support for it . . ."

2. The Open-Ended Question

"What's it like to be a nurse?" Taken too literally, this type of question can have you chasing all over the landscape. Regard it as an invitation to tell an anecdote that contains one of your bumper stickers. "Well, one of the things we do in hospitals is prevent major complications like bedsores that can cause the patient terrible suffering and sometimes even lead to death, and can cost between $4,000 and $70,000 to heal."[1,2]

3. The Double-Bind Question

By confronting you with two untenable options, these questions are a classic catch-22.

An example: "Did you become a nurse because you didn't have what it takes to get into medical school, or because you're just too nice to be a doctor?"

Without repeating the question, one answer would be: "I became a nurse because I wanted to apply my intelligence to caring for the sick and vulnerable. I work on a surgical unit where, among other things, I make sure that patients don't develop pneumonias, blood clots, or wound infections after their operations . . ."

4. The Erroneous-Assumption Question

Like the double-bind question, this query throws negative material at you. The challenge is to quickly dispense with the negative and turn to the positive.

A Canadian radio interviewer once interrupted a guest who was describing the burdens being placed on nurses with: "So if nurses don't get enough respect, why don't they just all move up the food chain and become doctors?"

To which the guest responded: "In my view, nurses are already at the top of the food chain. Think about it, if all the nurses become doctors, who would provide 24-hour care of the sick?"

Never be afraid to challenge erroneous assumptions or misinterpretations of nursing. You are being interviewed because you are the expert, and therefore it is your role to correct mistaken ideas about nursing. Be prepared to do so.

Several years ago, nurses being interviewed by journalist Bill Moyers for a documentary series, "Healing and the Mind," seemed taken aback when Moyers misidentified their work.

In the documentary, Moyers observed nurses working with fragile premature infants and their teenage parents at Parkland Memorial Hospital in Dallas and then talked with the nurses about what they were doing. Clearly impressed, Moyers nonetheless demonstrated at the end of the segment how even the most intelligent and sensitive people can be confused about nursing. "You're *more* than nurses, you're *more* than technicians," he exclaimed. Then placing their work in the context of innovations in medicine, Moyers declared: "That's what *medicine's* about today."

Moyers's response was startling. But imagine the effect the nurses might have had on millions of viewers if they had been ready for a predictable misinterpretation. They could have politely, but firmly, responded: "No, Bill, what you have just seen is the very essence of *nursing*."

5. *The Absent-Party Question*

The interviewer may use a comment made by a general or specific absent party to inject controversy or discredit your arguments.

An interviewer might say, for example: "Many people are now saying that nurses have become too vociferous in their demands." To which you might respond, "Most people tell us quite the contrary. They are glad that nurses are standing up for patient care."

A variation of the form might be: "I have a friend who teaches chemistry at a prestigious university and he says that nursing students are the dumbest ones in his class."

This technique is insidious because you know neither the person nor

---

Your Turn

Practice doing an interview with a friend or colleague and then critique it, paying attention to the following:

- Are you speaking in ordinary language?
- Are you describing your work briefly and concretely?
- Are you conveying your enthusiasm?
- Are you expressing a strong point of view?

Interview Tips

- Find out in advance what the interview will be about.
- Find out how much time you will have.
- Prepare three "bumper stickers."
- Don't be a captive of the question. Bridge from the interviewer's question to the points you want to make.
- Use anecdotes, personal stories, statistics, sparkling language.
- Avoid jargon, technical terms, and alphabet soup (i.e., initialisms and acronyms).
- Tell the truth; don't exaggerate to win an argument.
- Don't repeat a negative question or offensive words.
- Know in advance what you will not divulge. Whether it is personal or has to do with your institution or profession, know how far you are willing to go and go no further.
- Assume everything is on the record. Don't comment if you don't want your comment to be aired.
- If you don't know something, say so. Then talk about what you do know.
- Be cooperative and communicative.
- Enjoy your experience on air.

what he really said. Yet, the absent party is set up as an authoritative commentator. To this statement, you might reply that you have not heard the comment and then describe the rigors of nursing education—"Sorry I haven't heard that one. But in nursing school we learn pharmacology, anatomy, and pathophysiology not to mention family health and how to communicate with patients and families."

6. *The Loaded-Preface Question*

An interviewer might pack a lot of information—some of it inaccurate or provocative—into a question. He might say, "I know your organization doesn't represent many people and has not established a track record in this area. What is its mission in this campaign?"

Take a mental breath and use the question to describe the importance of your organization and its key role in the current issue. "Our organization represents 70,000 RNs. We've just done a study that documents how violence in the workplace harms patients and exacerbates the nursing shortage."

7. The Irrelevant or Non-Sequitur Question

Depending on the tone of the show, an interviewer may incorporate a statement that has no bearing on the subject, such as, "My mother-in-law just loves the nurses on *ER*."

Use this bland statement to make a point: "Yes, nurses who work in emergency rooms are great. In fact, they do a lot more than is shown on that show . . ."

8. The Direct-Accusation Question

How about getting hit with this? "You're complaining about violence against nurses. What about all those nurses who kill their patients?"

You might reply by saying: "There aren't many nurses in that category, but workplace statistics indicate that more must be done to protect *nurses* from violence." Whatever else, do not repeat the phrase "nurses who kill their patients."

Nurses and other caregivers are often criticized when they "break frame" by doing something that seems out of synch with their conventional image such as asking for something for themselves or going on strike. Journalists may imply that nurses are being selfish or hiding behind patient care to get something for themselves, as in the question: "Are you really trying to protect your patients, or are you just trying to protect your job?"

A picket-line interview during a strike might produce: "Why are you abandoning your patients? Isn't your job to be at the bedside no matter what?"

Because nurses don't want to be perceived as selfish and uncaring, they tend to spend time trying to prove how unselfish and caring they are. A better tack might be to state forthrightly:

"We certainly do want to protect our jobs. That's because our job is to save your life."

Or, "A hospital's job is to care for patients and to support and sustain the people—professional nurses and other staff—who provide that care twenty-four hours a day. Because hospitals have cut too many nursing jobs, staff nurses are frequently asked to work two back-to-back, ten-hour shifts. The nurse may be exhausted and have no time to go the bathroom or take a lunch break. Studies now show that these conditions lead to errors that can harm patients."

9. The Inconsistency Question

This type of question suggests that you are unable to make up your mind and thus can't be trusted.

An interviewer might say, "Nurses complain that they have to do too much non-nursing work, but now they're saying they don't want more nursing assistants to help them."

To which the response might be, "Nurses are doing too many non-nursing activities like transporting patients, answering phones, or cleaning up. We want nursing assistants to help with that, not to give patients baths, medications, or monitor their vital signs."

10. The Question You Don't Know How to Answer

Sometimes interviewers will ask you questions you simply can't answer. If you're an oncology nurse, an interviewer could come from left field and ask you a question about the treatment of diabetics or the latest proposal for health care reform. If you know about diabetes or have an opinion about the latest health care reform proposal, voice it. If you don't, don't take a stab at it. Simply say, "That's an interesting question, but it's not my field. You might want to talk to a nurse who specializes in diabetes," or "You can get a lot of good information on health care reform by talking to people at the American Nurses Association." Then, use the question to bridge into what you do know about.

Call-in Shows

Thanks to the myriad call-in shows that are on television and radio, you can use the electronic media to make your point even if you are never invited to

Beware of repeating negative statements. While it's a normal response for people to repeat the negative to refute it, you may inadvertently give it more weight than it deserves. If an interviewer asks you about "nurses who kill their patients," and you say, "Nurses don't kill their patients," the listener has just heard the words "nurses...kill...patients" twice.

When people are under stress they might even introduce a negative suggestion themselves, as Richard Nixon did in 1973 in the statement that became emblematic of his unraveling presidency: "People have got to know whether or not their President is a crook. Well, I'm not a crook."

If other people make allegations, simply refute them. Don't raise new ones yourself.

appear on a show. If you are at home, at work, or driving in the car and you hear people discussing health care, listen carefully. If you're thinking, "I have something to say about that topic," punch in the number and express your point of view. People who call in to shows are generally not asked to give their last names. So if you're worried about retaliation, this is a perfect forum. Some shows take e-mailed questions and comments as well, and the host reads them on the air. If you can't get through or don't want to make a call, your view may still be aired.

We've been on a number of shows where nurses have called in spontaneously. Some have recounted heart-wrenching experiences. Some have talked about the work they do with patients. Others have discussed their research. Most have significantly advanced the discussion.

The show doesn't have to be on nursing to allow you, as a nurse, to contribute. It can be about health care reform, legislation, a political candidate's stand on issues, women and gender, or education—whatever topic provokes and inspires you to interject your experience and expertise. If you are listening and feel that something should be added, you're just the one to do it.

Chapter 12

Promoting Nursing Research

On October 22, 2002, the *Journal of the American Medical Association* (*JAMA*) published a landmark study that found a link between high hospital patient-to-nurse ratios and patient deaths.[1] Over the next few days, news reports about this study were published and broadcast by a wide range of media. For example, on October 23, under the headline "Study Links Workloads of Nurses to Patient Risk," the *Boston Globe* carried a 1,059-word report that led with: "The more surgical patients assigned to a hospital nurse, the greater those patients' chances of dying, according to one of the largest studies to date on the relationship between nurse workloads and patient deaths."[2] Three days later the *New York Times* hailed the significance of data establishing this link in an editorial headlined "Dying for Lack of Nurses."[3] In the following months, the study, "Hospital Nurse Staffing and Patient Mortality, Nurse Burnout, and Job Dissatisfaction," was reported and commented on in all manner of media, not just in the United States but throughout the world.

How did this study, conducted by Linda Aiken and her colleagues at the University of Pennsylvania School of Nursing, receive widespread coverage?

Not by accident.

First, this study was bound to attract some attention because it was published in one of the most widely read medical journals in the world. Additionally, *JAMA* highlighted the importance of the subject by running an accompanying editorial commenting on the practical implications of the study's findings on nurse staffing. Significantly, the study was among those chosen by *JAMA* for special promotional treatment, which means that thousands of credentialed journalists and media relations specialists were alerted to its existence and could access both a news release describing the findings and the actual *JAMA* article as much as five days in advance of publication.

At the same time, other stakeholders in the research were working in advance of publication to promote the study. The University of Pennsylvania

School of Nursing prepared its own advance news release and reached out to its media contacts. Another news release went out from the National Institute of Nursing Research (NINR), which funded the research.

Nursing unions and professional nursing associations were quick to recognize the import of the study for their agendas and thus promoted it in news releases, newsletters, and other media. Although other studies (some by the same researchers) had documented the problems of nurse staffing, this one could be particularly influential. Its huge scope (data was analyzed from surveys of 10,184 staff registered nurses and the outcomes for 232,342 patients from 168 hospitals) was unusual. The track record and credibility of the researchers, as well as the reputation of the journal in which it was published, made it noteworthy. Finally, it was pertinent to the efforts of nurses' unions to improve hospital working conditions through legislative remedies.

In short, this study was of interest to working nurses, managers and administrators, unions, professional associations, educators, policy makers, workplace business consultants, health care journalists, physicians, legislators, and patients—that is, if they knew about it. As it turned out, the study was communicated through so many avenues, one can say without fear of contradiction that it is one of the most widely known and cited pieces of nursing staffing research in the world.

Traditionally, nurses have been invisible in media reports on research findings. Research by nurses on nursing care issues is radically underreported. Nurses usually do not appear as central participants when medical studies are reported or when journalists cover the process of medical research. Most people who read the newspapers, watch TV, or look up health reports on the Internet get the impression that medical and biomedical research is carried out by physicians and that all the major advances in understanding disease is a doctor-only affair. Few people, for example, know that nurses often run trials testing new medications or treatments.

Patients, families, and the health care system in general can only reap the benefits of research done by nurses if that research is disseminated and publicized beyond the nursing community.

The growth of nursing research is a story of both achievement and unfulfilled potential. After much lobbying from the nursing community, the U.S. National Institutes of Health (NIH) set up a National Center for Nursing Research in 1986 with an initial budget of $16 million. The center was upgraded to a full-fledged institute, the National Institute for Nursing Research (NINR), in June 1993. In fiscal year 2004, eighteen years after its founding as a center, the institute reached a budget of $135 million. Nurses participate in studies funded by other institutes, such as the one with the highest level of funding, the National Cancer Institute. But the NINR provides important research grants to nursing schools. It remains, however, the institute with the lowest level of funding in the NIH. Its allotment was less than one-half of 1 percent of the NIH budget of $28 billion.

The NIH is part of the U.S. Department of Health and Human Services and receives its funding from the federal government. The amount the NIH and its member institutes will get is worked out in interplay between Congress and the President. These decisions are influenced by lobbying and by the personal interests of the decision makers. A former presidential appointee who reviewed the NIH budget for the White House told us there is no question that money flows more readily to those who make the case for the relevance of their research. For example, alternative and complementary practitioners have not been highly regarded by the medical profession. But they have followed in the public relations footsteps of medicine by successfully mobilizing patients and the public to pressure politicians for money for research on alternative remedies. In 1999, the NIH established the National Center for Complementary and Alternative Medicine. Likewise, vigorous PR for nursing research can only enhance the funding process.

Public communication is also required if research findings are to be incorporated into practice. "Whether it's to change policy or enhance practice, our research is meant to be used," University of California nursing home expert Charlene Harrington told us. "It has to go beyond nursing publications. If we're trying to influence policy, we have to publish in policy journals like *Health Affairs* or *Medical Care*. And we have to reach out to the mainstream media, no matter where our work is published. If we keep this work a secret within nursing, neither practice nor policy will change."

Medical Journals Have Paved the Way

Although medical research is now a huge part of health coverage, only a few decades ago doctors had little incentive to communicate with reporters and the lay public. Until health care costs soared and research funds began to shrink, the idea that physicians had to be accountable to the general public was foreign to most MDs. Patients were far more passive in their relationships with their doctors. Medical organizations discouraged doctors from talking with reporters, equating this with advertising, an activity that used to be associated with quacks and patent medicine salesmen.

Over the past thirty years, several factors made it essential for physicians to communicate with the public. Insurers and government were no longer willing to write blank checks for health care services, and demands for reform of the system were increasing. If doctors were going to influence the funding and delivery of health care, they had to be willing to take their case to the public. At the same time, competition was growing for research funds, and patients were seeking more information from their doctors. In the United States, medical organizations did a turnabout. They dropped their bans against advertising, encouraged physicians to raise their public profiles, and taught them how to use the media effectively.[4]

Today, funders require applicants to have a plan for communicating their findings. "Funding agencies are eager to see that research results are disseminated to appropriate scientific, professional, and lay audiences," says Ross Koppel, a medical sociologist at the University of Pennsylvania's department of Sociology and Center for Clinical Epidemiology and Biostatistics. "They require a dissemination plan that typically involves presentations to professional meetings; publication in refereed journals; releases to popular venues like newspapers or magazines if appropriate, and, if possible, book-length manuscripts for wider audiences. To reach wide audiences, funders today want researchers to be able to talk about their work in ways that nonspecialists and laypeople can understand," Koppel told us.

Not all medical researchers are happy about pressure to communicate, nor do all appreciate the coverage—and competition for coverage—that results. Nonetheless, a critical mass engages in the process. Sixty percent of medical reporters surveyed for a special report on the relationship between journalists and physicians described doctors and medical researchers as highly accessible, and 38 percent said doctors were somewhat accessible. A survey of medical researchers found that 86 percent of them felt that news reports based on their research were accurate.[4]

For many years, the widely quoted bioethicist Arthur L. Caplan has been urging doctors to learn how to express themselves so that they can gain public support. He even teaches his students at the Center for Bioethics at the University of Pennsylvania how to write for popular audiences. Caplan told nurse executives attending a University of Pennsylvania conference that they must talk to the media both to inform the public about current health care issues and to influence the democratic process of decision making. He urged nurses to "take tough positions, advocate your views, and don't be wishy-washy."[5]

Medical journal editors have paved the way for nurse researchers willing to follow this advice. They have convinced journalists that dry, seemingly incomprehensible study reports can be fascinating and worthy of media and public attention. They have made research findings reader-friendly for reporters who, in turn, have learned how to translate that research into understandable, everyday language.

Although George Lundberg, a former recent editor of *JAMA* is generally credited with making medical research a media staple, the editors of *JAMA* have been recommending studies for news coverage since the 1930s. In the 1940s, *JAMA* editor Morris Fishbein provided the Associated Press in Chicago with advance page proofs of the journal with the caveat that no information was to be released until the journal's publication date.[4]

These days, news about health and medical developments swell midweek because of the orchestrated embargo system established by *JAMA* and adopted by the *New England Journal of Medicine (NEJM)*—the only two weekly medical journals in North America. To have time to prepare their stories, reporters can get advance copies of the journals. But they must agree to hold their stories until the nominal publication date, thus giving subscribers a chance to at least skim their journals before newly published findings hit the airwaves.

JAMA, which has a Wednesday publication date, releases its embargo at 3 P.M. Tuesdays (central time) to permit radio and television to break research stories then and newspapers to run their stories on Wednesday morning. The *New England Journal*, which publishes on Thursdays, does the same a day later. This system guarantees that "nobody can have a scoop. Nobody can jump the gun. Everybody has time to do it right," Lundberg has explained.[4]

Until the advent of the Internet, the media relations specialists for the journals published by the American Medical Association mailed press releases describing selected studies to thousands of journalists worldwide. Today qualified reporters and freelancers can register electronically with individual medical journals to gain access to embargoed material or sign up with the much larger EurekAlert!, a global news service operated by the American Association for the Advancement of Science (AAAS), for access to "embargoed and breaking news, peer-reviewed journals, experts, and other valuable resources."[6]

EurekAlert! is a boon to public information officers (PIOs) at universities and other research institutions who are trying to communicate with journalists and the public about research at their institutions. According to its Web site, "PIOs from hundreds of organizations worldwide use EurekAlert! to distribute science, health and technology news, [the names of] experts, and other resources to reporters."

A Web site of this sort is extremely valuable to journal publishers because few, if any, have the resources to fund a media operation on the scale of the AMA's. The editors of *JAMA* and of the nine AMA archives journals (e.g., *Archives of Internal Medicine*) select studies for media promotion sometimes weeks in advance of publication. Each week, the PIOs for the journals prepare media releases for three to five potentially newsworthy studies to be published in *JAMA* and usually one or more for a study in one of the archives journals.

The journal editors keep an eye out for those rarer studies that are rich in human interest or visual potential. These can be the subjects of video news releases (VNRs). A VNR offers television stations everything they need to do a report: a complete narrated feature, including interviews and dramatic visuals, that can run as is; a script if a station wants to use all or part of the feature but have its own reporter narrate; or sound bites and visuals for those who want to do their own report but need illustrations.

The VNRs are fed by satellite to television stations in North America and elsewhere. A signal embedded in the VNR allows a monitoring organization to see how widely it has been used. According to the AMA, scores of stations each week take excerpts out of the VNR to illustrate their own reports or use it in its entirety.

Using sophisticated public relations techniques is standard operating procedure in medical research. This is why most journalists see medicine as cutting-edge, dynamic, and the source of stories that must be covered. Journal editors may not always say so, but they actively court the news media. In 1990, *JAMA* even changed its publication date from Friday to Wednesday, a day earlier than the *NEJM*. *JAMA* editor Lundberg candidly admitted news coverage was one consideration for the change after reporters complained that Friday was a busy news day and that it was hard to do follow-up stories. *JAMA* chose Wednesday after surveying reporters to find out what day would be good for them.[4]

Newspaper and television coverage of medical and health studies varies widely. Some studies get boiled down into a paragraph for inclusion in health news columns. Others may get full-blown treatment on the front page or the top of the newscast. Some never see the light of day. Some independent-minded reporters resent the AMA's newsworthiness evaluation. They claim that they toss the news releases and read the journal themselves to decide what to report on. The reports that annoy the AMA are those that are so truncated that they neglect to cite *JAMA* or another AMA publication as the source.

To get the best coverage, the AMA goes out of its way to accommodate the media. Its rationale for its huge investment in media and public communication is that a large part of the organization's mission is public health education.

It is now established practice for medical researchers to engage in personal communication with journalists. Public relations specialists at research institutes, foundations that fund research, university medical schools, and hospital PR departments all try to get their researchers to talk about their work.

Doctors and other medical researchers can be assertive themselves in reaching out to help promote, and fund, specific research. Some even hire their own PR representatives. After the late actor Christopher Reeve suffered his severe spinal cord injury, researchers asked Reeve to help raise public awareness and money for spinal cord injury research. Reeve's physicians helped him to reconstruct the medical treatment he received so that he could write his book, *Still Me*. Reeve became an effective lobbyist for funds and the most visible bridge between the research community in this area and the public.

One could legitimately ask: Did nurse researchers ever approach him? Did nurses enlighten him about what they did for him during his original

How to Encourage a Reporter to Cover Nursing Research

Approach #1

Researcher: Hello. I am [full name], a nurse researcher at the University of…I've been following coverage of health care research that you've run over the past several months in the *Daily Bugle.* My colleagues and I are concerned because coverage tends to focus exclusively on medical studies and excludes important work done by nurse researchers.

Reporter: Sorry you don't like our coverage. But it isn't our job to cover professions. We cover good stories. By all means call when you have one.

Approach #2

Researcher: Hello. I am [full name]. I'm a researcher on cardiac care at the University of…School of Nursing. We have a very important study that we think will help save people's lives after they have had heart attacks. I hope this will interest you and provide material for a good story.

Reporter: What kind of researcher are you? Are you a nurse?

Researcher: Yes, I'm a nurse and a PhD on the faculty of…I study…

Reporter: We've already done stories on treatments for heart attacks.

Researcher: And I've seen them. But what they're missing is how people deal with heart attacks when they have them. Our studies show they're never going to get the treatment you described unless they recognize that they need quick medical attention. Many people don't respond to their symptoms and don't go to the emergency room and may die or suffer serious heart damage as a result. That's what our scientific research is about. We've studied why people delay getting treatment when they've had a heart attack and what will get them to go to the hospital quickly.

Reporter: I've never heard of nursing research. Is this what you do?

Researcher: Precisely. What's important to people isn't just what happens in the operating room or in the doctor's office. It's the care they receive when they get sick, how they respond to being sick, and how they live during or after an illness. That's the missing story in health care.

and other subsequent hospitalizations and ask him to speak to general audiences about the value of his nursing care? Do nurses approach wealthy patients and ask them to speak up for nursing research? Most important, do they do systematic outreach to those journalists who are their conduits to a broader public?

Journalists and Nursing Research

Many of the same journalists are unaware that nursing research even exists.

A lot of journalists have told us that they would "love to hear from nurse researchers" and do stories on their work. But that they don't get much usable material from nurses. "They seem to be new to the idea of peddling their work to the media," a radio journalist told us.

When she wrote about health care delivery and public health for the *Los Angeles Times*, Julie Marquis said that she rarely received material from nurse researchers until she was asked to speak on one of Sigma Theta Tau's media panels. After telling participants that she would like more information about nursing, she began to receive more. She told us she found material on the nursing shortage, nurse staffing, and health care delivery particularly useful. As journalists usually do, she became aware of nursing research through personal contacts.

"I would be very receptive to stories about important research done by nurses," said Richard A. Knox, a medical reporter for U.S. National Public Radio. "But since we have our hands full reading the major medical and scientific journals, someone has to call our attention to important studies if they want us to report on them."

Knox said he uses EurekAlert! to monitor announcements about studies. But when we asked him if he gets material or calls from nurse researchers or their organizations, he replied, "Very little."

We asked if he receives material from the National Institute for Nursing Research. "No," he replied.

For journalists "a good story" is what is paramount. They claim they don't care what initials follow a researcher's name, as long as it's "good copy" from a credible source. A study is newsworthy because it has value to patients or to the health care system, not because it was conducted by nurses.

If nursing research, however, is to receive the support it deserves, researchers will have to reach out to journalists so they understand that nurse scientists investigate a broad range of health and health care questions either within their own discipline or as participants in interdisciplinary studies. Their studies could be concerned with patient care, medical cures, health promotion or disease prevention, or with health care policy and systems of health

Your Turn

Log on to EurekAlert! and search for news releases in a clinical area that interests you or ones that contain the key words "nurse" or "nursing." Observe how they are written to make the findings understandable and interesting to a general audience. Pick out three studies from recent clinical nursing journals. Some can be found online; many are available in nursing school libraries. Translate the titles and abstracts into ordinary language. You can try your hand with the abstract below from the *Western Journal of Nursing Research:*[7]

Exercise and Functional Tasks among Adults Who Are Functionally Limited

This study compared the efficacy of 16 weeks of either resistance training, aerobic walking, or combined resistance training and aerobic walking on the performance of functional tasks among adults age 65 years and older with limited functional ability. One hundred thirty-one older adult individuals were randomized into four groups: resistance training, aerobic walking, combined resistance and aerobic walking groups, or a nonexercise control group. Each of the exercise groups documented 70 percent compliance with their respective exercise intervention, which included three weekly exercise sessions. At baseline, and 8 and 16 weeks following baseline, all participants completed six assessments of their functional ability. Analysis of covariance indicated that all three exercise intervention groups significantly improved measures of functional ability, with the resistance group demonstrating the most consistent gains over the six measures. These findings indicate that older adults who are functionally limited can improve their functional ability through a variety of types of exercise.

care delivery. Nurses who work with patients also participate in research by collecting and recording clinical data for studies of experimental treatments and various other interventions. It's essential for the public to know nursing practice is based on what has been learned from research studies.

Working with Institutional PR People

Some nursing schools and nurse researchers have incorporated public communication outreach into the budget of their school or research project.

When Claire Fagin became the dean of the University of Pennsylvania School of Nursing in 1977, one of her top priorities was addressing the invisibility of the school. "I made a deal with the Hospital of the University of Pennsylvania to use their PR staff to work with the School of Nursing," Fagin told us. "This reflected the hospital's high level commitment to promoting nursing. For a while it went very well. The hospital hired a very good PR specialist who had a mandate to work with the school."

After about five years, the hospital's priorities changed. They reduced their staff. "I decided the School of Nursing had to hire its own PR person, which we did on a part-time basis," Fagin says. Since the mid-1980s the school has employed its own communication professional. Joy McIntyre, who has been instrumental in promoting the school's nurse-staffing research, has held the post for six years.

Charlene Harrington, a professor at the University of California at San Francisco' (UCSF) School of Nursing is an expert in nursing home workforce issues. She explains that she works with the public relations office at UCSF to arrange press briefings and to construct news releases when research studies appear. "You may have to help PR staff write the press release, but they're looking for things to promote," she told us.

At McMaster University in Ontario, Gina Bohn Browne and her colleagues have integrated media work into their program. The McMaster System-Linked Research Unit on Health and Social Services Utilization compares the effects and costs of comprehensive care delivered by those in various disciplines. To inform those who can make use of this research, Browne and her colleagues created a plan to disseminate research findings to the media, patients, health care practitioners, policy makers, other researchers, and the public. Browne's group even hired a PR firm to put two of the unit's project reports into "digestible form" and get them out to the media.

Nurse researchers who want to promote their work may encounter resistance in their institution. Some faculty members may argue that popularizing research can oversimplify, mislead, or overstate what is actually known. Kathleen Dracup, dean of the School of Nursing at UCSF, elaborated for us on this problem: "Scientists are very reluctant to talk about the little nuggets that come from research that make a difference to people's lives. This is because, as scientists, they always want to replicate their findings before urging a change in practice. But then the problem becomes: When is there ever enough data? When can you ever feel comfortable taking the message to the public? We have to get over the tendency to wait too long."

Nursing research will be seen as a dynamic enterprise in the same league as medical research only if researchers are willing to comment, critically at times, on work by other researchers and stand up for their own findings when debate occurs. When journalist Ellen Ruppel Shell was researching how

JAMA and *NEJM* make decisions about which studies to publish, she looked for nurses knowledgeable about therapeutic touch to discuss a controversial experiment done by a nine-year-old girl for her fourth grade science fair that *JAMA* published discrediting the therapy.[8] The child, Emily Rosa of Loveland, Colorado, designed an experiment in which a therapeutic touch practitioner (she recruited twenty-one) and she were separated by a screen. "Then," as the *New York Times* reported, "Emily decided by flipping a coin, whether to put her hand over the healer's left hand or the right hand. The healer was asked to decide where Emily's hand was hovering. If the healer could detect Emily's human energy field, he or she should be able to discern where Emily's hand was. In 280 tests involving the twenty-one practitioners, the healers did no better than chance. They identified the correct location of Emily's hand just 44 percent of the time; if they guessed at random, they would have been right about half the time."[9]

Emily wrote up the experiment with her mother, Linda Rosa, a nurse who belonged to a local group critical of therapeutic touch, another member of that group, and the head of a nonprofit group named Quackwatch in Allentown, Pennsylvania, that posted information about questionable medical practices on the Internet. By publishing their report, *JAMA* kicked up a storm of controversy over its standards for evaluating research as well as over the healing practice itself.

Shell, who is also a journalism professor and co-director of Boston University's Center for Science and Medical Journalism, told us she wanted experts to discuss the therapy, which is affiliated with nursing, and the implications of such an article being published in a prestigious medical journal. "I wanted to get into the issues, but I couldn't because I couldn't get a nurse to talk to me about it on the record," Shell said.

While the impetus to shy away from a hot potato is understandable, to be taken seriously as health professionals, nurses must be willing to debate practice issues both within the pages of nursing journals and in the general media.

"Nurse researchers must assume the responsibility and authority that go along with being professional," Ruppel-Shell says. "Researchers can't say they have to ask someone for permission in order to comment. They can't hide behind the hierarchy or institution. They have to have the courage of their convictions and be forthcoming, otherwise freedom of speech is gone."

Journalists point out that while you can ask a reporter to read back your quote, you appear naive if you ask a reporter to show you a copy of their story so that you can vet it before it goes to press. Reporters don't make deals like that. Indeed, they will expect you or your PR officer to do much of their legwork for them. In this area of health and medical research, reporters have grown accustomed—perhaps too accustomed—to being spoon-fed. They may want you to send them not only your new study but all the studies you have done on the subject. They probably will want to talk to patients who have benefited from the research. They may want to shoot footage and interview people in your hospital. They may expect you to arrange it. They may want you to provide the names of other people they can talk to about the subject, including those who differ from you. They may want you to propose policy solutions or practical tips for patients that they can use in their story. You will have to decide how much time and energy to put into promotion. Assistance from PR staff can be essential.

Hiring Outside PR Help

In the winter of February 2000, reporters at major media outlets received the following news release:

News
Release

New Study Supports "Family Presence" in Emergency Departments: Research Demonstrates Numerous Benefits during Life-Saving Procedures

New York, NY, February 17, 2000—In 1994, Theresa A. Meyers, RN, trauma case manager at Parkland Memorial Hospital in Dallas, Texas, made a split-second decision that went against her hospital's usual practice, and ignited a firestorm of controversy. Her actions—letting the parents of a dying boy into a critical care area while medical personnel tried to save him—focused attention on this controversial practice and have been debated ever since.

Now a study released in the February issue of the *American Journal of Nursing*, on "family presence" in the emergency department (ED) during invasive procedures (IP) and cardiopulmonary resuscitation (CPR), confirms that family members, nurses, and physicians support the practice as positive and beneficial. Largely as a result of the study, Parkland Memorial Hospital implemented a policy and now offers the option for family presence during IP and CPR throughout the hospital.[10]

With this dramatic lead, the *American Journal of Nursing* (*AJN*) initiated a bold approach to publicizing nursing research. It hired a public relations firm to distribute news releases on its "family presence" report to hundreds of local and national print and radio outlets. Additionally a two-minute video news release (VNR) filmed at Parkland hospital and supplementary video material went out to television stations. Public relations staff followed up with phone calls to journalists and producers, pointing out the story elements inherent in this research and its potential to transform hospital practices. They also offered to arrange interviews with researchers. The *AJN* got another shot at coverage by notifying journalists of a Web cast on the study scheduled for February 29 during which the authors would answer questions submitted online or phoned in on a toll-free number.

Newspapers throughout the United States picked up the story. *USA Today* did a cover story. Cable News Network (CNN), which is seen throughout the world, shot a feature. Shortly after its release, the VNR aired seventy-five times in forty-five markets, reaching an estimated 5.7 million people.

As a result of this promotion, the family presence study attained a high level of visibility. In the process, it may have raised the profile of nursing research itself, making a significant contribution to new efforts to publicize research conducted by nurses. The study, like so many others, was also valuable to patients and families. That was certainly the intention of *AJN*'s editor-in-chief. In her editorial in the February issue, Diana J. Mason announced that the *AJN*, the official publication of the American Nurses Association, would be publishing (and publicizing) "compelling, original research that can transform practice."

Mason accepted the position of editor-in-chief in 1998 only after *AJN* publishers Lippincott Williams & Wilkins pledged to support her intention to editorially strengthen the journal, make it more relevant and credible, and promote it not just within nursing but in the broader health care and public communities. Although she says she had to fight hard to get what she regarded as a modest budget, she was determined to follow promotional models established by medical journals. Her publisher was pleased with the attention the family presence study received. The feedback indicated that the general public was now more aware of changing emergency department protocols and so were a greater number of nurses, physicians, and other care givers. They hadn't learned about the issue through the journal's publication but through the mainstream news media. Mason had succeeded in finding the right study to promote. Because of its outreach, the *AJN* is the most frequently quoted nursing journal in the news media.

Few research studies in nursing or medicine have as many strong news values as this one did. It featured a heroic working nurse, Theresa Meyers, who bucked the system to allow a mother and father to be with their dying fourteen-year-old child. It had controversy and conflict—some of the physicians, nurses, and administrators at Meyers's institution at the time, and a large percentage of medical residents in general, opposed the presence of family members during invasive procedures and especially during CPR. The study was attractive because it refuted conventional wisdom: Those family members who were permitted to stay were not disruptive and tended to appreciate, rather than judge, the work and life-saving attempts of the clinicians.

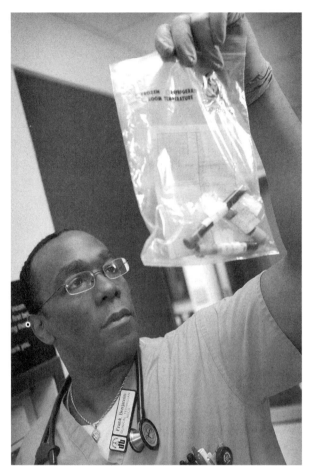

Photo by Keith Weller. Courtesy of the American Association of Colleges of Nursing.

The study had impact for members of a broad general audience who might imagine themselves in this tragic situation. They learned that 97 percent of the family members who were permitted to stay felt they had a right to be present and said the experience was important and helpful. The research seemed to convince nurses, physicians, and others on the interdisciplinary team that relegating families to waiting rooms during a code or invasive procedures might be too severe.

The *AJN*'s foray into high-test media relations is an excellent example of what can happen when nurses who conduct research tell the world about their studies and discuss the applications of their work. Over a two-year period, Jane E. Brody, longtime health columnist for the *New York Times*, used *AJN* articles as the basis for four of her columns. One of them was a 2003 special report called, "Facing Up to the Inevitable, in Search of a Good Death."[11] The article noted that the cases it described had been reported in an *AJN* series on end-of-life care. It also quoted nurse experts from that *AJN* series, Rose Virani, a research specialist at the City of Hope National Medical Center in Duarte, California, and Elizabeth Ford Pitorak, director of the Hospice Institute and the Hospice of the Western Reserve in Cleveland and featured a photograph of Pitorak.

However, apart from their association with a nursing journal, the article, typically, never mentioned that their discipline is nursing. Three other persons cited were clearly identified as physicians through the use of the honorific "Dr." The *Times* style is to restrict the use of that title to MDs, and to use Mr. or Ms. with others, including PhDs. To make nursing visible, it is important for researchers to stress that they want their nursing credentials mentioned.

Selecting Studies and Making Their Implications Clear

To promote nursing research, select studies that will interest a wide public. If you want to go to a mainstream media outlet, ask yourself if your study affects a broad swath of its audience. Studies on cancer pain, heart disease, or care of sick children, the elderly, and nursing homes obviously do. Research

Highlight Why Your Research Is Important

A nurse in Australia recently described her master's degree research project to us. "My research is about trying to reduce baby's pain during heel pricks in the neonatal ICU," she said. "Our long-term babies may have 30, 40, 100 heel pricks during their admission. So we are trying to reduce their crying and pain during the heel-prick procedure by giving them sucrose on their tongues during and after the procedure."

As far as it goes, this brief description makes the research project seem worthwhile but there is nothing compelling or important about it. It's nice. When we asked the researcher to elaborate further, we discovered that the impetus for the project was not the fact that babies cry when they get a needle stick but that they can become so distressed they could actually die. This significant piece of information was missing from her description. When asked more questions, a very different—and far more compelling—picture of the research emerged.

"The heels of very sick babies are pricked to test their blood. We prick them on their heel, which is a very sensitive part of their body, without using an anesthetic. The conventional wisdom has been that babies don't feel pain or that if they do, they forget it. As nurses we know that babies obviously do feel pain. They cry in high-pitched voices and screw up their faces and kick their legs out. Their heart rate increases to 200 beats per minute. They begin to pant. When babies are very sick—particularly babies with heart conditions—they can become blue and some have had a cardiac arrest during the heel-prick procedure. Although it's rare, there have been babies who have died. I worked with a baby who arrested and died, which prompted me to do my study. What they go through in an ICU can affect their growth and development in later years. So if we can do anything to reduce their pain during the heel-prick procedure, it can have a very significant effect while they are on and when they get off the unit."

that affects a smaller segment of the population might be a story if it has good news values.

Explain how the findings could save lives, and how many; save money, and how much; prevent suffering, and what kind; change the way care is given, and how.

When discussing a study on delays in getting treatment after a heart attack, for example, talk about how many people this problem affects. Describe the kinds of health problems such delays create. Calculate the differences in the cost between treating someone early versus treating someone who has delayed getting help. Draw attention to the additional burden of care borne by family members for the patient who delays such treatment.

If you have written a book on an important topic, send a complimentary copy to key journalists. Try to alert journalists to the publication of the book well before its release date.

Translate Your Research into Ordinary Language

We asked two internationally known researchers, Kathleen A. Dracup and Sean P. Clarke, to give us two summaries of their work—one in "research-ese" and one that would be more attractive to the public or the media. (Dracup does research in cardiac care and is co-editor of the *American Journal of Critical Care* and dean of the University of California San Francisco School of Nursing. Clarke is a prominent nursing workforce researcher and is associate director of the Center for Health Outcomes and Policy research at the University of Pennsylvania School of Nursing.

First Summary in Research-ese—Kathleen Dracup

We conducted a research study to identify predictors of delay behavior in patients who experience an acute myocardial infarction. A logistic regression revealed the following factors to be important characteristics affecting time to seek treatment: advanced age, low income, low educational level, embarrassment about calling for help, fearing what might happen in the future, and worrying about troubling others. These predictors can be used to tailor appropriate patient education interventions.

Second Summary in Ordinary Language

People who seek treatment immediately when they experience the symptoms of a heart attack are more likely to survive, have fewer complications, and have better outcomes than people who delay getting that treatment. Unfortunately, many people wait hours or even days after they first experience symptoms before they go to the hospital.

Nurse researchers who conducted studies in the United States and Australia found that individuals are more likely to delay getting treatment if they are older, poor, and less educated. We also found that people who had a second heart attack delayed just as long the second time as the first.

Why do people delay getting help? Here are a few reasons. Some people felt embarrassed about calling for help. Some feared what might happen if they had to go to the hospital, or worried about troubling others.

We're now testing an intervention to reduce the delay by encouraging patients to seek treatment immediately. This research can be life saving—particularly for people at high risk for having heart attack and for those who may delay treatment if they do. The public needs to know about the benefits of immediate treatment. It's simple: If you want to save your life, minutes count!

First Summary in Research-ese—Sean Clarke

Our study combined patient outcomes data from an administrative claims database with primary survey data and secondary data about hospital characteristics. Risk-adjusted surgical mortality in Pennsylvania hospitals was significantly positively associated with mean patient-to-RN staffing ratios. A one-unit increase in patient-to-nurse ratios was associated with an odds ratio of 1.07 in the fully adjusted models. It was further found that the odds of nurse burnout scores exceeding established norms for medical personnel and of nurse job dissatisfaction increased similarly with higher patient-to-nurse ratios. These results suggest a need to study the relationships of staffing to outcomes in other areas and in other populations and for healthcare leaders to carefully review the safety implications of staffing variability across hospitals.

Second Summary in Ordinary Language

We know that, for various reasons, hospitals hire and use staff in different ways. They can end up assigning different numbers of patients to nurses on average even when the types of patients are quite similar. Until a few years ago, we knew very little about whether this made any difference to how patients fared or how nurses felt about their jobs.

In 1999, registered nurses (RNs) working in hospitals across Pennsylvania were asked to complete questionnaires and indicate how many patients they were responsible for on the last shifts they worked. The average patient loads for registered nurses in each hospitals were calculated. Information about the types of hospitals was also used (how many beds were in each, for instance) as well as information from the state about all patients admitted to the hospitals for common surgeries.

Your Turn

Look through your specialty's journals or think about the research that you do. Which studies have the news values we describe in chapter 6 (timeliness, prominence, currency, impact, conflict, scandal/wrongdoing)? Which are newsworthy? Select those that are and then reduce them to a paragraph that you could pitch to a public relations professional or newspaper reporter.

On average, nurses in Pennsylvania hospitals cared for anywhere from about 4 to 8 patients on their last shifts. It was found that every additional patient in an average nurses' workload was associated with a 7 percent increase in the risk of death within 30 days for all the patients, after important differences were taken into account. This translated to a 31 percent increase in the risk of mortality for patients in hospitals with the lowest staffing levels.

Nurses in hospitals with higher workloads were more likely to be dissatisfied and to be burned out (or exhausted by their jobs). Although a lot of things affect whether nurses leave their jobs, being dissatisfied and burned out at work are often important predictors.

Next steps include seeing whether these connections between staffing in hospitals and how well patients and nurses do are found for other time periods, in other states, and across countries. We also want to know whether they apply to hospital patients who don't have surgery. This study should make hospital leaders and politicians think carefully about how staffing levels may affect public safety.

Using Meetings to Promote Nursing Research

Professional meetings provide wonderful promotional possibilities. Nursing groups hold meetings in every large city in the United States and Canada. These conferences often are held in cities that are home to local, and perhaps national, media outlets. Before arranging a national or regional meeting, organizers could take a tally of the researchers who will attend, get copies of their work, and devise promotional strategies.

Here's the procedure. Send news releases to journalists who cover the areas that will be discussed. Call them to inform them of specific research findings that will be presented at the conference. Give them background information and encourage them to attend the sessions where pertinent research will be presented. If they can't come to you, tell them you'll be glad to bring the researcher to them. If researchers will be attending but not present-ing, arrange interviews with them. Ask a select group of researchers if they would be willing to meet with journalists. Request summaries of their re-search for distribution to the press.

Do not assume that because you post a release about your meeting on a Web site that anyone will see it or attend your meeting because of it. Make personal contacts and use the Web as a supplement to those contacts.

Be sure to give the names of any journalists you expect to attend to the people at the registration desk. Never ask a journalist to pay a registration fee. A journalist would attend as an observer, not a participant. Make sure there is a packet of conference materials waiting for the journalist. A PR rep-resentative or someone else knowledgeable about the proceedings should be available to greet the journalist and see if he or she has any questions. Be available to introduce him or her to speakers upon request, but don't hover or act like the reporter needs a keeper.

If a political candidate plans to deliver a major policy speech at the con-ference, the media probably will come. But they won't necessarily stay around to explore nursing issues unless it is clear to them that there is another story to cover or unless they think the reaction of the conference participants might be newsworthy. If a journalist is a guest speaker at the meeting, ask him or her to meet with a select group of nurse researchers who can talk about new developments.

It would be worthwhile for small groups of leading researchers to make annual visits to health care journalists at major newspapers, magazines, and television outlets in such cities as New York, Washington, D.C., Los Angeles, Chicago, Toronto, Ottawa, Vancouver, and Montreal. A PR specialist could help them to set up these "dog and pony shows" and prepare presentations on current research and its impact on health and illness.

Encourage Nursing Journals to Do More Outreach

If journals are too small to have full- or part-time PR staff, perhaps a group of journal editors could start a cooperative project to promote articles from their journals. They could track who uses their releases and who doesn't and then call those outlets that have not used the research.

Nursing journal editors have told us that many publishers balk at spend-ing money to promote nursing research. Some have told us that companies that own and publish medical as well as nursing journals sometimes have a double standard. They pay physician-editors a fee to edit the journals and provide administrative and promotional support for them. "We aren't paid a cent for our work," one editor of a nursing journal told us. "Plus, we have to pay for the postage to send out articles to peer reviewers."

Given the relevance of nursing and nursing research, these biased attitudes and practices should not be tolerated, and nurses should be willing to make them public. Top researchers and nursing leaders should meet with publishers to discuss discriminatory patterns and insist on steps that would end them.

Look for Ongoing Opportunities to Promote Your Research

Lots of research gets done in interdisciplinary teams, but nursing and its contributions are often invisible. This is why it's so important that the publicity promoting such studies clearly shows that nurses were contributors to the study and that there is a nursing aspect to the issue. Nurses are part of, not apart from, the medical system and they are, not surprisingly, also involved in medical research and innovation. Nurses usually play a critical role in experimental protocols. They help to select subjects, collect and analyze data, and decide who stays in—and who will need to leave—a study. Nurses also administer and evaluate the treatments being given. Yet, in most cases, studies on experimental medical treatments and procedures omit nurses' role. Nurses should insist that their research function be highlighted and that they be included as sources of information when these studies are promoted. This means, however, that nurses must be willing to claim the credit due them, talk to reporters about their contributions and insights, and not defer to doctors when asked about their role.

Reporter: I understand that you were involved in a research study on *X* new cancer treatment. Could you tell me about your role?

Nurse: Oh, I'm really not able to talk about that. You should really ask the doctor.

Versus

Nurse: You know, patients receiving this experimental treatment suffer from terrible nausea and vomiting. It's my job to monitor and manage their symptoms and decide whether they can tolerate the treatment.

Certain subjects will reappear in the news. Researchers can take studies that are even a few years old to reporters if they illuminate a timely or hot issue in the news. It is not only timeliness, but the way research is packaged that influences coverage.

A good place to present your research is at conventions and meetings of associations of journalists who cover health care. You might approach conference organizers and suggest a presentation on why nursing research matters to the public.

Foundations, disease associations, and international organizations sponsor conferences for journalists on specific health problems, social issues, and health policy problems at which MDs and PhDs present overviews of recent research. Get into the network and convince the PR people who plan these programs to highlight nursing as well as medical research.

There are a number of university-based journalism fellowship programs that give journalists an opportunity to study for a semester or year. These fellowship programs arrange presentations from experts in various fields. You could be invited just by virtue of being visible in the media in connection with a timely issue like health care legislation. This is another venue where presentations can be proposed. Practically every school of nursing that conducts extensive research is situated in a university that has a communication or journalism school or department. Some journalism schools have science/health/medical writing courses, and a few have graduate programs in this area. Public relations programs may also have a track for those students who want to go into health or science PR. Nursing researchers can go to these departments and ask to do class presentations on cutting-edge research.

Tell the Story in Various Ways

You can also promote your research in what you might consider to be unconventional ways. The *American Journal of Nursing* news release on the benefits of "family presence" in the ED grabbed attention through a dramatic story about a nurse's personal experience. Many journalists undoubtedly were drawn to the story of a nurse taking a risk to do what she considered the right thing for her patient and his or her family. This nurse would be an excellent subject for a general or woman's magazine profile.

Once papers pick up on a study like family presence, researchers, or members of the Emergency Nurses Association (which developed guidelines for the study), can keep the story alive by writing op-eds, letters to the editor, or other kinds of articles on their own experiences with families in treatment rooms. Debate over the issue would be equally compelling.

Women's and self-help magazines are an avenue for discussion of all sorts of human-interest subjects. Once the first wave of reporting on research has crested, it's time to expand the audience by producing articles that help patients and family members turn theory into practice. Some researchers may want to write these articles themselves. An organization concerned with these developments can find a nurse writer or pitch the story to an editor who will assign an article to a staff or freelance writer.

In the case of the study on delaying treatment after a heart attack, for example, an excellent prospect for a women's magazine would be a piece on how to deal with a loved one who may have suffered a heart attack. The title might be "Ten Things You Need to Do to Keep Your Husband Alive after He's Had a Heart Attack." A similar spin-off on family presence could be "Ten Things You Need to Know When Your Child (Spouse, Parent) Goes to the ER."

Using Research to Strengthen Advocacy

Research is an essential tool in any campaign or struggle waged by nurses for better working conditions, staffing, improvements in patient care, and increases in institutional and societal resources needed to support quality care. The campaigns we described in chapter 9, for example, contained a research component. The media, policy makers, and health care administrators require documented research to demonstrate the importance of nursing care to patients and the conditions necessary to support nursing.

Any organization fighting for better patient care and better treatment of RNs will need research to underpin its arguments. "If you don't have the data, you will have trouble supporting your arguments," says Charlene Harrington. "To win, you need a combination of sound statistical research and anecdote." To be effective, Harrington says, there must be more contact between nursing researchers and patient, consumer, and nursing groups working for improvements in clinical practice and health care policy.

In their twenty-first century fight for safe-staffing ratios, the Massachusetts Nurses Association and other nurses unions are using studies that document a connection between higher levels of RN staff and lower levels of pneumonias, urinary tract infections, blood clots, falls, bedsores, and deaths to make their case. So are professional organizations, such as the American Nurses Association (ANA), to promote alternatives to legislated staffing ratios. The ANA has been using the growing body of nursing workforce and outcomes research to lobby for national legislation that would require hospitals to post the number of RN's providing direct patient care on each shift and require hospitals to develop staffing systems that would end the widespread practice of stretching nursing staff through high patient loads, mandatory overtime, and the floating of unprepared nurses to specialty units.

The Canadian Federation of Nursing Unions (CFNU) worked with other groups to influence regional health authorities and hospital administrators that had been replacing RNs with licensed practical nurses and unlicensed assistive personnel. "We wanted to convince them that RNs were the best buy for the money because we have a diversity of skills and knowledge allowing us to provide a better range of services," Debra McPherson, acting president of the CFNU, told us. "But of course, they weren't going to take our word for it. They felt that we were guarding our turf and our jobs."

Politicians and administrators, the CFNU leadership knew, would be swayed only if research documented the cost- and care-effectiveness of registered nurses. The union approached Judith Shamian, then vice president of nursing at Mount Sinai Hospital in Toronto and a researcher involved in an international project on nursing workforce and outcomes, spearheaded by University of Pennsylvania researchers Linda Aiken and Julie Sochalski.

"We asked Judith Shamian and her colleague Donna Thomson to put together a review of all the literature on the cost-effectiveness of nurses," said McPherson. "We knew they had to be objective and report everything they found, even if it didn't support our arguments. We told them up front that we accepted that. We felt it would be useful to know what didn't support our argument because it would point to the gaps in research that we could address in future projects." Shamian and Thomson produced a thirty-six-page study and accompanying slide presentation entitled, "The Effectiveness and Efficiency of Nursing Care—Cost and Quality."

"Nursing unions in this country are very effective because they have done two things," Shamian, who became executive director of nursing policy for Canada's federal department of health, told us. "While they represent the interests of nurses they are also strong advocates for a publicly funded health care system and equity for all Canadians. Secondly, there is agreement that nursing has to play a significant role in any discussion about the future of the health care system. This basic understanding has allowed us to look at where different groups agree and disagree and figure out how we can collaborate." By using research findings, professional associations and unions can present arguments that are based on evidence rather than emotional appeal, Shamian said.

Chapter 13

Conclusion

As we conclude this book, we feel that we have come full circle. We began thinking and writing about nurses and public communication during the nursing shortage of the late 1980s. We're concluding this revised edition as societies around the globe face an even more serious and potentially more intractable shortage of nurses. The common thread that connects these shortages is the lack of public understanding about what nurses actually do and the contributions they make to health care systems.

We've presented strategies and techniques that will help nurses explain their work. Nurses throughout the world are encountering challenges to their professional practice and integrity and recognize that they must take action to address them. This inevitably involves public communication.

In Switzerland, for example, the Swiss Nurses Association launched a major visibility campaign in 2005. Pierre-André Wagner, a nurse and a lawyer who directs the Association's legal department, eloquently described why a call to action is needed now in the following declaration.

> The Swiss Nurses' Association proclaimed 2005 "The Year of the Visibility of Nursing Care." What is the aim of this campaign? In Switzerland, as well as in most other countries, nursing care is under siege. Unfortunately, many nurses are not aware of how alarming our situation is.
>
> Why is a profession that is supposedly so respected, according to the opinion polls, in such jeopardy? In Switzerland, we see the intensity of the threat to nursing when prominent politicians suggest that health care costs can be safely cut by replacing every other nurse with a cheaper nurse substitute.
>
> This crisis is due to a number of factors. For a long time, we nurses were left alone to do our work as we deemed fit. We seemed to benefit from a broad consensus about its usefulness and worth. Even though the pay wasn't enough, health care systems seemed to recognize the need to pay for

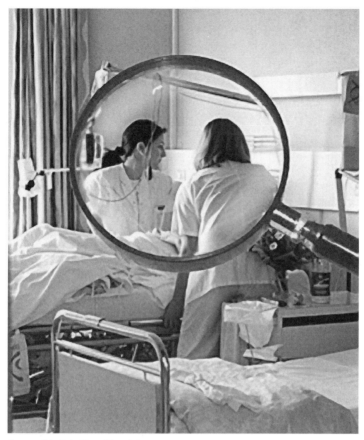

Courtesy of the Swiss Nurses' Association.

nursing care. Today's political addiction to market values has dramatically changed this: budget cut after budget cut is meant to artificially starve the state and make it less able to provide and finance a health care system accessible to all.

What does this mean? All of a sudden, we nurses are confronted with an alien rhetoric—cold, dry, hard, utilitarian dollar-speak that we, as nurses, have been proud not to be used to. However, today, people for whom money is all that matters, demand that we justify our utility, our market value, our very existence.

I can tell you that I have long hated this market discourse and I certainly don't like it much now. However, I believe that there might be a beneficial side to it. The more I think about the (in)visibility of nursing care, the more I have come to believe that market rhetoric and action presents us with a challenge worth accepting, and one that we, as nurses, are up to meeting. In order to accept this challenge, however, we must recognize that behind it lies another challenge, one that scares me much more.

We will only get what we ask for if we ourselves strongly believe that we deserve it. That is where I am assailed by serious doubts. Do we ourselves really believe in our competence, in our knowledge, strength, power and potential? Our worst enemy in the battles ahead is our timidity, our (false) humility.

I believe that we need not be afraid of the "money-discourse." This discourse offers an opportunity to our profession—if we are brave enough to seize it. You want to talk dollars and cents? Okay. Do you know how much it costs, on average, to heal a bedsore? Or treat a blood clot?

If you don't, how can you respond when the Health Minister of the State of Zurich tells us she wants to save money by having nurses turn their patients less often in order to reduce nurse staffing. Although this suggestion seems laughable, we need to take such proposals seriously. They show that even the upper echelons of the political establishment are unaware of:

- What a registered nurse basically does,
- What her or his work accomplishes,
- And why, for goodness sake, it takes a registered nurse to do it.

Where do people like the health minister get these ideas? They may have them because, in spite of the considerable evolution of our profession since the era of Florence Nightingale, the way we perceive ourselves, and thus the way we speak of our work, has remained quite "Victorian." To get the resources she needed to care for soldiers in the Crimea, Florence Nightingale used a discourse that emphasized the moral superiority of her female nurses and the salutary role that these women of virtue could play in the hospital. Unfortunately, this discourse has, over time, become a liability that is threatening to break the back of our profession by making nursing practice appear insignificant.

If we are to address the threats we face, we must consider two critical problems:

1. Out of pride or (false) humility, we are reluctant to talk about our work to "strangers."
2. And when we do, the terms we use just do not capture its complexity. Instead we fall into a pretentious, pseudo-scientific jargon that constitutes the most obvious symptom of a professional inferiority complex.

In any case, our (total or relative) difficulty articulating what we do shows that we are undergoing a grave identity crisis. Are we ourselves persuaded of our work's worth? Are we ourselves even aware of it? Are we, at the least, able to describe the essence of our practice?

At the 2004 congress of the United Kingdom's Royal College of Nursing, the Exeter branch dared to ask whether nurses had become "too posh to wash?" This question was, of course, meant as a provocation. I really believe that the time has come to ask similar questions here in Switzerland. I do know nurses who feel they are "too posh" to give direct, hands-on care to patients. On the other hand, many nurses show utter contempt for the medical, technical side of nursing. These antagonisms do not make any sense to me. The truth is that as the first health care assistants are knocking at the door, nursing care, as a whole needs to be rehabilitated. It has become a matter of life and death for our profession to show those who pay us—politicians, health insurers, citizens and taxpayers—that in order to fulfil the mandate society has bestowed upon us, much more is needed than to be born female, or to be sweet, caring and diligent.

This will be hard work indeed. It means fighting against deeply rooted stereotypes. It requires explaining that bathing a patient means much more than helping him have a bath; that talking to a patient means much more than chatting with her; that when we have a coffee or do some errands with her, we aren't trying to cheat the taxpayer, but rather are helping the patient overcome a depression by teaching her how to connect to the outside world. It is necessary to explain that often it is the quality of our observation, the correctness of our interpretation, and the swiftness of our reaction that will prevent a complication, allow the patient to remain at home, or save his life.

Visibility is not an option. It is an obligation. If we fail to make our work visible, we are betraying our mission, our patients present and future, and society itself. Society entrusts its most vulnerable members to us—the sick, the wounded, the newborn, the dying. Society therefore is duty bound to provide us with whatever we need to accomplish this mission. But in order to do so, society needs to know what we do and what we need. It is our responsibility to tell our story in a way that illuminates what nurses really do, why it is so important, and why it is worth funding.[1]

Although this could be a call to action for nurses worldwide, it raises a critical issue about the divisions within nursing. If nurses act to promote nursing what kind of nursing do they promote? Today we see instances of competing agendas threatening to divide the profession and undermine the message.

Many RNs want to make visible the challenges and complexity of caring for the sick—the work that most nurses have done and always will do. They want to build a basic understanding and respect for hands-on nursing. Appreciation for nurses who do other work such as research, teaching, primary care, and management could and should be incorporated into this fundamental concept. This is different from nursing "speaking with one voice." It means mobilizing a multitude of nursing voices and mass communication to challenge conventional (mis)understandings of caregiving work to significantly improve the conditions of that work so that the best and the brightest do not feel compelled to flee the bedside, or nursing.

Others favor a different approach. They want to downplay the traditional work of nurses as hands-on caregivers in order to highlight the work of those who appear to be more detached from the care of the body. Some nursing leaders appeal to potential nursing students by insisting that nurses today are more technologically skilled than ever before. Thus, they suggest, erroneously, that nurses in the past weren't as technologically and scientifically advanced as the systems in which they worked. They are tempted to emphasize only the avenues that lead nurses away from the care of the sick. We are told that the nursing degree could be a launching pad to a career as a nurse attorney, or nurse entrepreneur, or CEO of a hospital, or health policy maker. The message of this sales pitch is clear: Borrow the social legitimacy of another profession or occupation to hide the lack of status of nursing. In this approach, nursing is a career path not a career.

We don't think you can trick people into becoming nurses or into valuing nurses. If our society does not understand what the core member of the profession does in her or his work in hospitals, clinics, nursing homes, schools, homes, and hospices, it cannot really value nursing however "elevated" or "advanced." If we don't want to pay for the care of the sick and vulnerable, the aging and the dying, anyone with the word *nurse* in his or her professional title will ultimately be diminished by their connection to the sick, dependent, and vulnerable.

Selling the nurse as anything but a nurse also sells the public short. In more than a decade and a half of writing about nursing, we have been struck by how receptive people are to stories about the work of nurses when nurses describe how their work saves lives, prevents suffering, and saves money. However, when nurses refer to themselves as "just a nurse," they diminish both themselves and their work. This phrase, uttered unthinkingly, grates on some nurses to the extent that they want to distance themselves from the very word *nurse*.

Suzanne Gordon wondered what would happen if this phrase were "spun" so that it illuminated the richness and importance of nursing. She conceived of the script on the following page for a nurse recruitment campaign.[2] Many nurses regard "Just a Nurse" as a poem and have posted it in their workplaces. Some nurses have added stanzas of their own. You are invited to do the same.

Just a Nurse

by Suzanne Gordon

I'm *just a nurse*. I just make the difference between life and death.

I'm *just a nurse*. I just have the educated eyes that prevent medical errors, injuries, and other catastrophes.

I'm *just a nurse*. I just make the difference between healing and coping, and despair.

I'm *just a nurse*. I just make the difference between pain and comfort.

I'm *just a nurse*. I'm just a nurse researcher who helps nurses and doctors give better, safer, and more effective care.

I'm *just a nurse*. I'm just a professor of nursing who educates future generations of nurses.

I'm *just a nurse*. I just work in a major teaching hospital managing and monitoring patients who are involved in cutting-edge experimental research.

I'm *just a nurse*. I just educate patients and families about how to maintain their health.

I'm *just a nurse*. I'm just a geriatric nurse practitioner who makes a difference between an elderly person staying in his own home or going to a nursing home.

I'm *just a nurse*. I just make the difference between dying in agony and dying in comfort and with dignity.

I'm *just a nurse*. I'm just the real bottom-line in health care.

Wouldn't you like to be *just a nurse,* too?

References

REFERENCES TO INTRODUCTION

1. Bernice Buresh, Suzanne Gordon, and Nica Bell, "Who Counts in News Coverage of Health Care?" *Nursing Outlook,* 1991. 39(5): 204–208.
2. Bernice Buresh, and Suzanne Gordon, eds., *A Journalist's Guide to Nursing Sources.* 1994, Women, Press & Politics Project.
3. Suzanne Gordon and Sioban Nelson, "An End to Angels." *American Journal of Nursing,* 2005. 105(5): 62–69.
4. *The Woodhull Study on Nursing and the Media: Health Care's Invisible Partner.* 1998, Sigma Theta Tau International Honor Society of Nursing.
5. Suzanne Gordon, *Nursing against the Odds.* 2005, Ithaca: Cornell University Press. 204–205.

REFERENCES TO CHAPTER ONE

1. Bernice Buresh, Suzanne Gordon, and Nica Bell, "Who Counts in News Coverage of Health Care?" *Nursing Outlook,* 1991. 39(5): 204–208.
2. *The Woodhull Study on Nursing and the Media: Health Care's Invisible Partner.* 1998, Sigma Theta Tau International Honor Society of Nursing.
3. Jennifer Steinhauer, "Hospitals Battle Insurers over Refusal to Pay for Portions of Patient Stays." *New York Times,* October 19, 1999: p. A19.
4. Center for Nursing Advocacy. http://www.nursingadvocacy.org/create/create.html. Accessed May 20, 2005.
5. David W. Moore, "Nurses Top List in Honesty and Ethics Poll." 2004, The Gallup Organization.
6. Nancy Dickenson-Hazard, "New Harris Poll Is Sobering Wake-Up Call for Profession." *Excellence in Clinical Practice,* 2000. 1(4): 2.
7. Suzanne Gordon, "Necessary Nursing Care." *Nursing Inquiry,* 2000. 7(4): 218.
8. Linda H. Aiken, S. P. Clarke, D. M. Sloane, Julie. Sochalski, et al., "Hospital Nurse Staffing and Patient Mortality, Nurse Burnout, and Job Dissatisfaction." *Journal of the American Medical Association,* 2002. 288(16): 1987–1993.

9. Jack Needleman, Peter I. Buerhaus, S. Mattke, M. Stewart, et al., "Nurse-staffing Levels and the Quality of Care in Hospitals." *New England Journal of Medicine,* 2002. 346(22): 1715–1722.

10. *Health Care at the Crossroads: Strategies for Addressing the Evolving Nursing Crisis.* 2002, Joint Commission on the Accreditation of Health Care Organizations.

11. Mary A. Blegan, Colleen J. Goode, and Laura Reed, "Nurse Staffing and Patient Outcomes." *Nursing Research,* 1998. 47(1): 43–50.

12. National Advertising Council, *If Caring Were Enough.* 1990, National Commission on Nursing Implementation Project (NCNIP).

13. *A Nationwide Survey of Attitudes toward Health Care and Nurses.* 1990, Peter D. Hart Research Associates, Inc.

REFERENCES TO CHAPTER TWO

1. Linda H. Aiken, S. P. Clarke, D. M. Sloane, Julie. Sochalski, et al., "Hospital Nurse Staffing and Patient Mortality, Nurse Burnout, and Job Dissatisfaction." *Journal of the American Medical Association,* 2002. 288(16): 1987–1993.

2. Amartya Sen, *Development As Freedom.* 2000, New York: Anchor Books.

3. Florence Nightingale, *Notes on Nursing: What It Is and Is Not.* 1969, New York: Dover.

4. Patricia Benner, *From Novice to Expert.* 1984, Reading, MA: Addison-Wesley.

5. Isabel Marcus, "Dark Numbers: Domestic Violence, Law, and Public Policy in Russia, Poland, Romania, and Hungary," unpublished manuscript.

6. Suzanne Gordon and Sioban Nelson, "An End to Angels." *American Journal of Nursing,* 2005. 105(5): 62–69.

7. Sioban Nelson, *Say Little, Do Much.* 2001, Philadelphia: University of Pennsylvania Press. 237.

8. Susan M. Reverby, *Ordered to Care: The Dilemma of American Nursing, 1850–1945,* 1987. Cambridge: Cambridge University Press.

9. Sara Ruddick, *Maternal Thinking: Toward a Politics of Peace.* 1989, Boston: Beacon Press.

10. Laurel Thatcher Ulrich, *A Midwife's Tale: The Life of Martha Ballard, Based on Her Diary, 1785–1812.* 1990, New York: Vintage.

11. Patricia Benner, Christine A. Tanner, and Catherine A. Chesla, *Expertise in Nursing Practice.* 1996, New York: Springer.

12. *Nurses: Always There for You.* 2000, International Council of Nurses: Geneva, Switzerland.

13. For an example, see Andrea Rock, "How Hospitals Are Gambling with Your Life." *Reader's Digest,* September, 2001: 151–164.

14. Mary Cadwalader Jones, Claire M. Fagin, and Donna Diers, "Becoming a Nurse: Two Views, 1900 and 2000." *New York Times,* 2000.

15. George Anders, *Health against Wealth: HMOs and the Breakdown of Medical Trust.* 1996, Boston: Houghton Mifflin.

16. Sandra P. Thomas, *Transforming Nurses' Stress and Anger: Steps toward Healing.* 2nd ed. 2004, New York: Springer. 318.

17. Jeannie Chaisson, "Asking the Right Questions." *Technology Review,* October 1992: 47.

REFERENCES TO CHAPTER THREE

1. Suzanne Gordon and Elizabeth M. Grady, "What's in a Name?" *American Journal of Nursing,* August 1995. 31–33.
2. Crystal Lindaman, "Talking to Physicians about Pain Control." *American Journal of Nursing,* 1995 (January): 2–3.
3. Arthur Kleinman, *The Illness Narratives: Suffering, Healing, and the Human Condition.* 1988, New York: BasicBooks.
4. Linda H. Aiken, S. P. Clarke, D. M. Sloane, Julie Sochalski, et al., "Hospital Nurse Staffing and Patient Mortality, Nurse Burnout, and Job Dissatisfaction." *Journal of the American Medical Association,* 2002. 288(16): 1987–1993.
5. J. Needleman and P. Buerhaus, "Nurse Staffing and Patient Safety: Current Knowledge and Implications for Action." *International Journal for Quality Health Care,* 2003. 15(4): 275–277.
6. Erving Goffman, *Asylums: Essays on the Social Situation of Mental Patients and Other Inmates.* 1961, New York: Doubleday Anchor Books.
7. National Institute for Occupational Safety and Health (NIOSH), *Violence: Occupational Hazards in Hospitals.* 2002, Department of Health and Human Services, Center for Disease Control and Prevention: Cincinnati. Publication 2002-101. http:www.cdc.gov/niosh/2002-101.html. Accessed September 8, 2005.
8. American Nurses Association Center for Ethics and Human Rights, "Code of Ethics for Nurses—With Interpretive Statements." 2001, Provision 4.2. http://www.nursingworld.org/ethics/code/protected_nwcoe303.htm#4.2. Accessed September 8, 2005.
9. John Seabrook, "The White Dress." *The New Yorker,* March 18, 2002: 122–127.
10. *American Heritage Dictionary of the English Language, fourth edition.* 2000, Boston: Houghton Mifflin Company.
11. Erving Goffman, *The Presentation of Self in Everyday Life.* 1959, Garden City, N.Y.: Doubleday Anchor Books.
12. Celia Davies, *Gender and the Professional Predicament in Nursing.* 1995, Buckingham: Open University Press.

REFERENCES TO CHAPTER FOUR

1. Christopher Reeve, *Nothing Is Impossible.* 2002, New York: Random House.
2. Institute of Medicine, *Keeping Patients Safe: Transforming the Work Environment of Nurses,* ed. Ann Page. 2003, Washington, DC: National Academy Press.
3. *AACN Standards for Establishing and Sustaining Healthy Work Environments: A Journey to Excellence.* 2005, Aliso Viejo, CA: American Association of Critical-Care Nurses.
4. Margarete Sandelowski, *Devices and Desires: Gender, Technology, and American Nursing.* 2000, Chapel Hill: University of North Carolina Press.
5. "ICN Code for Nurses: Ethical Concepts Applied to Nursing." 1973, Geneva: International Council of Nurses.

REFERENCES TO CHAPTER FIVE

1. Institute of Medicine, *To Err Is Human: Building a Safer Health System,* ed. Linda T. Kohn, Janet M. Corrigan, and Molla S. Donaldson. 1999, Washington, DC: National Academy Press.

2. National Diabetes Statistics, 2005, National Diabetes Information Clearinghouse (NDIC), a service of the National Institute of Diabetes and Digestive and Kidney Diseases, http://www.diabetes.niddk.nih.gov/dm/pubs/statistics/#13. Accessed May 28, 2005.

3. "All about Diabetes," American Diabetes Association. http://www.diabetes.org/about -diabetes.jsp (accessed May 28, 2005).

4. Ellen D. Baer, Claire M. Fagin, and Suzanne Gordon, *The Abandonment of the Patient: The Impact of Profit-Driven Care on the Public.* 1996, New York: Springer.

5. Institute of Medicine, *Keeping Patients Safe: Transforming the Work Environment of Nurses,* ed. Ann Page. 2004, Washington, DC: National Academy Press.

6. Institute of Medicine, *Nursing Staff in Hospitals and Nursing Homes: Is It Adequate?* ed. Gooloo S. Wunderlich, Frank Sloan, and Carolyne K. Davis. 1996, Washington, DC: National Academy Press. 560.

7. Courtney H. Lyder et al., "Quality of Care for Hospitalized Medicare Patients at Risk for Pressure Ulcers." *Archives of Internal Medicine,* 2001(161): 1549–1554.

8. Susan Skewes, "Skin Care Rituals That Do More Harm Than Good." *American Journal of Nursing,* 1996. 96(10): 33–35.

9. John A. Heit, W. M. O'Fallon, T. M. Petterson, C. M. Lohse et al., "Relative Impact of Risk Factors for Deep Vein Thrombosis and Pulmonary Embolism: A Population-Based Study." *Archives of Internal Medicine,* 2002. 162(11): 1245–1248.

10. Sanjay Saint, R. H. Savel, and M. A. Matthay, "Enhancing the Safety of Critically Ill Patients by Reducing Urinary and Central Venous Catheter-Related Infections." *American Journal of Respiratory Critical Care Medicine,* 2002. 165(11): 1475–1479.

11. Sanjay Saint, "Prevention of Nosocomial Urinary Tract Infections," in *Making Health Care Safer: A Critical Analysis of Patient Safety Practices,* Evidence Report/Technology Assessment, No. 43, Agency for Healthcare Research and Quality, http://www.ahrq.gov/clinic/ptsafety/chap15a.htm (accessed May 28, 2005).

12. Anne E. Rogers, W. T. Hwang, L. D. Scott, Linda H. Aiken, et al., "The Working Hours of Hospital Staff Nurses and Patient Safety." *Health Affairs,* 2004. 23(4): 202–212.

13. Suzanne Gordon and Bernice Buresh, "Finding the 'I' in the 'We.'" *American Journal of Nursing,* 1996. 96(1): 21–22.

14. Suzanne Gordon, *Life Support: Three Nurses on the Front Lines.* 1997, Boston: Little, Brown.

15. Milt Freudenheim, "As Nurses Take On Primary Care, Physicians Are Sounding Alarms." *New York Times,* 1997. pp. A1, D4.

16. Barry Morley, "The World Is Loud but Nurses Remain Silent." *Australian Nursing Journal,* July 2005: Australian Nursing Federation.

REFERENCES TO CHAPTER SIX

1. National Health Council, *21st Century Housecall: The Link between Medicine and the Media— Key Survey Findings.* 1998. http://www.nationalhealthcouncil.org.

2. Frank Luther Mott, *American Journalism: A History 1690–1960.* 3rd ed. 1962, New York: Macmillan.

3. John Hohenberg, *Free Press, Free People.* 1973, New York: The Free Press.

4. Tony Case, "No Dearth of Health Care Coverage." *Editor & Publisher,* October 1, 1994: 14–15, 37.

5. Kaiser Family Foundation, "E-Health and the Elderly: How Seniors Use the Internet for Health Information." January 2005, http://www.kff.org/entmedia/7223.cfm (accessed May 10, 2005).

6. John Hohenberg, *The Professional Journalist: A Guide to the Practices and Principles of the News Media.* 1978, New York: Holt, Rinehart & Winston.

7. No author, "No Flier Miles for Airborne Germs." *New York Times,* March 22, 2005, D7.

8. Nicholas Bakalar, "Finding Medical Destiny on the Family Tree." *New York Times,* March 22, 2005, D7.

9. Robin Marantz Henig, "At War with Their Bodies, They Seek to Sever Limbs." *New York Times,* March 22, 2005, D6.

10. Joel Dresang, "Life Support: The Need for Nurses." *Milwaukee Journal-Sentinel,* February 23–24, 2003.

11. Paul Hemp, "Witness to Courage." *Boston Globe Magazine,* February 5, 1995.

12. Darcy Frey, "On the Border of Life." *New York Times Magazine,* July 9, 1995.

13. "Special Health Issue: The New Healers." *US News & World Report,* January 31–February 7, 2005.

14. Melvin Mencher, *News Reporting and Writing.* 2nd ed. 1981, Dubuque, IA: Wm. C. Brown Company.

15. Lawrence K. Grossman, "Can TV News be Saved?" *The Brook,* Publication of the State University of New York at Stony Brook, 2005. 5(2): 12–13.

16. Arthur Caplan, "How Old Is Too Old to Have a Baby?" MSNBC Commentary, January 24, 2005. http://www.msnbc.msn.com/id/6862098/. Accessed April 5, 2005.

REFERENCES TO CHAPTER SEVEN

1. Todd Hunt and James E. Grunig, *Public Relations Techniques.* 1994, Fort Worth: Harcourt Brace. 47.

2. Hayward Zwerling, "When It's My Time, Let Me Go." *Boston Globe.* March 27, 2005, p. K10.

3. Ross Koppel, Joshua P. Metlay, Abigail Cohen, Brian Abaluck, et al., "Role of Computerized Physician Order Entry Systems in Facilitating Medication Errors." *Journal of the American Medical Association,* 2005. 293(10): 1197–1203.

4. Linda Morton, "Researcher Finds Complaints against Press Releases Are Justified." *Editor & Publisher,* May 8, 1993. pp. 52, 42.

5. Bernice Buresh, "Healthcare Forms New Media Partnership—Nursing Must Participate." *Revolution,* 1998. 8(1): 68–75.

6. *The Woodhull Study on Nursing and the Media: Health Care's Invisible Partner.* 1998, Sigma Theta Tau International Honor Society of Nursing, key findings available at http://www.nursingsociety.org/media/woodhullextract.html (accessed August 1, 2005).

7. Bernice Buresh, "The Missing Voices in Coverage of Health." *Nieman Reports,* Fall 1999. pp. 52–55.

8. Jeannie Chaisson, "Nursing Stories Journalists Fail to Cover." *Nieman Reports,* Fall 1999. pp. 55–56.

9. Bernice Buresh and Suzanne Gordon, "Fighting Scapegoat Journalism." *American Journal of Nursing,* 1995. 95(7): 19–21.

REFERENCES TO CHAPTER EIGHT

1. Suzanne Gordon, *Nursing against the Odds: How Health Care Cost Cutting, Media Stereotypes, and Medical Hubris Undermine Nurses and Patient Care.* 2005, Ithaca: Cornell University Press.

2. "Patient Perspectives." *The Campaign for Nursing's Future* (VHS), 2002, Johnson & Johnson.

3. Suzanne Gordon and Sioban Nelson, "An End to Angels," 2005. *American Journal of Nursing,* 2005. 105(5): 62–69.

REFERENCES TO CHAPTER NINE

1. Lois Monteiro, "Nightingale and Her Correspondence: Portrait of the Era," in *Florence Nightingale and Her Era: A Collection of New Scholarship*, ed. Vern L. Bullough, Bonnie Bullough, and Marietta P. Stanton. 1990, New York: Garland.

2. Clea Benson and Lisa Rapaport, "Judge Tells Hospitals: Raise Nurse Staff Ratio." *Sacramento Bee*, March 5, 2005.

3. Jackson Lewis. "Schwarzenegger Attempts to Halt Scheduled Decrease in Nurse-Patient Ratios." Legal Update, December 9, 2004, http://www.jacksonlewis.com/legalupdates/article.cfm?aid=680 (accessed August 1, 2005).

4. Dan Glaister, "Schwarzenegger Meets His Match." *The Guardian*, April 15, 2005.

5. Robert Salladay, "Nurse Is Asked How She Got into Screening." *Los Angeles Times*, February 23, 2005.

6. Australian Nursing Federation media release, "Nurses Launch TV Ad Campaign to Preserve Nurse Patient Ratios." April 13, 2004, http://www.anfvic.asn.au/ (accessed August 1, 2005).

7. Australian Nursing Federation media release, "Victorian Nurses Save World's First Ratios Again." May 4, 2004, http://www.anfvic.asn.au/ (accessed August 1, 2005).

8. Barry Adams, "Protecting Our Patients." *Newsweek*, November 16, 1998: 17.

9. Massachusetts Nurses Association news release, "Chronology of Communications between Barry Adams RN and the Massachusetts Board of Registration in Nursing (BORN)." November 30, 1999.

10. "State Faults Youville in Overdose Death of Patient: News of Probe Comes as Ex-Nurse Who Alleged 'Serious Patient Safety Issues' Files Wrongful Termination Suit against Hospital." *Boston Globe*, March 19, 1997.

11. Canadian Nurses Association, "A Submission to the House of Commons Standing Committee on Finance and the Minister of Finance." September 1998. p. 2.

12. Registered Nurses Association of Ontario, "Media Advisory: Government on Right Track—But Not Fast Track—to Boost Full-time Work for Ontario RNs: RNAO Survey."

June 14, 2005, http://www.rnao.org/media_room/releases/MR_050614_70_Percent_Report_released.asp (accessed September 26, 2005).

13. Doris Grinspun, "Untie Nurses' Hands: SARS Is a Full-Time Fight." *Globe and Mail*, May 30, 2003. p. A17.

14. Ontario Ministry of Health and Long-Term Care, "Diseases: Severe Acute Respiratory Syndrome (SARS)." Fact sheet, April 2004, http://www.health.gov.on.ca/english/pub lic/pub/disease/sars.html (accessed September 24, 2005).

15. Susan M. Poutanen, Donald E. Low, and Bonnie Henry et al. "Identification of Severe Acute Respiratory Syndrome in Canada." *New England Journal of Medicine*, 2003. 348(20): 1995–2005.

16. Elaine Carey, "SARS One Year Later: Still a Mystery." *Toronto Star*, March 5, 2004. p. A1.

17. Kevin Donovan and Tanya Talaga, "SARS: The Chain of Errors." *Toronto Star*, September 20, 2003. p. A1.

18. Elena Cherney and Mark Heinzl, "Toronto Nurses Claim Warnings Weren't Heeded in SARS Sequel." *Wall Street Journal*, May 30, 2003. p. B4.

19. Ontario Nurses Association, "Updated Guidance to Members, Local Coordinators, Bargaining Unit Presidents and Joint Health and Safety Committee," June 17, 2003.

20. "SARS War's Unsung Heroes." *National Nursing Week*, a supplement to the *Globe and Mail*, May 12, 2003. p. N1.

21. Tom Blackwell, "'Do Not Let Her Death Be Wasted on Fear.'" *National Post* (Canada), July 5 2003. p. A3.

22. Caroline Mallan and Theresa Boyle, "Patients' Rights at Stake in Public Inquiry: Eves." *Toronto Star*, June 10, 2003. p. A7.

23. Registered Nurses Association of Ontario media release, "Registered Nurses Association of Ontario to Premier Ernie Eves: Conduct Full Public Inquiry into SARS Outbreak." June 9, 2003, http://www.rnao.org/media_room/media_releases_2003.asp (accessed March 20, 2005).

24. The SARS Commission Mandate, http://www.sarscommission.ca/ (accessed September 20, 2005).

25. Registered Nurses Association of Ontario media release, "RNAO Releases Final Report on SARS Outbreak as RNs Mark the One-Year Anniversary of the Loss of Two Colleagues in the Line of Duty." June 29, 2004, http://www.rnao.org/media_room/releases/MA_040629_SARS_Report.asp (accessed September 24, 2005).

26. Colin Perkel, "Family of Nurse Killed by SARS Can Sue Ontario Government for Negligence." *The Canadian Press*, August 23, 2005.

27. Reynolds Holding and William Carlsen, "Epidemic Ravages Caregivers: Thousands Die from Diseases Contracted through Needle Sticks." *San Francisco Chronicle*, April 13–15, 1998.

28. J. Jagger, E. H. Hunt, J. Brand-Elnaggar, and R. D. Pearson, "Rates of Needle-stick Injury Caused by Various Devices in a University Hospital." *New England Journal of Medicine*, 1988. 319(5): 284–288.

29. J. M. Lee, M. F. Botteman, N. Xanthakos, and L. Nicklasson, "Needlestick injuries in the United States. Epidemiologic, economic, and quality of life issues." *American Association of Occupational Health Nurses Journal*, 2005. 53(3): 117–133.

30. Center for Nursing Advocacy, "Inject Me: Skechers Tries on the Stereotypes with Christina Aguilera as 'Naughty and Nice.'" August 2004, http://www.nursingadvo cacy.org/news/2004aug/skechers.html (accessed March 15, 2005).

31. Center for Nursing Advocacy, "Procter & Gamble Pulls Clairol Shampoo Commercial

and Apologizes to Nurses." June 11, 2003, http://www.nursingadvocacy.org/news/2003jun11_clairol.html (accessed March 15, 2005).

32. Kaiser Family Foundation, "The Impact of TV's Health Content: A Case Study of *ER* Viewers." June 2002, survey snapshot available at http://www.kff.org/entmedia/upload/Survey-Snapshot-ER.pdf (accessed August 1, 2005).

REFERENCES TO CHAPTER TEN

1. Mark Jurkowitz, "A Drawbridge of Letters." *Boston Globe,* May 29, 1995, p. 13.
2. Mark Jurkowitz, "Getting Through to the Globe." *Boston Globe*, October 30, 1995.
3. Lee Rainie and John Horrigan, "A Decade of Adoption: How the Internet Has Woven Itself into American Life." January 25, 2005, Pew Internet & American Life Project, http://www.pewinternet.org/PPF/r/148/report_display.asp (accessed May 20, 2005).
4. Robert B. Semple Jr., "Op-Ed at 20." *New York Times*, September 30, 1990. p. 4A.
5. Jeannie Chaisson, "Asking the Right Questions." *Technology Review*, October 1992. p. 47.
6. Suzanne Gordon, "The Importance of Being Nurses." *Technology Review*, October 1992.

REFERENCES TO CHAPTER ELEVEN

1. Courtney H. Lyder et al., "Quality of Care for Hospitalized Medicare Patients at Risk for Pressure Ulcers." *Archives of Internal Medicine*, 2001(161): 1549–1554.
2. Joseph V. Agostini, Dorothy I. Baker, and Sidney T. Bogardus, "Prevention of Pressure Ulcers in Older Patients," in *Making Health Care Safer: A Critical Analysis of Patient Safety Practices*, Evidence Report/Technology Assessment, No. 43, Agency for Health Care Research and Quality, http://www.ahrq.gov/clinic/ptsafety/chap27.htm (accessed May 28, 2005).

REFERENCES TO CHAPTER TWELVE

1. Linda H. Aiken, Sean P. Clarke, Douglas M. Sloane, et al., "Hospital Nurse Staffing and Patient Mortality, Nurse Burnout, and Job Dissatisfaction." *Journal of the American Medical Association*, 2002. 288(16): 1987–1993.
2. "Study Links Workloads of Nurses to Patient Risk." *Boston Globe*, October 23, 2002.
3. "Dying for Lack of Nurses." *New York Times*, October 25, 2002. P. 34.
4. Rita Rubin and Harrison L. Rogers Jr., *Under the Microscope: The Relationship between Physicians and the News Media.* 1995. A publication of the Freedom Forum First Amendment Center.
5. Arthur L. Caplan, "University of Pennsylvania Health System Invitational Conference for Nurse Executives." June 11, 1999. Philadelphia.
6. EurekAlert! http://www.eurekalert.org (accessed September 26, 2005).
7. Robert Topp, Debra Boardley, Amy L. Morgan, Mariane Fahlman, et al., "Exercise and Functional Tasks among Adults Who Are Functionally Limited." *Western Journal of Nursing Research*, 2005. 27: 252–270.

8. Linda Rosa, Emily Rosa, Larry Sarner, and Stephen Barrett, "A Close Look at Therapeutic Touch." *Journal of the American Medical Association*, 1998. 279(13): 1005–1010.
9. Gina Kolata, "A Child's Paper Poses a Medical Challenge." *New York Times*, April 1, 1998. P. A1.
10. Theresa A. Meyers, Dezra J. Eichhorn, Cathie E. Guzzetta, et. al., "Family Presence during Invasive Procedures and Resuscitation: The Experience of Family Members, Nurses, and Physicians." *American Journal of Nursing*, 2000. 100(2): 32–43.
11. Jane E. Brody, "Facing Up to the Inevitable, in Search of a Good Death." *New York Times*, December 30, 2003. Pp. D5–D6.

REFERENCES TO CONCLUSION

1. Pierre-André Wagner, Swiss Nurses' Association. Delivered at the annual general assembly of the Neuchâtel/Jura branch of the Swiss Nurses' Association, March 15, 2005. (Translated from French by the author.)
2. Suzanne Gordon, " 'Just A Nurse.' " First published in *Nursing Management*, United Kingdom, September 2001. 8(5): 6.

Index

Adams, Barry, 186, 188–91

advocacy campaigns: and Center for Nursing Advocacy, 15, 132, 200–203; and needlestick injury prevention, 196–200; and Nightingale, 179–80; and nursing research, 183, 270–71; and nursing shortages, 1; and SARS in Ontario, 191–96; and staffing legislation, 179, 181–86; and whistleblower legislation, 186–91

agency of nurses, 29–33, 37, 40, 54, 63, 66–68, 82. *See also* voice of agency

Aiken, Linda, 151, 249, 271

American Association of Critical-Care Nurses (AACN), 68–69, 131, 140

American Association of Nurse Anesthetists (AANA), 163, 164

American Journal of Nursing (AJN), 154, 260–62, 269

American Medical Association (AMA), 37, 140, 253, 254

American Nurses Association (ANA): and advocacy campaigns, 190, 191, 202; and image of nursing, 16, 226; and news releases, 120, 152; and nursing research, 261, 270; and public relations professionals, 166; and Schiavo story, 138–40

American Nurses Association (ANA) Code of Ethics, 55, 120, 139

Anders, George, 37

anecdotes: audiences for, 102–3; construction of, 82, 83, 95; and descriptions of nursing practice, 6, 23, 82, 90, 93, 95–102; facts and statistics in, 90–91, 92; hot topics for, 103–5; and jargon, 84, 88–90; makeovers of, 89, 95–102; and nursing research, 270; painting a picture, 83–88; painting whole picture, 93–95; painting yourself into picture, 91–93; and television appearances, 228–30, 240

anonymity, 32–33, 36–37, 51, 53–55

Associated Press (AP), 124, 252–53

Australia, 44, 160, 176, 179, 187–88, 206

Australian Nurses Federation (ANF), 187–88

Bégin, Monique, 191

Benner, Patricia, 30, 33

Bernays, Edward L., 165

Blakeney, Barbara, 138, 151

Blendon, Robert, 126

blog sites, 130, 204, 205, 211–14

body language, 23, 54, 61–63, 75, 236

books, 127–29

Boston Globe: and Adams, 190; columnists of, 123; editorial page of, 122; and health coverage on sample day, 113–16; and Nurses of American campaign, 155–56; and nurse-to-patient ratio, 249; and nursing shortage stories, 160; and op-ed pages, 223–25; and reader responses, 206; and Schiavo story, 114, 140; and sources, 131

Boston Women's Health Collective, 110

Boylston, Zabdiel, 109–10

British Broadcasting Corporation, 124

British Columbia Nurses Union (BCNU), 169, 171

Brody, Jane E., 117, 262

Browne, Gina Bohn, 258

Buresh, Bernice, 20, 35, 77, 157, 240, 241–42

Bush, George W., 115, 130, 138, 139, 184, 213–14

Bush, Jeb, 213–14
Business Record, 225, 226–27

California, 179, 181–86, 187, 196–200
California Nurse, 182–83
California Nurses Association, 153–54, 181–86, 200, 270
Campbell, Archie, 194–95
Campo, Rafael, 127
Canada, 44, 47, 67, 160, 191–96, 230, 271
Canadian Association of Schools of Nursing (CASN), 147, 152
Canadian Federation of Nursing Unions (CFNU), 271
Canadian Medical Association Journal, 128
Canadian Nurses Association, 160, 167, 191–92
Caplan, Arthur L., 134–35, 252
caring aspect of nursing practice: and agency of nurses, 67; and clinical judgment, 86–87; and medical and technical focus, 69–70, 167; and painting whole picture, 93; and professional image, 18, 19, 20; and professional self-representation, 48, 58; and public communication skills, 72, 73, 74; and public relations professionals, 176; and television appearances, 233–34, 239; and virtue script, 33, 34–35, 169; and visibility of nursing, 275–76
Carlsen, William, 196, 197, 199
Cassell, Eric, 127
Cellucci, Paul, 191
Center for Nursing Advocacy, 15, 132, 200–203
Chaisson, Jeannie, 40–41, 93, 157, 220
China, 192
Chu, Kwan Sui, 192
Clarke, Sean P., 264–66
Clifford, Joyce, 155, 175
Clinton, Bill, 117–18
Cohen, Jamie, 199
columnists, 113–14, 120–23, 153, 180, 215–16, 262
communication. *See* public communication; public communication skills
Connelly, Paddy, 84
Connors, Kathleen, 80

Dalton, Cindy, 228–31, 240
Davies, Celia, 63
Davis, Gray, 182, 183, 184

Day One, 162, 163, 164
Dayton, Ellen, 197, 199
DePaolis-Lutzo, Mary, 164
Dickinson-Hazard, Nancy, 156
Di Giacomo, Kelly, 186
Donnelly, Judith, 85–86
Dowd, Maureen, 114
Dracup, Kathleen A., 175, 258, 264–65
Dresang, Joel, 121
Drummond-Webb, Jonathan, 233
Dugan, Judy, 155
Duke, Paul, 218–20

editorial pages, 122, 183
Emergency Nurses Association, 156, 269
Eves, Ernie, 193, 194
expertise of nurses: and anecdotes, 82, 98; awareness of, 17; and clinical judgment, 26, 35–36, 42–44, 67, 82, 85–87, 94, 103; compelling narratives of, 220; and internalized knowledge, 87–88; and interviews, 125; and journalists, 1, 11, 131, 136, 140, 177; and letters to the editor, 122, 206, 208–9, 227; and nurse/physician relationship, 69–70; and nursing research, 6; and professional self-presentation, 43, 49, 58; and public communication skills, 71; and salaries, 13; and television appearances, 230–31, 232, 233, 235, 244. *See also* knowledge script

Fagin, Claire, 81, 155, 156, 227, 258
features. *See* human interest and features
Ferguson, Carole, 206, 208
Fernald, Phoebe, 71–72
Fishbein, Morris, 252–53
FitzPatrick, Lisa, 188
Foster, Scott, 166
Franklin, James, 110
Frey, Darcy, 122–23
Fukui University, 77
Funk, Marjorie, 222–25

Gilbertson, Michelle, 209
Goffman, Erving, 49, 63
Goodman, Ellen, 114, 232
Gordon, Suzanne, 26–27, 30–31, 32, 77, 170, 228–30, 276–77
Gotbaum, Rachel, 116
Grady, Elizabeth M., 47, 91
Great Britain, 44, 179–80, 209–11
Grinspun, Doris, 192

Grossman, Lawrence K., 126, 130
Grunig, James E., 137

Hale, Claire, 209–11
Harrington, Charlene, 251, 258, 270
Hart, Peter, 20
Hawaii Nurses Association, 166
Hayano, Masako, 77
Health Affairs, 128, 251
health care administration, 12–13, 17, 28, 97–99
health care business, 114–16, 123, 160, 182
health care information, 1–3, 11, 109–13, 118
health care institutions: cultural practices within, 55–58; inviting reporters to, 156; and naming practices, 45, 48–51, 55–58; and nurse-to-patient ratios, 13, 183, 184; and nursing practice, 103, 119; and nursing shortages, 160; and public communication skills, 78–81; and public relations professionals, 173–77; restructuring of, 3, 181, 191–93, 195; and safer needles, 197; and television appearances, 234; and violence, 52–53, 54
health care policy, 109, 112–15, 119, 122
health care resources: allocation of, 2, 12–14, 17, 110, 166, 272–75; and nursing stereotypes, 4, 27, 110, 169
health care workers: nurses confused with, 44, 56, 58; and nurses' professional self-presentation, 43; and personal safety, 52–54; as replacement for nurses, 13, 17, 70, 181, 182, 271, 272; respect for, 60, 99–100; and safer needles, 197, 198; and SARS, 192; whistleblower protection for, 188, 195
Hemp, Paul, 122
Herbert, Bob, 123
Herbert, Sidney, 179
Hersher, Judy Holzer, 186
Holding, Reynolds, 196, 197, 199
Hubbell, Steve, 128, 129
human interest and features, 114, 117–18, 121, 122, 153, 269–70
Hunt, Todd, 137
Hurt, William, 127
Hurwitz, Joan, 166, 191

"ICU" documentary, 233–34
Idelson, Charles, 186
Image: Journal of Nursing Scholarship, 222–23
Independent, 210–11

India, 114, 116
Institute of Medicine (IOM), 68, 90
International Council of Nurses (ICN), 36
International Council of Nurses (ICN) Code for Nurses, 75
Internet: and book reviews, 127; as health information source, 109–11, 130; and letters from public, 204–5; and media strategies, 7, 138, 140, 141; and medical journals, 253; monitoring of, 120, 129–30; and nursing research, 250
interviews: and advocacy campaigns, 195, 199; and bridging technique, 240, 242–48; etiquette of, 238–39; and journalists, 131, 165; and negative coverage, 163; preinterviews for radio and television appearances, 232; preparation for, 231; and public relations professionals, 173; and silence of nurses, 3, 5, 182; and television appearances, 125, 235; tips for, 245

Jamieson, Kathleen Hall, 20
Japan, 25, 77–78
jargon, 84, 88–90, 97, 240, 274
Jenner, Edward, 110
Johnson, Ruth, 89
Johnson & Johnson Campaign for Nursing's Future, 168–69, 170
journalists and journalism: and anecdotes, 84; and angle of story, 159–60; and blog sites, 211; and coverage of nursing, 1–3, 11, 16–17, 118; and deadlines, 132, 134; and definition of news, 118–20; and expertise of nurses, 1, 11, 131, 136, 140, 177; function of, 111, 112; and health care information, 109, 110; and images of nurses, 200–201; Internet's impact on, 130; and medical journals, 252–54; and networks of relationships, 137–38; and news conferences, 158–59, 183, 198; and news/entertainment distinctions, 112; news releases for, 145–52; and news values, 114–15, 118, 142, 208; nurses' presentations to, 156–57; and nursing research, 249, 250, 255–57, 259–60, 266–69; and nursing stereotypes, 6, 15–17, 203; and public communication skills, 6, 23; and public relations professionals, 168, 172–73, 175, 177; and research news, 116; and sources, 1–3, 131–38, 140, 143; and virtue script, 33–34, 35, 36; written materials for, 144. *See also* news media

Journal of the American Medical Association (JAMA), 116, 120, 128, 142–43, 249, 252–54, 259
Jurkowitz, Mark, 205, 206, 211

Kaiser Family Foundation, 111, 202
Kalisch, Beatrice, 201
Kaplan, Madge, 133
Kesey, Ken, 51
Kevorkian, Jack, 103
Kleinman, Arthur, 48, 127
knowledge script, 4, 17, 21, 42–44, 49, 58, 65, 87–88. *See also* expertise
Knox, Richard A., 256
Koppel, Ross, 55, 142–43, 252
Kuehl, Sheila James, 183

Lake, Nancy, 34
Laroza, Nelia, 194, 195
Lesmond, Joan, 195
letters to the editor, 113, 122–23, 140, 168, 183, 204–11, 227, 269
Lin, Tecla, 195
Lindaman, Crystal, 47
Logan, Jean, 225–27
Los Angeles Times, 155, 256
Lown, Bernard, 127
Lundberg, George, 252, 253, 254
Lydon, Christopher, 240
Lynaugh, Joan, 18, 46, 180

MacKinnon, Sine, 196
Maclean's, 123, 215
magazines, 26, 123–24, 126–27, 159, 204–5, 216, 269–70
Maraldo, Pamela, 155
Marcus, Isabel, 32
Marquis, Julie, 256
Martineau, Harriet, 180
Marville, Betsy, 213–14
Mason, Diana J., 154, 230, 261
Massachusetts Nurses Association (MNA), 131, 153–54, 155, 188–91, 270
McCarthy, Karen, 143, 160, 167
McInaney, Maureen, 174–75
McIntyre, Joy, 258
McNamara, Eileen, 123
McPherson, Debra, 271
media kits, 145, 158, 168, 198–99
media strategies: assembling written materials, 144–45; and audience determination, 141–

42, 167; and broadcast releases, 152–53; broadening story's impact, 159; and distribution, 153–54; establishing rules of game, 164–65; and meetings with editorial boards, 154–56, 183, 199; and negative coverage, 161–64; and news conferences, 158–59; and news releases, 145–52; and news sense development, 118–20; and newsworthiness, 142–43; and nurses' outreach lags, 138–40; nursing organizations, 157–58; opportunity awareness, 143–44; and phone calls, 154; pitching your story, 159–61; presentations to journalists, 156–57; and radio and television, 7, 125; and source-originated news stories, 137. *See also* public relations professionals
Medical Care, 251
medical journals, 110, 251–56
medical paternalism, 7, 110
men in nursing, 7, 13–14, 32, 74
Meyers, Theresa A., 260, 261
Mezibov, Dan, 172
Migden, Carole, 199
Milwaukee Journal-Sentinel, 121, 146, 207
Monteiro, Lois, 180
Moralejo, Lisa, 209
Morieson, Belinda, 187
Morley, Barry, 104–5
Morley, Ben, 104
Morley, Grace, 104
Moyers, Bill, 244

National Institute of Nursing Research (NINR), 180, 250–51, 256
National Labor Relations Board (NLRB), 189, 190
National League for Nursing (NLN), 155
National Public Radio, 26–27, 204, 256
Nelson, Sioban, 32, 207
New England Journal of Medicine (NEJM), 115, 116, 120, 128, 142, 197, 253–54, 259
news media: and breaking news, 113–14, 117, 122, 168; and definition of news, 118–20; and health care business, 114–16; and health care coverage, 111–13; and health care policy news, 112–15; and human interest and features, 114, 117–18; monitoring of, 120–24; positive versus negative coverage, 15–17; and research news, 116–17; and source-originated news stories, 137; and visibility of nursing, 2, 3, 5, 14–15, 16. *See also* journalists and journalism; media strategies

newspapers: and advocacy campaigns, 181, 183, 199; and book reviews, 127; and health care information, 113; on Internet, 204–5; and medical journals, 254; monitoring of, 120–23; and news releases, 146; and nursing research, 261; weekly newspapers, 141, 146, 215. *See also* op-ed pages

news releases: and advocacy campaigns, 203; audience for, 141; body of, 151–52; broadcast releases, 152–53; components of, 148–50; distribution of, 153–54; format of, 146–47; and media strategies, 145–52; and medical journals, 253; news values of, 119–20, 142; and nursing research, 249–50, 258, 266–67; and public relations professionals, 168; video news releases, 253–54, 260, 261

news syndicates, 124

Newsweek, 123, 186, 191, 215, 218–19

New York Times: and advocacy campaigns, 181, 186; and columnists, 123; and documentary evidence, 133; and health coverage on sample day, 113–17; and images of nursing, 36, 94; and nurse-to-patient ratio, 249; and nursing research, 262; and nursing shortage stories, 160; and op-ed page, 215, 216, 227; and Rosa, 259; and visibility of nursing, 14–15, 16

New York Times Magazine, 123

New York Times Sunday Magazine, 121

Nieman Reports, 157

Nightingale, Florence, 30, 35, 36, 58, 179–80, 274

Nightline, 124

nurse managers, 60, 94–95, 188, 189

nurse midwives, 12, 89, 90, 180

nurse/physician relationship: and agency of nurses, 31–33, 37, 66–68; and body language, 61–63; and competency of nurses, 162, 174; and fear of physicians' anger, 68–70; and internalized knowledge, 87–88; and medication errors, 142–43; and nurses' professional self-presentation, 45–47, 56–57; and nursing practice, 67–68; and nursing research, 268; and patient care, 62, 88, 91, 123; and public relations professionals, 174; and use of term "girl," 60

nurse recruitment, 19–20, 276–77

Nurses' Day/Week, 28, 34–36, 143

Nurses of America (NOA) project, 1, 3, 155

nursing administration, 4, 100–102, 175–77, 183, 186, 188–89, 234

nursing education: and advocacy campaigns, 180; and anecdotes, 99–100; and caring aspect of nursing practice, 169; costs of, 206; and doctorates, 38; and health care resources, 13; and news releases, 147; and nursing shortages, 160–61; and professional self-representation, 56; and public relations professionals, 175; standardized requirements for, 4

nursing journals, 120, 128–29, 222–25, 267–68

nursing organizations: and advocacy campaigns, 194; and journalists, 2, 3, 11; and media strategies, 119–20, 142, 157–58; meetings as form of outreach, 157–58; and news releases, 152, 153, 177; and Nurses of America project, 1; and nursing research, 250, 266–67; and nursing shortages, 160; and professional image, 28; public communication duties of, 22; and public relations professionals, 171–73; and Schiavo story, 138–40; and virtue script, 169

nursing practice: and acceptance of thanks, 70–72; and agency, 29–31, 66–68; and anecdotes, 6, 23, 82, 90, 93, 95–102; complexity of, 26, 66–67, 84–85, 96, 99, 178; conflict in discussion of, 78–81; description of, 65–66; and fear of physicians' anger, 68–70; and interviews, 3; and journalists, 16–17, 136; medical and technical aspects of, 18, 20, 39, 64–66, 69–70, 93–94, 100, 167, 177, 234, 276; and nursing research, 257, 270; and nursing stereotypes, 27, 275; and personal image, 17–18, 27; practice narratives, 5, 177; and professional image, 18–21, 27, 28, 142, 234; and public communication skills, 21, 64, 65–66, 72–73; and public relations professionals, 174, 175; responding to comments on, 73–75; and television appearances, 233–34. *See also* caring aspect of nursing practice; patient care

nursing profession: and asymetrical power relationships, 45–46; credibility of, 1, 163; devaluation of, 38–39, 72, 73–75; divisions within, 275; improving image of, 129; inaccurate representations of, 200–203; labeling within, 94–95; as largest health care profession, 1, 4, 21–22; religious and secular influences on, 31, 32; and resource competition, 4, 27. *See also* nursing practice; nursing stereotypes; professional self-representation; visibility of nursing

nursing research: and advocacy campaigns, 183, 270–71; example of medical journals, 251–56; and expertise of nurses, 6; highlighting importance of, 263; and journalists, 249, 250, 255–57, 259–60, 266–69; and keeping story going, 161; and nursing journals' outreach, 267–68; ongoing opportunities for promotion, 268–69; and public relations professionals, 257–62, 267, 269; selecting studies to promote, 263–64; telling story in various ways, 269–70; translating into ordinary language, 264–66; visibility of, 11, 249, 250, 255–56, 268

nursing shortages: and advocacy campaigns, 1; angle of story, 160–61; and columnists, 121; as hot topic, 103; images of, 36; and images of nurses, 200, 272; and letters to the editor, 209–10; nurse-to-patient ratio, 5, 12, 19, 28, 84, 148–50, 174, 177, 179, 181–88, 249, 270–71; and nursing stereotypes, 19–20; and public relations professionals, 175; and restructuring, 192, 195; and unions, 160, 177; and visibility of nursing, 5, 28

nursing stereotypes: and angelic images, 16, 17, 36, 40, 169; and body language, 62; and health care resources, 4, 27, 110, 169; and journalists, 8; "just a nurse" stereotypes, 4, 151, 276–77; and letters to the editor, 206–7; and mass media, 6, 15, 16, 17, 203; and nurse as title, 51–52; and nursing practice, 27, 275; and nursing shortages, 19–20; and public relations professionals, 168, 178; replacement of, 13; and television appearances, 233, 234, 239; and virtue script, 33, 40

Ontario Nurses Association (ONA), 192, 193, 194–95

op-ed pages: and advocacy campaigns, 183; contents of, 215, 216; and media kits, 199; and nursing research, 269; and physicians, 220; placement of, 122; placing in publications, 221, 225–27; and public relations professionals, 168; revising nursing journal article for, 222–25; and Schiavo story, 140; writing of, 216–18

opinion sections, 121–23, 204–5

Palmer, Helen, 153

patient care: and advocacy campaigns, 179, 182, 188–90; anecdotes concerning, 83–88; and approachability of nurses, 48; complexity of, 19, 26; enthusiasm for, 75; and hospital nursing, 14–15; and media strategies, 142; news media's coverage of, 112, 117; and nurse/physician relationship, 62, 88, 91, 123; nurses' advocacy for, 119, 181; and nursing education, 161; and nursing research, 270; and professional image, 18–21; and restructuring, 3; and three Rs, 14, 27–28; and visibility of nursing, 5. See also nursing practice

patients: activism of, 110; and advocacy campaigns, 181–83, 186–87; as audience of nurses, 6, 22, 65, 141; and clinicians, 7–8; confidentiality of, 75–78; and expertise of nurses, 12; and nurse/physician relationship, 67–69; and nurses' personal safety, 52–54; and nurses' right to privacy, 54–55; and nurses' voice of agency, 29; and nursing practice, 18–19, 25, 26, 27, 65, 78; and professional self-presentation, 42–48, 58–59, 61–62; relationship with physicians, 48, 56, 61, 251; as sources, 2, 119

Philips, Jean Ann, 233

Phipps, Marion, 30–31

physicians: book publishing of, 127–28; credited by journalists, 144; fluctuation in population of, 161; and medical journals, 267; and nurses' professional self-presentation, 42, 43, 45, 46–47; nurses teaching of, 13, 26; and nursing practice, 19, 26, 27, 33, 37; and op-ed pages, 220; and power positions in hospitals, 32–33; and press coverage of health and health care, 12; professional image of, 17–19, 36–37, 45, 167; and public communication, 251–52; and public relations professionals, 173, 174; relationship to patients, 48, 56, 61, 251; and research, 250, 251, 254–55, 262; and safer needles, 197; as source for journalists, 2, 140, 174, 175; and television appearances, 232, 233, 234–35. See also nurse/physician relationship

Pimentel, O. Ricardo, 211

Pitorak, Elizabeth Ford, 262

professional self-presentation: and appearance, 23, 35–36, 42, 58–63, 236–37; and first name use, 46–51, 53–58; and name identification, 44–46; and naming practices, 42, 45, 47–51, 55–58; and nurse as title, 42, 46–47, 51–52, 54, 56; and nurses as "girls," 59–60; and public communication skills, 23, 43

Public Broadcasting System, 124, 125, 126

public communication, 22–23, 197–98, 251–52

public communication skills: and accepting thanks, 70–72; and agency of nurses, 66–68; and conversational openings, 64–65, 72–73, 83; development of, 7, 21; and enthusiasm, 75; fears/inhibitions concerning, 4, 5–6, 23–24, 25, 68–70, 78–81; and news media, 3; and nursing practice, 21, 64, 65–66, 72–73; and patient confidentiality, 75–78; and "publics," 6, 22, 43, 64–65; and responding, 73–75. *See also* anecdotes

public relations, 112, 251, 254. *See also* advocacy campaigns

public relations professionals: and breaking news, 168; and clinical workplace, 173–77; and communication specialists, 167, 172, 174, 175; as consultants, 170; guide to selection of, 178; and internal and external communications, 171–73; and medical journals, 254; and meetings with editorial boards, 155; and monitoring news media, 120; and nursing research, 257–62, 267, 269; press contacts of, 141–42, 167–68; and public communication skills, 3, 7; and quotes for news releases, 151; and source-originated news stories, 137; as sources, 131; and television appearances, 234; and virtue script, 168–69

Quill, Timothy, 116–17

Rabkin, Mitchel, 175

radio, 7, 125–27, 134, 146, 152–53, 204, 247–48. *See also* television and radio appearances

Raphael, Sally Jesse, 232–33, 234

Reeve, Christopher, 66–67, 118, 254–56

Registered Nurses Association of Ontario (RNAO), 191–95

registered nurses (RNs): and advocacy campaigns, 183; and conflict in public communication, 80; cost-effectiveness of, 271; credentials of, 151, 262; and Iraqi prisoner abuse scandal, 120; labeling of, 94; layoffs of, 181, 191, 195; and nurse/physician relationship, 37, 68; and nursing research, 270; and professional self-presentation, 44–46, 56–57, 59–60, 62; recruitment of, 20, 187; and staffing, 13

Reuters, 124

Reverby, Susan M., 33

Richler, Mordecai, 123

Roberts, Leslie, 229–30

Rogers, Anne, 226

Rosa, Emily, 259

Rosa, Linda, 259

Rosenbaum, Ed, 127

Rosenberg, Neil, 146

Rosseter, Robert, 173

Royal College of Nursing, 274–75

Ruddick, Sara, 33

Russell, William Howard, 179

Salant, Richard, 125

Sandelowski, Margarete, 70

San Francisco Chronicle, 133, 137, 196–200

SARS, 191–96

Scharfenberg, Kirk, 131

Schiavo, Terri, 113, 116, 138–40

Schildmeier, David, 167, 168, 189–91

Schwarzenegger, Arnold, 184, 186, 187

Semple, Robert B., Jr., 215, 216

Sen, Amartya, 28–29

Service Employees International Union (SEIU), 133, 178, 184, 196–200

Service Employees International Union (SEIU) Nurse Alliance, 198, 199–200

Service Employees International Union (SEIU) Nurse Alliance of Florida, 211–12, 214

Shamian, Judith, 271

Shell, Ellen Ruppel, 258–59

Sigma Theta Tau International, 131–32, 156, 256

silence of nurses: ending of, 21–22; and external communication plan, 173; as international problem, 8; and interviews, 3, 5, 182; and nurse/physician relationship, 68, 69; and nursing practice, 66; and public communication skills, 4, 76–80; as threat to profession, 28; and virtue script, 39; and willingness to communicate, 23–24

Simpson, Kate, 104

Snyder, Marie, 189

Sochalski, Julie, 271

Storr, Janie, 84–85

Strunk, William, Jr., 151

Summers, Sandy, 200–201, 203

Swartz-Lloyd, Tony, 174, 175

Sweeney, Susan, 92–93

Swiss Nurses Association, 272–75

Sykes, Kim, 176

Takayama, Masumi, 77–78

Takayama, Shigeko, 77–78

Tannen, Deborah, 60

Technology Review, 40–41, 220

television: and advocacy campaigns, 199; and book reviews, 127; and broadcast releases, 152–53; call-in shows, 125–26, 247–48; communication techniques for, 7; and feedback on Web sites, 204; and medical journals, 254; monitoring of, 120, 124–25; and news conferences, 158; and news releases, 146; popularity of, 113; and sound bites, 125, 134; and video news releases, 253–54, 260, 261

television and radio appearances: anecdotes for, 228–30, 240; and appearance, 236–37; basic rules for, 231; and bridging, 240, 242–48; and expertise, 230, 232, 235, 244; and feeling in control, 231–35; and interviews, 125, 235; setting ground rules, 57–58, 238; tone of voice and interview etiquette, 238–39

Thomas, Sandra P., 39–40

Thomson, Donna, 271

Tohoku University College of Nursing, 77

Twigg, Di, 100–102

Ulrich, Laurel Thatcher, 33

unions: and advocacy campaigns, 182, 190, 196–200; and anecdotes, 97; and journalists, 11, 131; and nursing research, 250, 270; and nursing shortages, 160, 177; and painting whole picture, 94; and public communication, 22; and public relations professionals, 177–78; and support for exposing system problems, 80

University of California San Francisco (UCSF) School of Nursing, 175, 258

University of Pennsylvania, 84–85, 148–50

University of Pennsylvania, Center for Bioethics, 134, 252

University of Pennsylvania School of Nursing, 249–50, 258

USA Today, 15, 123, 261

U.S. Congress, 113, 115, 126, 138–40, 251

Valentine, Nancy, 155

Virani, Rose, 262

virtue script, 4, 17, 21, 27–28, 32–36, 40, 168–69, 274

visibility of nursing: and caring aspect of nursing practice, 275–76; and letters to the editor, 208; and news media, 2, 3, 5, 14–15, 16; and nurse/physician relationship, 70; and nursing research, 11, 249, 250, 255–56, 268; and nursing stereotypes, 234; and professional image, 11, 27, 28; reservations about, 25, 27; and silence of nurses, 8, 22; and Swiss Nurses Association, 272–75

voice of agency, 5, 24, 29–33, 39–41. *See also* agency of nurses

Wagner, Pierre André, 272–75

Wahl, Barb, 193, 194–95

Wall Street Journal, 115, 122, 123

Warner, Yvonne, 194

whistleblowers, 137, 186, 188–91, 194–95

White, E. B., 151

Wilhite, Wilson, 163

Williamson, Andrew, 176

Wilson, Pete, 182, 200

Wilson, Rand, 178

wire services, 124, 126

Wittenberg, Anne, 175

women's movement, 60, 110

Woodhull Study on Nursing and the Media, 15–16

working conditions: and advocacy campaigns, 191–96, 199; and anecdotes, 84; and medication errors, 92; and National Labor Relations Act, 80; and nursing research, 250, 270; and nursing shortages, 160; and unions, 177, 178; and virtue script, 36, 39

Wright, Gail Leondar, 126